THE
TEN-YEAR
CLUB

THE TEN-YEAR CLUB

A Decade of Infertility and Us

LOUISE LINDIN

GREY BARNABY
GREAT BRITAIN

Published by Grey Barnaby (Great Britain)
www.greybarnaby.com

Northern Sky, written and performed by Nick Drake,
is taken from the album *Nick Drake – A Treasury*
(www.brytermusic.com)
and reproduced by kind permission
of Warlock Music/BMG Rights.

Cover image: © Piotr Marcinski/Shutterstock
Cover logo: © iLoveCoffeeDesign

PB ISBN 978-0-9929595-0-0
eBook-ePub ISBN 978-0-9929595-1-7
eBook-eReader ISBN 978-0-9929595-2-4

Typeset in Adobe Garamond Pro

To find out more about our authors and books visit
www.greybarnaby.com for author interviews and extracts.

For anyone who knows the pain of infertility

INTRODUCTION

I APPROACHED THE FINAL months of 2012 with enough trepidation to power a meteorite. It wasn't because I believed, like a surprising number of earthlings, that the world would come to an abrupt end when the Mayan Long Count Calendar 'ran out', on December 21, 2012. It was of no consequence to me if it happened or not. Whether the sun fell from the sky or the moon imploded, December 2012 threatened the end of *my* world for entirely different reasons. Shortly before Christmas, around the time of the predicted apocalypse, I would join the Ten-Year Club. I had imagined so many worst-case scenarios but I had never imagined this: after ten years of trying to start a family, I would still be childless. Doomsday or not, I remained at the mouth of an endless black hole, one that had threatened to draw me in, batter me in its vortex and ultimately obscure my view of the future. What was in that dark place? I was too afraid to look. When I tried to imagine a future without a family, I felt clammy and sick, breathless and panicked. I didn't want that future to exist; nearly a decade on and I still could not accept that it might.

I'm fairly sure I was another person altogether before I joined the Ten-Year Club. I was certainly optimistic enough to sit in a Pizza Express in central London and debate with my partner of only four months what we might call our children. The year was 2002 and the choices, lightly made between a Fiorentina pizza and a chocolate brownie, were Ava for a girl and Flynn for a boy. However, in the ensuing decade, the world has been filled with other people's Avas and Flynns; there would be too many of them now for us to keep those names and feel in any way original. After 120 cycles, 120 conceptions that never happened, we know what we would call a son, but somehow we don't talk about girls' names anymore. Those are harder to agree on and, anyway, it is too late now to have two children; one seems a miracle, two beyond all realms.

Another thing I can remember about me before I joined the Ten-Year Club: I would have written this book differently, with one breakthrough following another, all chronological and tidy. But infertility does not present itself to you as a timeline neatly drawn. It is like a 'washing machine' wave on Bondi Beach; one minute you're admiring the shimmering, cloudless sky, the next a rogue wave has sucked you in. It will relentlessly churn you around and around, and sometimes, when you can't feel your legs and your face is grazing the sand, you wonder if you will ever breathe again. That's when it becomes so insidious. It will let you grab a tiny breath, a little gulp of hope, enough to keep you alive for another minute or so, and then the whole tortuous cycle will start up all over again. By the time it's over, you will either have drowned or you will emerge, raw and half-choked, and it will be a long, long time before you know which way is up.

So, this is not a 'how-to' manual, where thoughts happen in straight lines and cause and effect perfectly follow one another in a beautifully choreographed dance. How could it when infertility boils down to the bare fact that the action of unprotected sex has not produced the expected effect of pregnancy? That absence of order, of A following B, silently builds from unsettling to unnerving to destabilising and, before you know it, you are dealing with sheer chaos of both thoughts and emotion. Sometimes I'm just glad to see that night still follows day – at least some things are where I expected them to be.

❦ ❦ ❦

A decade might have passed, but I never did become an expert on either fertility or infertility; all I know is how one of them makes you feel. I wanted to write honestly about that, about what it does to a person, and to a relationship, when you are struggling not to become involuntarily childless. Despite our battle with prolonged infertility, I know we did not have the worst of it. I'm conscious of those couples who have suffered devastating pregnancy losses or cycle after gruelling cycle of failed fertility treatments. I was not as brave as those women and men who faced these things; I admire the strength of each and every one of them and wish they could all, finally, be free of infertility.

This book tells our story alone, but it doesn't mean we're proud of it. We know that neither of us reacted to infertility in a likeable or pleasant or particularly rational way. We got nearly everything wrong. We blundered and stumbled and turned on each other. At times, it felt as if parts of the medical establishment had turned on us. We had so many arguments that, halfway through this book, it felt exhausting just writing about them. It was tempting to sugar-coat it a little, both for my own relief and yours, to skim over the worst of ourselves and of infertility. But I couldn't paint over the dark stains in that generic fertility-clinic shade of white, to provide relief where there was none. I wanted to show what really happens to a life, and the characters within, when infertility sneaks up on you. Some of it is difficult to read, some of it is unsettling, some of it is ridiculous, but all of it is real. This is what it feels like to be in the Ten-Year Club.

* All names and some locations have been changed to protect those who did not ask to be written about, but everything within happened.

* For reasons that will become obvious, this book is in no way intended to be a source of medical advice.

ONE

I DON'T REMEMBER THE first time I actually 'tried' to make a baby. It was something we just naturally fell into, more an agreement that we wouldn't try *not* to have a child, an understanding that if it happened, it happened, and we'd both be happy about it. I do know that I was definitely 'trying' on New Year's Day, 2003. How long ago, how unexpectedly old-fashioned, 2003 seems now – no Facebook, no Twitter and most of us using our mobile phones for calls or texts only. These ordinary little observations are the evidence, as if I needed it, of how much time has passed.

A decade ago, it was New Year's Day and the rest of my life lay ahead of me, bursting with promise. A month earlier, my partner Chris and I had taken up residence in our first flat together, in northwest London. We were ninety seconds from the tube station at West Hampstead and five stops from the heart of the city. It suited us, the proximity to everything that bustled. On that first day of the year, Chris and I laughed and 'tried' for conception and laughed some more, content with the shelter of our duvet, and of each other, while outside it rained ice. We were halfway through 'trying' a second time when the doorbell rang. It was one-thirty in the afternoon; there was nothing to do but laugh even harder as we hauled the duvet right over the top of our heads. We were having too much fun to let the harping and honking of the doorbell interrupt us.

It rang again. And again. Who did we know who was so damn persistent?

"Blast!" Chris lifted a shoulder so that part of his face poked out from the duvet. "It might be important."

"Not *that* important," I replied, grabbing his shoulder and pulling him back down into the warmth, possibly a little too firmly.

Joy. It was quiet once more; whoever it was had obviously given up and gone off to find a more interesting way to spend their New Year's Day.

Under the duvet, things moved on. We were about to reach the point at which a pregnancy might become possible when we heard a tap, tap, tapping on the kitchen door. This was alarming, not only because it must really be something important, but because the kitchen, like our bedroom, was at the back of the house – had our visitor seen us through the floor-to-ceiling windows as they crossed the garden? Could they see us now?

We flattened ourselves against the mattress as if rolling-pinned to the sheets. Now there was calling as well as tapping, but the voice was drowned out by the rain. Chris slid off the bed and wriggled across the floor on hip and elbow, like a lopsided action man toy, before peeking through the window.

"Oh! It's Vanda and Amy."

My sister and her teenage daughter, visiting from the southern hemisphere. As far as we knew, they were in Edinburgh recovering from the effects of Hogmanay the night before.

"We'll have to let them in," he added unnecessarily. "They're soaked."

"I can't go." I emitted the whispered version of a horrified shriek. "What if something runs down my leg?"

"Well, at least they won't see that," and he gestured hipwards, at his own evidence of our attempts to procreate.

"For Pete's sake, can't you hit it with a cold teaspoon? Isn't that what they do in hospitals?"

I sprayed a dose of perfume and grabbed a dressing gown before heading for the door. "Um, sorry," I said when I finally opened it. "We were fast asleep, big night last night."

My sister and my niece entered the kitchen dragging saturated overnight bags and looking like mutinous hypothermia victims. "I thought I'd cook us a roast dinner for New Year's night," Vanda said evenly, shooting me a look that said, 'I know exactly what you've been doing and my teenage daughter does too.'

It's important to me now that I can remember New Year's Day 2003 so clearly – it's my touchstone of how we used to be, who we each were, before this thing overtook us. We could be carefree, we did have fun! Sometimes you forget, sometimes you need to be reminded. And when you do remember, the question that lurks unanswered is this: can I ever be that person again? Will I ever – all the time, not just for one day – be someone who knows that lovemaking is natural and funny and free, and not just a heartbreaking means to an end?

※ ※ ※

On the face of it, there was not much to suggest Chris and I would make a well-matched couple. We were opposites in every category you cared to name. I grew up on a farm in the southern hemisphere; I had ridden horses since I was eighteen months old and, on the back of my Welsh Mountain pony, roamed freely across several hundred acres of land owned by our neighbour. I was off on my own doing this from the age of five. Unsurprisingly, there was the odd incident – I once rode to the top of an extinct volcano and then realised it was too steep to get back down again; on another expedition, I tried to lead my pony over a bog, only for him to gradually sink so deeply into the cloying mud that much of his body was submerged. The pair of us were eventually hauled out by our farmer friend, who seemed uncharacteristically shaken, and I trotted off home to explain why my grey pony now appeared black. When it came to physical boundaries, I had very few.

7

On a farm, you are free to climb trees, have cow-pat fights, raise all manner of animals, spot tadpoles and eels in creeks. However, beyond that, I had another advantage – I was the youngest of six children and my parents had got a lot more relaxed about things by the time I came along.

However, much darker constraints were waiting in the wings. When I was seven years old, I watched, stricken and mute, as my father collapsed and died in one of the paddocks where I usually ran free. He had been chopping firewood and suffered a heart attack while stopping for a cold drink and a chat with my mother, my brother and me. So many things might have gone so differently, were it not for that day in March 1976. Although I had just witnessed an event that would traumatise most adults, my father's actual death was perhaps not the thing that shocked me the most. The thing that upset me above all else was seeing my mother cry – Mum, who could use a chainsaw, build fences, clear a wasp nest, see off marauding possums with a shovel, drive tractors and trucks. I had never seen Mum weakened, never seen her look lost for a moment. I'm not sure I even knew that adults cried. It was her tears that really underlined for me how terrible things were; I began fretting and worrying at that point and, in some ways, I've never stopped.

After we lost Dad, I was raised in a single-parent household on state benefits, supplemented by the money Mum earned cleaning other people's houses and assembling fruit boxes for one cent a box. We had never been wealthy, but we had been stable; now nothing was certain. We moved house because we could not afford to stay in the old one, I changed schools and wore second-hand 'Granny' shoes that the other kids laughed at. From the age of eleven, when the last of my brothers and sisters left home, it was just Mum and me. It was as if a bomb had exploded on the day my father died and bits of shrapnel were now embedded in everything. But the largest piece of collateral damage is that I cannot remember what it is like to grow up in a family unit. That is part of the reason why, as I battle infertility, the idea of a family is forever tantalising, and why it is so painful to realise that it seems destined to remain out of reach.

As my childhood unfolded in the southern hemisphere, the man I would eventually decide to start a family with was on the other side of the world, living a life not only literally but metaphorically poles apart from my own.

Chris and I did have one thing in common – he also grew up in the country, but in a six-bedroomed manor house with an actual name rather than a mere rural delivery number. He lived there with his parents, his younger sister and an aunt who ruled her own self-contained wing of the mansion. His father commuted to his office in London, while his mother ran the home with the help of two 'dailies', one in the morning and another in the afternoon. A gardener came every Saturday to help maintain the expansive grounds, Chris's Granny came for lunch every Sunday and there were endless parties around the pool in summer and family tennis matches in the garden. His father also owned a boat, moored nearby, and they would sometimes sail to France on it, or often just putter around the harbour.

The other thing we had in common: Chris also experienced a life-changing event when he was seven. He awoke one day to the eagerly-received news that he and his parents were going to stay in a hotel. He did not stop to question why his sister was not joining them; he was too busy wondering if there would be ice cream sundaes or perhaps swishy circular doors in the lobby, which you could chase round and round in. It was a good twenty minutes after he had been deposited at the 'hotel' and his parents had disappeared entirely that Chris realised the horrible truth: he was at boarding school. And his mother and father had not even stopped to say goodbye. So, aged seven, and still unable to tie his shoelaces or make a bed, he involuntarily left home. He was too unruly, it had been said, for his village primary school; it was two years after his arrival at prep school that the reason for this was uncovered – he was dyslexic, unable to make sense of the books on his desk or the chalk marks on the board. In the meantime, he did not let this hold him back – he drew darkly imaginative pictures and avoided bullying by becoming the class joker, even if that did mean being beaten with a cane twelve times in one term alone.

All of these formative events lay far behind us when we met at work in London in early 2002. It was a Saturday job and I already knew of Chris, if only by name, because some of my weekday colleagues had worked with him before.

"Stick with Chris, he'll look after you," one of them advised when I expressed nerves about my first day in a new office. "He's a good guy." He paused before adding a caveat: "He can flirt for England, mind."

This proved a correct assessment, although it might have been closer to the mark to say that Chris could flirt for England, Wales, Scotland and Northern Ireland. He even managed to do this while working to four daily deadlines (and for a boss who would throw rubbish bins across the office if you failed to meet them). It made no odds to me – Chris wasn't my type. I don't know why I started bringing up his name in after-work conversations with friends, I don't know why I wondered what it would be like to have him holding my hand when I fell ill a couple of months later, I don't know why I eventually kissed him while sitting on a wall admiring the lights of Tower Bridge. I think the master flirt put a spell on me.

Whatever the case, I had certainly not stopped to consider all of the differences looming between us; if anything it was the things that set us apart that made us so intriguing to each other at the beginning.

Our first 'date' was a seven-and-a-half hour phone conversation that ran on through the night until we finally hung up at 5am. This was a novelty for me. The type of men I knew, the ones with similar backgrounds to my own, were more the strong, solid, silent type; that and the jocular type, the ones who went through life using humour to avoid real intimacy. Now here was a man who could not only flirt for England but converse for his country as well. The conversation ranged freely from our own lives to travel, history, sport and spiritual matters too. It was interesting, funny and even educational. I knew I had met someone different. However, there was one more major difference I didn't yet know about. And as we later battled infertility, through argument after agonising argument, it would be the thing that I repeatedly threw back at him. The thing that meant we should never have been together in the first place.

Two

U<small>NTIL THE POINT JUST</small> before I began trying to have a family, I had done a fairly good job of keeping to the script. Without being aware of it, I had taken my cues from the actions of those around me and I had done the right thing; I had done what was expected.

Even in the seemingly progressive 1980s, when I was a teenager, I knew that the worst thing I could do in life was to get pregnant. The shame would have been unbearable and, as far as I understood it, my future would be instantly and brutally cancelled. That is why I can still remember, thirty years later, the name of the one girl at my secondary school who was unfortunate enough to endure a teenage pregnancy – she wasn't in my year, she wasn't a friend, in fact I had never even spoken to her, but the scandal was such that her name has always stuck in my mind. She disappeared, abruptly, midway through the winter term and never returned to school.

Back then, she was the walking evidence that, if you let a boy's bits anywhere near you, then pregnancy would certainly follow. I didn't really need this example, though – I had more than enough evidence in my own life. The thing hardly anyone knew about me was that I was adopted; I was the result of a teenage pregnancy myself. As far as I was told, which wasn't much, my seventeen-year-old birth mother was oblivious to my existence until the fifth month of my gestation. She had one very compelling reason for believing that she couldn't possibly be pregnant – she had not technically had sex, not only five months earlier, but ever. There had been a close call at a New Year's Eve party as 1967 rolled into 1968, however that was all it was. She knew the rules too – one slip could ruin your life. But there I was, and here I am – another reminder of how easy it is for conception to happen. Well, she might have been caught out but I was not going to be. I started taking the contraceptive pill during my late teens and, just for good measure, always used barrier methods of contraception as well.

Whereas my birth mother had proved how dangerously easy it was to fall pregnant, my adoptive mother proved how tough was the life that followed. She could even have been the template for the sacrifices made by women of her generation in order to raise children.

Mum married at eighteen, abandoning her vocational training halfway through to join my father on the family farm. Their first child was born a month after she turned twenty and three more followed in quick succession. My brother, Ray, the closest in age to me, was something of a surprise, arriving when Mum was thirty-six. By the time they adopted me, she was forty years old and had already been raising a family for twenty years of her life. After Dad died, when it was only Mum and me at home alone, I understood more than anyone just what she had given up to be a wife and mother. She was intelligent, practical, full of initiative, but she had no profession, no training, nothing that allowed her to further herself – it wasn't an option; the family came first. Now, with Dad gone, Mum had no career to fall back on, no way of making a decent living. I watched her struggle to make ends meet, I watched her cleaning other people's floors on her hands and knees and I made myself a promise – I would have a career, I would always have something of my own to fall back on.

All of these things, whether I was aware of them or not, contributed to my decision to wait until my early thirties to have a family. In fact, throughout my twenties, the negative messages about parenting and pregnancy were so ingrained that I would often tell people I did not intend to have children at all.

Two close friends unexpectedly fell pregnant and we drifted apart; to my shame, the drifting was more on my behalf than theirs. It was simple: I did not want anything to do with babies. I was at a loss to understand why anyone would think them adorable or cute – whereas I could almost faint with joy at seeing a baby animal of any species, any time I saw a human infant I got an overwhelming urge to leave the room before someone thrust the terrifying bundle into my arms. Whenever a colleague proudly debuted their new-born at the office, I would smile from a distance and then discreetly edge out of the door and into the canteen, where I would hide out until I was sure they had left. I think about this now and I don't recognise myself.

It meant nothing to me when a childless colleague expressed annoyance about routine demands from both friends and strangers as to when she and her husband were going to start a family. She giggled: "I say to them, 'Did you know that one in six couples is infertile?' That shuts them up."

If I cringed inwardly then, it was only because of the potential for awkwardness in those exchanges; now such a comment, carelessly thrown around an office, would break my heart. The colleague in question went on to effortlessly produce two children right on cue – like so many, she will never know, never *feel* the meaning of her little joke about fertility stats.

It is odd to realise now that I was once as oblivious to infertility, and its delightful array of knock-on effects, as most other people seem to be. In fact, it had already affected my own family and I had barely noticed.

Aged about ten, I overheard conversations between Mum and Vanda, my sister who is sixteen years older than me, and I gathered that there was some problem to do with having children. Once, after Vanda and her husband Paul had been teasing each other in cartoon voices, I watched Vanda turn to

Mum and sigh: "No wonder we can't have babies. We don't even talk like proper adults."

However, when I was nearly thirteen, Vanda and Paul had the first of their three children. Mum was thrilled. "I knew the vitamin E would do the trick," she beamed.

It turned out Vanda had been trying to conceive for two years – it finally happened not long after she began the vitamin E supplements that Mum had recommended.

Somewhere in my subconscious, I took all of this on board. When Chris and I started trying for our family, I thought two years might not be an unreasonable time to wait, and that if vitamin E had been the magic ingredient for Vanda, then it would probably be the same for me. It hadn't occurred to me that, sometimes, there is no magic ingredient.

❧ ❧ ❧

Having dutifully kept to the script, having ensured there were no 'slip-ups', I had been on the contraceptive pill for more than fifteen years by the time we decided to have a family. My monthly cycle, ever since the day it arrived, had been something to get through as quickly as possible, something that I sincerely wished would go away and never return. As a tomboy who climbed trees, played rugby and threw cattle dung at her brother, I was not one of those girls who welcomed the onset of womanhood. I paid it as little attention as possible and, when monthly cramps interfered with one of my many sporting competitions, I would blitz the enemy with whatever painkiller I could find, hardly stopping even to read the instructions. A doctor once prescribed some blue pills the size of Brazil nuts for the cramps; they were so bulky that I could hardly swallow them. I eventually discovered it was easier just to take the contraceptive pill each day; I barely noticed my cycle from then on, and that was exactly the way I liked it.

Whilst trying to beat my cycle into submission, I was treating the rest of my body with an equal measure of contempt. As a teenager at high school, I ate nothing at all until 4pm, when I would arrive home and scoff a slab of cheddar cheese topped with a thick dollop of golden syrup; at dinner I ate only meat and potatoes (all my life there had been an ongoing battle over the eating of vegetables; my mother finally surrendered when I was twelve). Later in my teens, when I experienced my first relationship break-up, I went for as long as five days without eating anything at all. This became the pattern – I would eat only when happy and content; any emotional upset at all and I would starve.

Then, still in my late teens and with the physique of a string bean, I moved 450 miles away from home, off the farm and into the city. No more horse riding, no more running across the paddocks to herd sheep, no more lifting hay bales for the cattle. Having discovered both city life and a pay packet, I morphed first from string bean to broad bean and onwards, meal after rich meal, into an engorged marrow of best-in-show proportions. Between the ages of nineteen and twenty-eight, I gained nearly forty kilogrammes (six-and-a-half stone). It turned out that, whereas I starved while miserable, I more than made up for it when life was good.

All of this mistreatment of my body, all of the dark and awful things I thought about the way it looked, the myriad ways I ignored its nutritional needs – none of this even entered my sphere of awareness; my body was just a thing that either looked okay (and made me feel okay) or looked dreadful (and made me feel dreadful).

Ten years ago, when I first started trying to conceive, all I thought about my body was that I wished I could trade it in for a more attractive one, preferably with a faster metabolism. Mine was such damn hard work. Five years earlier, at the age of twenty-nine, I had lost thirty kilogrammes (4st 7lb) through

16

both a frantic return to exercise and a drastic diet, which allowed only 30g fat per day, less than half the recommended daily intake. I did not use fresh food to achieve this goal – my weapon of choice was pre-prepared 'meals' in plastic containers, always cooked in the microwave. I might have returned to a blandly average size, but I was still as divorced from my body as it was possible to be. I had alternately starved and binged with both food and alcohol, I had shown a lack of interest in my monthly cycle that bordered on disdain, but I had turned thirty-four – it was time to take some vitamin E and make a baby. Why wouldn't my body be ready for it?

※ ※ ※

It was not exactly the best time to start having children. I had known Chris for less than a year and I had moved to the UK only two-and-a-half years earlier, leaving my own family an entire hemisphere away. I was still finding my feet, having all but started life over from scratch at the age of thirty-one. However, that was not the worst of it. The fact is, when I began trying to conceive, I was still unconsciously and inconveniently bound to someone else. Someone who wasn't Chris. This is the first in a long list of Things I Did Not Allow Myself To See after I suddenly found that my heart was set on having a family.

The truth was, when I thought I would never want children, it was always going to be another man who I spent the rest of my life never having them with. We were both twenty-one when we met, although we didn't so much meet as somehow recognise each other; the way we instantly fitted together, you would have thought we were two separate parts of one set. It was Jai who caused such a drastic physical transformation in my twenties, mainly because he made me totally and stupidly happy. So happy that, when we were both twenty-nine, we got married, as had long been expected, in a church overlooking the sea. That was the only reason I had frogmarched all that supposedly joyful weight back off my body; I would not proceed up the aisle looking like a floating cream bun.

When I imagined our life together, I saw travel, not babies; procreation, if it happened at all, was still years away. I wish I could conjure that feeling now, remember what it's like when fertility is just a random word with no great meaning. Or perhaps, if I'm going to make wishes, I should wish the opposite; that I had never been so indifferent to fertility in the first place.

It wasn't exactly a biological urge of a different sort that drove me to the other side of the world, but it was strong enough to feel like one. Jai would just as happily have settled where we were; I didn't notice. In the year 2000, we moved to London together, leaving behind our house – bought when I was only twenty-three – my well-paid job where I could likely have seen out the rest of my career, our two cars, our families and our friends. We arrived in the city with two backpacks, no jobs and nowhere to live.

More wishes: I wish I knew what happened next or that I had taken better note of what had happened before. Because, knowing what I know now, I would have stopped it immediately. I would have hit re-wind, I would have done whatever I could to change the fact that, by March 2001, I was living in London alone. After eleven years together, Jai and I had separated. My funny, strong, reliable, easy-going husband was gone. I thought it was a temporary break; he thought otherwise.

Jai left London for good in November 2003, without saying a final goodbye; I waved him off at Finchley Road tube station thinking he was going home to the southern hemisphere for only two months. We would have a drink together when he returned in the New Year – we had agreed that, whatever happened, our friendship would last for life. However, I have never seen Jai again, and the reason for this did not make itself sharply and painfully clear until I was already buckling under the weight of infertility.

THREE

As I neared my mid-thirties, it seemed a sense of urgency had sprung up from nowhere. I didn't necessarily have the primal urge that people describe when they snigger about ticking biological clocks, but I did have an increasing awareness that time was limited. Suddenly, from all around came the message: 'Get on with it, you don't have time to linger.' This deadline, this countdown to childlessness, is particularly unsettling because no one can agree on exactly how much time you have to work with. Ask the least optimistic and they will tell you that you'd better get going well before thirty-five, others say thirty-seven is the age of doom, and opinions are more divided than ever by the time a woman reaches her forties. The reality is that no one really knows at which time the clock will stop for each of us; the answer is written in every individual body. The message that seeps through, though, as you approach thirty-five is that time itself is about to become a *really big deal*.

Had I been twenty-five when I broke up with Jai, I would have done things very differently. In fact, this is true of many of the decisions I have made during my time in the Ten-Year Club. But deadline-induced pressure forces you to act, to make decisions that you might not otherwise consider, particularly so when the stakes are this high. Ten years ago, all of these observations were yet to make themselves clear to me; all I heard was that quiet voice: 'Now. You need to start now.'

I stopped taking the contraceptive pill in November 2002. One month earlier, I had turned thirty-four. I still looked, and felt, the same as I had during the 'slimmer' parts of my twenties; I was yet to even develop my first facial wrinkle.

The concept of ageing was still something that applied to other people – my understanding of what it would be like to age extended to getting wrinkles and having grey hair. I was blissfully unaware of all the unexpected little treats that a few extra years would have in store for me. I was blissfully unaware of a lot of things.

Chris and I agreed that, when it came to having a family, we would 'start trying without trying', we'd let nature take its course and see what happened. Ideally, we wouldn't conceive for another year or so anyway. However, given that we knew it might take a bit longer than for a couple in their twenties, we thought we'd better get a head-start on things.

We flew to Amsterdam for Chris's birthday in March 2003 and rented an impossibly cosy room in the gable of a boutique hotel, stuffed with antiques and curios and overlooking a placid canal. This would be a memorable place to conceive! On Chris's birthday, we wandered endless cobbled streets, drifting amiably in whichever direction we felt like heading; he ended the day getting comically drunk and we laughed until it hurt.

For our first anniversary a month later, we stayed at a bed and breakfast in a sleepy street in Henley-on-Thames; my first visit to Oxfordshire. *This* would be a memorable place to conceive! The B&B was run by an eccentric gentleman of seventy, who insisted that breakfast was at eight sharp, not a minute before or after. We hauled ourselves out of bed each morning and, still dopey, obediently gulped down our fried bacon and eggs before crawling back to our room for a nap. After we had properly gotten up for the day, we walked the banks of the River Thames, fell asleep in the long grass and awoke to find ourselves surrounded by resting ducks. We had that feeling, which we shared so often in the early days of our relationship, of being in a joyful bubble that no one else could pierce.

Not long after we had returned home to London, I lay on the couch and, rubbing my belly, glanced up at Chris and announced, "Guess what? I think we've done it!"

"What? What have we done?"

"Got pregnant, silly."

His face lit up into a beacon of delight.

"Really? But why? How do you know?"

"Well, I've never felt like this before," I explained. "My boobs really hurt and there's a twinge in my side – down here," and I gestured to an imaginary line running diagonally between hip and groin.

He lifted my feet from their resting place on his knees and enveloped me in a gentle hug. "I hope so," he said. "Nothing would make me happier." And then he quizzed me again about what I was feeling, and where, and what it could all mean.

For the next couple of weeks we daydreamed about the new life that awaited us, the life of a family. But then my period arrived, punctual as usual, and the daydreams ended. I was not pregnant.

＊ ＊ ＊

How can I describe my relationship with Chris as our first year together moved into a second? It's almost embarrassing to relay parts of it because, in many ways, we were not unlike two children. Here he was, in his forties, and me in my thirties, chasing each other around our flat, play-fighting, tumbling on the carpet, laughing uproariously at idiotic jokes that only we found funny. No one at the office where we still worked together would have recognised either of us: to them, I was vastly more gentle and mild-mannered than the type of colleagues they were accustomed to; Chris was a salt-and-pepper-haired professional, a crack shot on deadline, sometimes a bit bolshie, often incredibly charming.

The thing about Chris is that, underneath, he is not what you would expect. The first thing I noticed about him was the way he talked – when he speaks, even now, I still think it's the best voice I've heard. The dusky timbre is so unusual; it's as if the sounds he makes have an extra layer to them, almost as if his voice has been digitally enhanced. Sometimes I think he's upset about something when he's not because the way he pronounces his vowels can sound so precise, so short and uptight, compared to the languid, lazy vowels I grew up with in the southern hemisphere. Given all of this, Chris looks and sounds like a person who would be serious, straight, perhaps someone who wouldn't suffer fools (and certainly wouldn't laugh at their jokes). But he is actually one of the funniest people I know. He's a brilliant mimic – there's not a relative or colleague that he cannot do a side-splitting impersonation of, perfectly capturing their verbal and physical tics. In our early days together, we could spend entire afternoons in bed, taping Chris on a mobile phone as he reeled off one impression after another, and hooting helplessly when we played them back to ourselves.

Another thing I did not expect, given the driven and efficient Chris that I had seen in the office: in *real* life, he was incredibly and, sometimes infuriatingly, vague. His dressing-gown pockets bulged with unopened bills that he had poked in there when collecting the mail, and promptly forgotten about. He accidentally and randomly left his possessions strewn around London; his brief case on a tube station platform, his reading glasses atop a hedge outside a school, and, on the seat of a Jubilee Line train, a bag of South African delicacies given to me by a friend. Also hidden somewhere in the city was the brigade of umbrellas that had mysteriously disappeared from his grasp.

Given that he had been Mr Charisma, swaggering around the office, I accused him of false advertising on many fronts.

For one thing, I had mistakenly assumed that, because Chris had left home at seven, he would be as self-sufficient and independent as it was possible to be. However, his premature departure from family life had had the opposite effect; he was great at following orders issued by someone else, but had never really had the opportunity to think for himself, to use his initiative when it came to practical matters.

It was a shock when it gradually dawned on me that Chris was not entirely sure how his oven worked, or his dishwasher, or his mobile phone, and definitely not his washing machine. All of the crisp, tasteful shirts he wore to the office were only ever dry-cleaned and, for anything more taxing than changing a light bulb, he had always 'got people in'. Growing up on a farm in the southern hemisphere, I had never known anyone like this. Perhaps that was why I initially assumed Chris would not be fazed by practicalities; I should have taken more notice of the pyramid of used tea bags stacked up in his sink.

When I first visited him, I took a train to the countryside south of London and, as it pulled into the station, he ran along the platform, sweeping my suitcase from my hands before I had barely taken a step. When we reached his car, he walked to the passenger side and held the door open for me, closing it again when I was settled in the front seat.

When we later arrived at his home, it was arty and sophisticated, but not stuffy. It was full of pine furniture, kilim rugs, shelves of books and CDs and terracotta urns, bowls and pots that could all have been chosen by me. I thought it was just another marker of the way in which we matched each other. And at least all of this, he had done himself. I knew Chris cared about what I thought of it because there was a crisp new duvet on the bed and a matching towel set in the bathroom when I arrived. On the first morning I woke up there, he brought me breakfast in bed – croissants, pain au chocolat and fruit bread. Later, when we'd been so wrapped up in each other that we'd forgotten to eat anything else, he ate cornflakes in bed at midnight, splashes of milk speckling my dark hair as I nestled into his chest. The next day he sat me down in an armchair and said he wanted to play me a song. It was Nick Drake's *Northern Sky*:

> *I never felt magic crazy as this*
> *I never saw moons knew the meaning of the sea*
> *I never held emotion in the palm of my hand*
> *Or felt sweet breezes in the top of a tree*
> *But now you're here*
> *Brighten my northern sky*

There were tears in his eyes when it finished. "I still can't believe I found you," he said.

※ ※ ※

I've mentioned so many ordinary things about us because they are key to what came next, to understanding what happens to a relationship when it is blown off its foundations by infertility – and whether it is even possible to think about rebuilding once you've picked up all the pieces. For one thing, can you ever actually pick up all the pieces? When I lie in bed at night, staring into the darkness even though there is nothing to see, my biggest fear is that this will still hurt when I'm eighty. If I don't have children, then I won't have grandchildren either. There won't be anyone there to care if I am a sprightly, active eighty-year-old or a bed-bound ghost. I think a pathetic thought: who will look after me? Even as I think it, I know that those who do have children are not guaranteed that comfort themselves; maybe it would be even more heartbreaking to have kids who just plain don't care.

However, the other reason I worry about being old and alone comes down to disclosure at the start of our relationship – or rather, something Chris didn't disclose. I kept things from him, of course; we all do. For my part, I did highly immature things like pretending I did not have certain bodily functions – for eight months, and sometimes causing great discomfort to myself, I kept up the illusion that I was a person who never needed the bathroom. Unfortunately, that was dramatically dashed when I caught a stomach bug on holiday. Afterwards, I was almost pleased by the inconvenient turn of events; it's tiring trying to present the airbrushed version of yourself at all times. And vain. And a total waste of time. I hope I was pretty honest about the big things, though, the stuff that really matters. I even mentioned Jai quite often, probably too often.

But it turned out there had been a lie of omission at the beginning, a misunderstanding that was not corrected. When Chris and I met at work and furtively leaned around our computer screens to have whispered conversations between assignments, I took something he said and used it to calculate that he was forty-two. I was thirty-three and thought nine years was right at the upper limit when it came to an age gap. Sometimes I mentioned it in passing, that he was forty-two, sometimes I alluded to the fact that there was nearly a decade between us, but not quite.

Then, nearly two months into our relationship, we were walking along the seafront in Brighton. We strolled past a palm reader's booth, shielded from the world by a pair of unevenly-faded red velvet curtains, and immediately fell into a discussion about fortune tellers, clairvoyants and astrology.

"What about the Chinese zodiac?" I asked. "Do you know what animal you're supposed to be? Apparently, I'm a Monkey."

"Yes, I can see that," Chris replied as he looked me up and down. "It suits you."

I cuffed him on the arm. "Okay then, let's work out what year you are – you might not be so pleased with yourself when you find out. What year were you born again … 1959?"

There was a pause. Then Chris stopped walking.

"Look," he said. "About that. The thing is," and the words fell quickly, as if he wanted them out and done with, "I'm afraid I'm actually forty-seven. I didn't really know how to tell you." He looked embarrassed, self-conscious.

"Really? But why didn't you just say so?"

"I don't know. You seemed so young when I first saw you – I didn't want you to think I was some old fogey. Then you assumed I was younger and I suppose I was flattered, then embarrassed …"

I did what I always used to do when I was thirty-three; I rushed to make the other person feel better, without really stopping to consider the implications of what had just been revealed. "I'm not like that," I said, truthfully. "You're a person, not a set of numbers on a birth certificate."

He gave a rueful smile. "I thought you might leave me."

"Why would I dump you for being forty-seven? Don't be stupid."

And I meant it. But inside I was struggling with the idea of being with a man who was so much older than me. I worked it out: he was thirteen years and seven months old when I was born. He was already at secondary school. I felt momentarily nauseous, which didn't make a lot of sense as it was true that I didn't categorise people that way.

"I should have known you wouldn't be like that," Chris said. "But you can't tell when you first meet people, can you?"

"Honestly, it doesn't matter," I reassured him. "Just be happy that you might be forty-seven but you don't look it – or act it. Nothing near."

"Actually, I forgot," Chris muttered. "It was my birthday at the beginning of last month. I've, ahm, just turned forty-eight."

Fourteen years and seven months old when I was born, then. Eighty-five when I would be seventy-one.

My instincts had been reliable; somewhere inside the warning light had instantly flashed on. It's just that my brain is really slow on the uptake. Sometimes I *know* that something is wrong, but I can't put it into words; it's almost like my mind won't let me know it. Maybe that's what people do when they're in denial.

It's unlikely that I would have agreed to go out with Chris if I had known he was forty-eight, but, even though I couldn't put it into words that day, the number itself wasn't the problem. It was the fact that, by concealing the truth, he had taken away an initial choice that should have been mine. I might never have thought about it that way if it wasn't for infertility. But prolonged infertility forces you to look at all the things you don't want to see, about others and about yourself. The age issue did not disappear that day in Brighton; it was just temporarily buried by Chris's relief and my denial. Whilst in the Ten-Year Club, I would have many thoughts and feelings about it – some insightful, some irrational – but, really, if I had looked deeper at the start I would have realised that it was not so much an isolated incident as a stark pointer towards what was to follow.

FOUR

I DIDN'T SEE IT coming. How many people have said that after an accident or any other sudden reversal of fortune? "We never thought something like this would happen to us." It seems that none of us ever do, not really, not deep down. The irony is that I have spent so much of my life worrying about what might go wrong – then when it did go wrong, I wasn't prepared for it. Like a speeding car shooting a stop sign, infertility blindsided me. Just like that, it made my life messy and painful; it tore away any shred of security I thought I might feel about anything. I didn't see it coming. I didn't think it would happen to me.

If you had told me in 2003, while I was happily romping in an array of locations, that I would still be childless in 2012 – 2012! A whole new decade, a decade so far away in another time that it was the one Marty McFly travelled to in *Back to the Future II* – then I don't know what I would have done. I suspect I might have gone to bed and never got up again. Would it have been better to have known? Would I already have found a new path for my life to follow if I'd been aware that all my efforts were pointless? Or has it been kinder, less of a shock, to let the realisation sink in slowly? Who can say for sure, but I think I would rather have known; there is nothing more demoralising than chasing a future you will never have.

The thing about infertility is that it flings you from hope to despair and back again, over and over, and sometimes that constant shifting of the foundations feels worse than if you had just stuck with the despair in the first place. All that time ago, in 2003, I would have been horrified to know that I would still be trying to conceive in 2008 – surely that couldn't happen, surely we would find a solution before then? But 2012? Come on, you must be joking. *20-fucking-12*, that's what I think sometimes when the anger washes over me. I see 2012, I see 2003, I see all the time that passed and I want to tear up those godforsaken calendars and kick down all of those miserable, dark years. Even now, if I think about it too much, I just want to batter and punch something, to kick out until I can't breathe anymore. There are moments when I wish infertility had a face because then I could spit in it, I could hit it, I could shout at it, I could scratch every last bit of flesh off it – me, who has always played the gentle peacemaker, who has always broken up fights, me who now wants to beat the living daylights out of something. How did it change me this much?

❧ ❧ ❧

In 2003, I was thinking of pregnancy, not infertility. I stopped eating runny cheese 'in case it harmed the baby', I asked a pharmacist whether the spot cream I used was safe in pregnancy, I wondered where we should live when we had a child; I didn't think we could stay in London.

I even went to the doctor because I thought I was pregnant and had experienced implantation bleeding; he was a young locum and didn't know what 'implantation bleeding' was. I knew though, through very personal experience – the only reason I exist is because my seventeen-year-old birth mother continued to have what appeared to be 'periods' during the early part of her pregnancy. That knowledge has made infertility ever more confusing for me; even when it seemed my period had arrived, I could convince myself that there might still be a chance, I might still be pregnant. Like my mother, the one who conceived me too easily, too young, the one who might have snuffed out my life before it began if she had not taken five months to realise that I was there. If any urge drove me in 2003, it was probably the severing of those initial blood ties. I had keenly felt the loss, the sense of 'otherness' that arises when you are unable to look around your family and think, 'Yes, I see the similarities between us, I see where I fit in.' It had only recently occurred to me that I could compensate for that when I had a family of my own. I could not wait to have my own baby, to hold him or her close and, for the first time, to think, 'Wow, we share the same DNA, we are made of the same stuff.' This was my chance to experience 'family' the way that other people experienced it, to share it with my own child. Somehow, I felt it would help me to understand things I had not understood before.

It's stupid really, not to mention irrational, but I had always assumed that I would not be left childless – infertility would not happen to me because I had already been adopted; now things would even out and I would get to experience the birth family I felt I had missed out on. Maybe that is why, in 2003 and 2004, I had no real concept of what lay before me. I didn't see it coming. I didn't think it would happen to me.

᠅ ᠅ ᠅

Not thinking for a moment that this would become a decade-long challenge, I casually let it slip to some close friends and my sisters Jane and Vanda that we were trying to have a family. I purposely did not mention it to my mother because I wanted to surprise her; she had it in mind that I was a "career woman through and through" and that children were "not on the agenda", as she put it.

My sisters were thrilled with the news, though. Their own children were all young adults and they loved the thought of having babies and toddlers around again. "Oooh," said Vanda, "get on with it then. I can't wait to play aunty to your

31

little ones." I laughed. We were getting on with it as best we could.

At Christmas 2003, I went out for a drink with Dean, an old friend from home, first of Jai's and then of mine.

"So how's Granddad then?" he asked after a while. Dean always called Chris Granddad; I sometimes suspected he couldn't understand how I had ended up with someone so vastly different to Jai.

"He's great," I said. "Things are moving along, I suppose." Before I could stop myself, I added: "It's probably a bit early to say anything but we've decided to have a family ... well, we've been kind of trying but we're not really trying-trying, if you know what I mean."

Dean chuckled. "Nope! I don't know what you mean, but it sounds fun. Wow. Kids. Awesome news."

I also confided in my friends Lisa and Suzanne; the three of us had met at work in London and found that we shared not only Antipodean roots but the same birth year. Neither of them was remotely child-minded and had assumed I felt the same. They both looked surprised to discover I had become 'broody', as they described it.

Suzanne was living with her girlfriend and reported that they both found kids a noisy, irritating, messy pain. "I'll hold yours and say nice things about it," she said, "but don't expect me to do any babysitting."

Lisa shared an inner-city apartment with her boyfriend and enjoyed a legendary social life that she did not intend to give up in favour of having a family. "Great," she said, "I can be an aunty to your kids. I'll enjoy all the good bits then I can give them back to you." She paused, suddenly serious. "Good for you. I'm really glad you're happy."

Suzanne piped up again. "I think I should be the godmother, though."

FIVE

WHEN CONCEPTION DOESN'T GO to plan, life very quickly becomes an exercise in information gathering. One of the first – and most basic – things you will glean is advice about 'when it's time to see the doctor'. We all hope at the beginning that this time will never come. *Please don't let it happen to us.* But as the months tick by, the general guidelines play over and over in your mind: see a doctor if you have been unsuccessfully trying to conceive for more than a year; or for six months if you are over thirty-five. The more time that passes, the less confidently you can reassure yourself; it will be okay, it takes a while sometimes, not everyone fits into a set of guidelines, maybe it's just not the right time yet.

With my sister, Vanda, as my template – and knowing that I wasn't desperate to conceive *immediately* – I let two years tick by before really starting to worry that something was wrong, that it was not going to happen.

I was not one of those people who obsessed about every detail from cycle one. I didn't buy ovulation test kits (I'm not sure I even knew they existed), I didn't take a pregnancy test each month, I didn't fill the kitchen with pre-conception supplements; I just gave up alcohol and starting taking a multivitamin.

During the first few months, I bought a couple of small books about pregnancy: what to do and what not to do after you had conceived, what to expect during each stage of your baby's gestation. They are now buried at the bottom of a box in the loft; after ten years I don't need their mocking presence on my bookshelf.

During those first two years of trying to conceive, I can remember moments of extreme happiness. It helped that Chris and I travelled a lot – while blithely pursuing conception we had indulged in unprotected sex in both hemispheres and at several points in between.

I have a clear snapshot in my mind of our second anniversary; we were sitting by the river under Pulteney Bridge in Bath, Somerset, lounging against each other in the sun and watching the world go by on a weekday. I remember sitting there and thinking, I wish everyone could be this happy. That was in early 2004; we had been trying to start a family for more than a year.

By that time, I had begun to gravitate towards the 'health' sections of bookshops – I had not spent much time there before, expect perhaps to surreptitiously leaf through diet books. It had started about eight months in, when I was buying a magazine in WH Smith and stumbled across a book that asked the same question, there on the cover, that I often asked myself: *Why Am I So Tired?* Here, it seemed, was a possible answer. Written by a naturopathic consultant, the book outlined the symptoms of mild hypothyroidism, some of which included exhaustion, weight gain – and infertility. Here it was. This would be the key. This would be the vital piece of information that led to me getting pregnant!

The book even mentioned perpetually cold hands and feet, and wasn't Chris always shouting in shock every time I climbed into bed and tried to warm my painfully freezing hands on his back, which, like all of him, blazed with the ferocity of a furnace? He would jump violently, as if stung. "Argh! They're like ice blocks. *Please,*" he pleaded, "warm them up under the pillow first." It is yet another way in which we are opposites: Chris's metabolism is as hot and fast as mine is cold and slow.

When I read beyond the book's cover, it felt as if, finally, I had found something that gave a detailed and plausible explanation for the 'symptoms' I had long exhibited, but which so many doctors wave away under that catch-all of 'stress' or a hectic lifestyle. Why did I always feel more sluggish than 'normal' people, even if I had had nine hours' sleep at night – and why, after nine hours, did I wake up feeling groggy and hungover, worse than I had felt before going to sleep in the first place? Why did I feel nauseous if I had to wake up any earlier? Why did I gain weight even when I seemed to be eating less than those around me? Why couldn't I get pregnant?

I learned that thyroid hormones regulate metabolic rate, body temperature and cellular repair and, crucially, that in diagnosing a problem in this area there is a lot more to it than simply running the standard blood test for levels of Thyroid Stimulating Hormone. It was possible to fall within the normal range for TSH, but to still be affected by hypothyroidism. The book explained that levels of free thyroxine were often overlooked, but could be equally important.

The information resonated to such an extent that I did something I had never done before – I contacted the author's office and made an appointment with him, my first foray into private healthcare. Apart from the vitamins, this was my first conception-motivated expenditure. I cannot remember now how much it cost; if I had known this struggle with fertility was going to last for ten years, I would have started up an accounts book and noted it down: September 2003, thyroid consultation. What would I have done then if I knew how many pages of that notional account book would ultimately be filled up?

But everything was still shiny and new and, like the tourist that I have always remained, I was quite pleased to have a proper look at the renowned Harley Street, the venue for my appointment with the author.

I remember him being like a genial professor who had devoted years of his life to his specialist subject and knew what you would describe even before you described it. It was a relief not to have to rush the conversation, not to feel the pressure of having to sum up your symptoms, your feelings, your lifestyle in five minutes flat, as with so many visits to the doctors' surgery. We had a lengthy conversation, ranging across many areas. At one stage, he asked which season of the year was my favourite. This threw me, so I just said 'summer' because it reminded me of Christmases at home in the southern hemisphere.

He smiled. "Most of those with hypothyroid symptoms opt for autumn or spring. They tend to find winter too cold and summer too hot." When I thought about it, he was right. The summer of 2003 had reached record temperatures in London and, on the day it notoriously hit 38 degrees, I spent most of the time feeling like I was going to pass out – I eventually filled the bath with cold water and gingerly crawled into it several times in one afternoon.

By the end of our appointment, I had been referred for both a detailed thyroid profile and a test for candida over-growth. These tests were carried out at a private laboratory on Wimpole Street and would have filled entries two and three in my 'fertility account book'. When the blood test results came back, I was sure we had found the cause of our fertility problems, that this would be both the beginning and the end of our dealings with the healthcare profession. The author/naturopath wrote to say that my results fell within the normal reference ranges for thyroid function. However, my Free T4 level – at 13.6 – was too low. "To place these figures into context, M.E. patients [suffering a form of chronic fatigue syndrome] average 12.3 and symptom-free individuals average 16.9," he wrote. "At your age, an acceptable level would be 15-20 …"

He suggested three different supplements for adrenal and thyroid support – and that was how I found myself taking nine tablets a day, some of which contained bovine thyroid from New Zealand, along with my one multivitamin. Entry four for the account book. After several months of supplementation, I was retested: my T4 level had climbed to 14.9; I had almost reached the target. By now, 2003 had moved into 2004. I felt better within myself, more energetic, but I still was not pregnant.

My other life, the one I lived outside of fertility issues, kept ticking along; I took on a stressful new job and used up most of my newly-restored energy to deal with it. Factions of the almost exclusively male staff were aggrieved at my arrival; in taking the contract, I had unwittingly leapfrogged one of them, having clearly received preferential treatment by virtue of being a 'girl'. I was a thirty-five-year-old 'girl' with eighteen years' experience in my chosen profession; I ignored the sniping that went on just under the radar and tried not to notice that, when I sat down for dinner in the staff canteen, everyone else at the table would get up and leave. Why should I care about it? I would be pregnant soon; I would be taking maternity leave, possibly even a long-term career break, and they would see that I was no threat. I didn't want their testostcrone-fuelled jobs – all I really wanted was to be a mother.

೪ ೪ ೪

Something else happened in 2004 – it wasn't directly related to fertility but it knocked my confidence in its own way; somehow it added to the growing feeling that I was already a different person to the more carefree one who had casually started trying to conceive so many months before.

The event announced itself, like summertime thunder, in mid-August when I arrived at work to find an e-mail awaiting me from Jai. I had barely heard from him since he had disappeared from London the previous Christmas and I still couldn't understand why he hadn't returned. I had missed his friendship; we'd always agreed we were like 'family' and that the bond would never leave us. So an e-mail from him felt like a familiar, welcome thing. I ignored everything else in my inbox and opened it, eager to reconnect. There was an obligatory line or two of small-talk, which by its very presence emphasised the distance between us. Then came a revelation that hit so hard I reflexively clutched at my stomach. Tears instantly pricked my eyes. I held my breath and willed them away; I knew any sign of 'female' weakness would play right into the hands of my hostile male colleagues who still couldn't accept that a woman belonged in their midst.

"I wanted to let you know," wrote Jai, "that I've been seeing a bit of Dana since I got back. I don't know where it's going but I enjoy her company. I know what's coming next now you know this, but I'm sorry, I just had to tell you."

Dana. My best friend, the chief bridesmaid at our wedding. Dana, who said I was like a sister to her. Dana, who had spent days, months, years with us after I became her 'support person' when her mum was terminally ill. Dana, who I thought I knew almost as well as I knew myself.

I could hardly begrudge Jai a new relationship, but why – why? – could he not go out into the world and meet someone who had nothing to do with me?

I knew what she looked like first thing in the morning and last thing at night, I knew that she went to the gym daily, even when ill, and did her housework every Friday; I knew everything about her, or at least thought I had. I couldn't *not* imagine them together. Then a new fear hit: when I walked down the aisle at our wedding, was he really looking behind me, was he looking for her all along? She was slimmer, blonder and more compliant than me; of course he was.

Sometimes, when I was worrying about trying to conceive, I had kept the fear at bay by forcing myself to remember funny, warm things that had happened in my life. I often thought of Jai during those times – there had been barely a cross word between us during the first five or six years of our relationship and I could choose from seemingly endless memories of laughter-filled days to keep me going when I was struggling. Now I realised that Dana's arrival in our lives coincided almost exactly with the change in our relationship, with the stresses and strains that suddenly arose. How had I missed it?

The double-dose of betrayal took my breath away.

I sent Chris a text on the way home from work and told him what had happened. When the tube pulled in to our station, at about twenty past midnight, he was there waiting for me, as usual.

He enveloped me in a cocoon-like hug. "I'm really sorry, sweetheart," he said. "Those two are beyond the pale."

At home, I sat on the couch and cried, finally, Chris pulling me to his chest.

"She was the only one who ever said Jai and I shouldn't stay together – now I know why!"

"I know. I know," he soothed. "But it won't last you know, these things never do."

"I really cared about her," I stuttered. "I couldn't have looked after her any better when her mum was ill – and for years after she died."

"I know Lou, you were a great friend. It's not right."

Every time I came up with another Dana story, and there were dozens, Chris made suitably comforting comments: "Some people are just human parasites, I'm afraid. It'll come back around on her, you wait and see."

He must have wanted to turn out the light and go to sleep – it was after 1am and I was still outraged and upset – but Chris kept hugging me and delivering one of his pep talks, trying anything he could think of to make me feel better.

"It's because I'm too fat," I interjected dolefully. "She's skinny. And blonde."

39

"You mustn't say these things about yourself," Chris urged. "You're more beautiful than you know, and it's about time someone made you realise that."

"Well, Jai obviously doesn't think so," I grunted.

"I doubt that's even true," Chris said. "I've seen the pictures – Dana looks like a demented toothpick."

Finally, I stopped feeling sorry for myself and let out a giggle. "Anyway," I added, "her breath smells 'cause she never eats any carbs."

"I knew it," said Chris. "I could tell she was a stinky kind of woman."

This is how we were before we were overtaken by infertility, before it felt like a battle to survive, like when a ship is sinking and someone cries, "Every man for himself!" Before we had fallen into that trap, each focused on our own survival, we had always backed each other up, even when it wasn't particularly comfortable to do so.

Chris even went so far as to encourage me to remain friends with Jai.

"Give it time," he counselled. "You don't know what's around the corner. You've played a wonderful part in each other's lives, it would be a shame to throw away your friendship now. I think you'd regret it eventually."

He also pointed out that Jai had at least written to apologise and explain. "It's more than your so-called best friend has bothered to do."

I looked up at Chris, genuinely troubled to see me so upset, and he appeared every inch the tolerant and understanding father.

"Thanks," I whispered. "You'd be a lovely dad."

Later, when he fell asleep, arms still wrapped around me, I lay awake through the night thinking of nothing but two people who I used to know. The pain brought with it a warning whisper: should this hurt so much? If Chris was so very right for me that I had chosen him to be the father of my children, then why was I so shaken? It felt like one of the pillars holding up my life had just fallen.

If you were with the right person it wouldn't feel like this. I captured the inconvenient thought and smothered it before it could cause too much damage. I was good at that type of thing. I'd once done much the same with a silly, irrational suspicion that my best friend was a little too fond of my husband. And look how well that had turned out.

Six

BY JANUARY 2005, WE had been trying to start a family for more than two years. I had spent hours in bookshops devouring any information I could find about how to conceive. Chris would disappear to the sports section and relax with a cricket or rugby book while I studied and studied, trying to find the missing piece of the jigsaw. My thyroid levels were now all within normal ranges; if it wasn't that preventing us from getting pregnant, then what was it?

I bought a copy of *Women's Bodies, Women's Wisdom*, written by a doctor who also took into account the 'mind, body, spirit' connection when dealing with health issues. I wished someone had given me such a book when I was twelve. For the first time, I truly understood what my body had been miraculously achieving month after month while I gave it next to no nutritional support and berated it for not fitting into the right-sized clothes. It was embarrassing to realise the extent of my ignorance. I thought back to the conversation I had had with Chris on the couch that night after we returned from Henley, the 'I think I'm pregnant' one. I feel ridiculous when I think of that now; it underlined everything I didn't know. What had most likely happened that month was that I had noticed signs of ovulation for the first time since coming off the contraceptive pill; all those years on the pill and I never really knew what it felt like to ovulate. I had never properly understood the intricate workings of my cycle; for most of my life, all I had understood was that I wanted to be rid of it. Now, suddenly, I wanted – needed – to know everything about it. I started paying it a lot more attention, but even then there was still more to learn than I could imagine.

One thing was obvious, though – it was time to face the facts: we had spent two years 'trying without trying' and it was clear that we were not going to have a family without some help.

As always when it came to fertility, I was the one who initiated our first nervous visit to the doctor. Chris did not know much more about fertility and conception than he had when we started out more than two years ago; anything he knew had been passed on by me. Sometimes he seemed to take information on board, sometimes he didn't. He seemed so unconcerned about our fertility problems that you would almost think they were happening to someone else. I knew that if he had investigated further, if he had read the raft of stats and opinions about fertility and ageing, then he would have shown a greater sense of urgency. Still, he agreed it was time to see a doctor and, once I had made the appointment, instantly began fretting about the state of his sperm.

"What if I don't have any at all worth using?" he said. "I've always worried that it might not be up to scratch."

"Don't worry," I replied, "it's more likely to be something wrong with me."

Apart from registering with the surgery when we first moved into the area a year earlier, neither of us had ever visited our new GP. We had never been ill enough to bother and, besides, I felt that unless there were serious complications, it generally wasn't worth the effort – whatever bug I rolled up with, the blanket solution seemed to be a dose of antibiotics and I'm allergic to nearly every one of them. Prescription medication and I did not get along at all. So on the Monday when we first visited the GP, we were venturing into new territory in more ways than one.

We arrived early, discreetly tried to explain to the robotically stern receptionist that we were having a joint appointment, and perched anxiously on our waiting-room seats like two errant pupils sent to sit outside the headmaster's office. We watched an elderly man stagger in on his own, making slow and laboured progress towards the reception desk.

"Good afternoon," he said, his rasping voice betraying signs of exertion. "Now, it's rather a long tale, I'm afraid."

The receptionist showed no sign of recognition that someone was speaking to her.

"I telephoned earlier, you see …"

And eventually it emerged that there had been a mix-up with his heart medication; he had ordered an emergency prescription to replace the tablets he already should have taken that morning.

The receptionist finally acknowledged his presence. "Prescription collection is at 2pm," she said.

I looked up at the clock on the wall; it was 1.53pm. The elderly man looked nonplussed. "Oh," he said. "The fellow who brought me here by taxi was a bit early, you see."

"You're welcome to sit in the waiting area until 2pm," the receptionist intoned before turning her attention back to the file of notes she was reading.

The man surveyed the distance between the desk and the nearest chair and you could almost see him summoning the energy to force himself across the gaping chasm. It was obvious that it would take the full seven minutes until the magic hour of 2pm for him to cross the floor, sit down and then wrench himself back up again.

"Here," Chris offered warmly. "Let me help you," and he picked up a chair, carried it across the room and placed it down at the corner of the reception desk. The look he gave the receptionist said, 'Don't even think about complaining.'

When Chris sat back down again, I squeezed his hand and smiled. This was precisely why I wanted him to be the father of my children – he could be so gentle, he knew how to look after people when they needed it.

At one minute to two, a nurse appeared and called our names. We left the elderly man patiently waiting for the clock to tick forward one more notch and followed her up some stairs. We expected to be shown into an office, but she gestured to a set of chairs in the carpeted corridor that ran the length of the building. This was level two of the waiting game.

Seated once more, Chris's right knee bounced up and down, up and down, faster and faster; he did this in the office when working under pressure. Today, as at work, his face appeared calm, but his frenzied leg was telling a different story. Having reached this daunting place – the place at which you stop skirting around your problem and stare it straight in its ugly face – we each just wanted it over with. Finally, a door opened, a middle-aged man departed down the stairs and a minute or so later, a woman doctor peered into the corridor and summoned us in. This was it. We were here.

I did the talking, in a quiet monotone that didn't sound anything like my usual voice, thanks to the anxiety bubbling up my throat. The doctor didn't say much; there were some questions for me about whether I was having regular periods – I confirmed that I was – and that was it. Any further conjecture would have to wait until we had each undergone tests. There would be several blood tests for me, and a scan, which I very much hoped would not be internal. It felt like a pivotal moment for us to be there, discussing these things, but the doctor seemed indifferent to the swirl of emotions it was causing.

"You will also need to undertake a semen analysis," she half-mumbled, glancing towards Chris, who was yet to say a word.

"I have an explanatory form here, detailing what you need to be aware of," and she rifled through a drawer in her desk before handing it over. "I'll also give you a container to … um, collect the sample in." More rifling, but no plastic pot. "Sorry, we don't seem to have any. But you can get one from any pharmacy, they will know what you need."

The blood tests would be done through the GP surgery, the scan and sperm analysis at the local hospital. I asked when we should book the tests and the doctor's reply was sharp.

"Well, I wouldn't waste any time," she said. "You can't afford to muck around at your age."

Her words shot through me. "At your age", meaning 'old'; no one had ever said it in that context before.

The doctor looked to be in her mid-thirties herself; I supposed she must have already had her children, bang on schedule, at the optimum time. There was certainly a hint of superiority in the clipped tone of her voice; if we had wanted empathy or reassurance, we wouldn't find any here. The surgery itself, along with anyone we had met who worked within it, felt cold. I supposed that wouldn't matter in the scheme of things – the main issue was whether they could diagnose our problem and, beyond that, help us fix it. But it would not be the only time throughout the next ten years when I found myself wondering why the so-called 'caring' professions had attracted a fair share of people who didn't appear to care much at all.

We left clutching various bits of green and white paper documenting our next steps and immediately headed for the local park to clear the experience from our systems.

"Was it just me" asked Chris, "or did she look really embarrassed when she was talking about my sperm test?"

"Oh! I thought it was just me. I thought she looked seriously uncomfortable actually."

"She couldn't even look at me," he said. "What on earth was going on?"

"Maybe she's just not used to couples turning up together. Maybe she was overcompensating because she was worried you'd be embarrassed …"

"Maybe," he echoed, sounding doubtful. "And no collection pot. Does this mean I have to tell the whole of Boots that I'm having a sperm test?"

"No. Just say you want a pot for a urine sample."

"But how do I know it will be the right size? What if it's too small and I get the aim wrong? Then what do I do?"

"It will be the right size," I reassured him. "Just aim and fire."

"Hmm. Easy for you to say."

A harried-looking man in a crumpled suit strode past and I waited for him to scurry out of earshot.

"Well, at least no one's going to be looking at your bits. I've got a horrible feeling I'm going to be having a probe up my wotsit."

"A what?"

"An internal scan. Urgh. I don't even want to think about it."

"This whole thing is appalling," said Chris.

"Yep," I said glumly, "and just think of all those people out there who have had multiple rounds of IVF. Imagine what they've been through."

Please don't let it happen to us.

As we wandered through the park not really noticing the lush landscape that usually relaxed us, my stomach began to churn with fear. The doctor's words kept playing back and forth in my mind. "You can't afford to muck around at your age." For the first time, I felt rising panic about it. *You're too old. You're too old. You've left it too late.* I had turned thirty-six three months earlier.

Chris gave me a hug. "What would she know? Look at you – there's not a line on your face."

"That doesn't matter," I snapped. "It's about what state my *insides* are in. I might not have any eggs left for all we know, or they might be so old and damaged that they're useless. And do you know what happens to fertility rates after a woman turns thirty-seven? She's just said it pretty straight – I'm practically too old for this."

"Come on," Chris cajoled. "Don't give up yet. We haven't even had the tests. Let's just see what they show."

I walked home feeling like a different person to the one who had walked to the surgery earlier that day. Everything about me, both in mind and body, felt heavier.

Several weeks later, I had given blood, as directed, on days three and twenty-one of my cycle. The first test would measure my baseline level of Follicle Stimulating Hormone, which would give a pointer as to how many eggs I had left to work with. None of this was explained to us, I picked it up by reading yet more books. Through my reading, I had gleaned that, if baseline FSH is elevated, then it reflects a declining number of eggs – and possibly a decline in egg quality, too. The day twenty-one test, on the other hand, would check a range of things, including progesterone levels, and it should show whether I had ovulated or not. My thyroid hormone levels would also be checked again, but by now I knew the test would assess Thyroid Stimulating Hormone only, it would not extend to free thyroxine levels.

On the day I was due to phone the surgery for my results, I was at work in a near-silent office, surrounded by my male colleagues. I picked up the phone on my desk and dialled the number; I figured I would just say, "I'm ringing for my blood test results" and, if anyone did happen to overhear, they would be none the wiser about what I had been tested for.

The robotic receptionist answered. I gave my pre-planned opening spiel. "Test results are between 3pm and 4pm," she said before hanging up. I looked at the clock. 2.45pm.

Twenty minutes later, I tried again.

"Hello? I've been told to phone at this time to receive my test results."

I gave my name and the receptionist put me on hold. A click on the line signalled her return. "Yes," she barked. "It's confirmed – you have been immunised against rubella."

What? I knew that already. I clearly remembered lining up in our high school gym, rolling up my sleeve to receive the injection and seeing the girl behind me faint clean away before the needle had even touched skin. In fact, if I needed further proof of my immunisation, the needle mark was still clearly visible on my upper right arm.

"Eer," I stammered. "I don't think that's what I was being tested for."

"Oh? What results were you expecting?" she enquired.

I leaned as far into the phone as I could get. "I think," I whispered, "that the tests should show whether I have normal," and the whisper got even lower, "ovarian reserves. And also whether I'm … ov..ul..ating … or not."

I glanced quickly around; the men were all typing at their computers, reading newspapers or talking on the phone themselves. The receptionist put me on hold again, tinkly music and all, and returned a couple of minutes later.

"I have all of your results in front of me," she said, "and everything has come back as normal."

"My ovarian reserve is okay? And I'm ovulating?"

"Yes," she confirmed. "Everything is normal."

I hung up the phone, relieved. Time had not quite run out yet.

※ ※ ※

"What if the taxi comes and I'm not done?"

Chris looked as panicked as I had ever seen him. He was pacing the lounge wielding a sample pot.

"What if I do it too quickly and they all die before we get to hospital?" He peered sceptically at the plastic container for what seemed like the millionth time. "It really is a very small target, you know. What if I miss, what if the sample ends up all over the bathroom floor?"

"There's not going to be a sample at all if you don't calm down," I said.

"Exactly! That's what I'm worried about."

49

I looked at the kitchen clock. All we seemed to be doing lately was monitoring time. If I wasn't counting how many years might remain of my 'fertile' life, I was calculating what day of my cycle it was or how long it would be before I could receive my next test results.

Now, timing-wise, the utmost of precision was required. A taxi was coming at 8.45am and it would transport us, along with Chris's sperm sample, to a hospital twenty-five minutes away. To achieve clear results, the sample needed to be tested as soon as possible after collection and definitely no more than an hour afterwards.

Chris had been adamant that he was not, under any circumstances, undertaking sample 'collection' at the hospital. I didn't push him to change his mind; I knew what he was like in hospitals. It was the smell, he said. He couldn't take it. I had already warned him that he'd better be over that by the time I gave birth. I expected him to be there, not only that but sitting upright, not lying in a green-tinged heap in the corner.

On this occasion, though, we had a carefully strategised Plan B – he could collect his sample at home, preferably at 8.40am; the taxi was due to arrive at 8.45am and it should take twenty-five minutes to drive to hospital. Therefore, allowing time to walk it inside, we could have the sample at the lab within about forty-five minutes of collection. That was the idea, anyway. At the moment, it looked like the plan was about to fall apart at step one.

"I knew I should have bought you a magazine," I said.

Chris looked aghast. "You know that's not my thing at all," he growled. "It's so *seedy*."

It was true. While some men got their kicks from lads' mags and lapdancing clubs, Chris was of a more romantic bent; he liked carefully-chosen music, poetry, candlelight, luxurious surroundings, the whole shebang. Unfortunately, all he had was a sample pot and our bathroom. I wondered, momentarily, whether I should have moved the stereo in there. Music could always calm him down, change his mood.

"What's the time?" he asked, again.

"8.29. One more minute and you might as well go in there."

"Okay," he said. "Right … can I call you if I need help?"

I ignored his request. "Good luck!" I urged as he trudged down the hallway and shut the bathroom door.

Now I could let my own anxieties show. I turned up the radio and jiggled up and down on the spot in the kitchen, manically shaking my fingers, arms, legs and hands as, almost automatically, I tried to move the nervous energy out of my body. I obsessively glanced first at the clock and then outside at the street to see if the taxi had arrived. Back and forth, back and forth. Deep down, I didn't think he could do it. Deep down, I felt sick.

I heard a car and froze. *Please don't be early.* It drove past.

I filled my water bottle, placed it in my handbag, slicked on another layer of lip gloss and threw the tube in too, checked my wallet again for the cash to pay the taxi driver.

Above the morning chat on the radio, I heard the bathroom door open. *Oh no, he needs some 'help'.*

I poked my head out into the hallway. Chris was practically skipping towards me in his boxer shorts. Held aloft above his head was the pot – and there was something in it. He couldn't have looked more pleased with himself if he had won Olympic gold. It was 8.37am. Suddenly we both wanted the taxi to be early.

Chris hurriedly dressed, I checked the contents of my handbag one last time and we raced downstairs and out onto the street, eager to get step two of Operation Sperm Test under way. The sample pot, and its contents, was sitting snugly in the top pocket of Chris's jeans, being kept as close to body temperature as possible.

8.44. A black sedan pulled up outside our flat; we were at the driver's side window before he could undo his seatbelt, let alone exit the car or knock on the door. He was one minute early; I could have hugged him. On the journey to the hospital, Chris and I sat on opposite sides of the back seat, hands clasped together in the middle. Both sets of eyes were on the digital clock spelling out our progress on the dashboard display. I willed time to go slower and the traffic banked up all around us to go faster. We both worked nights; we had forgotten the joys of the morning 'rush' hour, when nothing much rushes at all. Every time our journey came to a halt, which was often, we shared an anxious glance. We didn't want to contemplate doing this again next week if we missed this crucial deadline.

We finally turned out of the main body of traffic and started to pick up pace down a side road I'd never noticed before. A shortcut. I could have given our driver another hug. I wondered if he had worked out why we were both so tense that we could barely speak to each other; would he have sniggered if he knew what we had stashed in Chris's pocket?

Houses, parks, schools, all went past the window in a blur as my thoughts raced ahead of us. Then suddenly, for the first time that morning, my mental gymnastics were brought to a halt – we were pulling into the main entrance of the hospital. It was eleven minutes past nine; the sample was about thirty-four minutes old. We paid the driver, who seemed taken aback to receive a robustly healthy tip, and surveyed the bank of signs in front of us.

Outpatients. No
Radiology. No.
Accident & Emergency. It felt like it, but No.
Oncology. No, thank goodness.
Cardiology. No.
Day surgery. No.
Maternity. Oh how we wish.

Neurology. No.

Physiotherapy. No, no and no.

Where was it? Where was the one department we wanted?

Chris followed the path around the corner of the main building. "Here!" he called, and I trotted over, taking in the sign that said 'Pathology' and the arrow pointing to another multistorey block across the car park.

We were over the tarmac and up the first flight of stairs in a flash. Just before we left the stairwell and pushed open the doors to pathology reception, I pulled a brown paper bag out of my handbag. I had brought it along to hold Chris's sample pot, to save him the embarrassment of handing it over with the contents on view for everyone to see. With pot in bag, we had finally reached our destination. Even better, there was no queue; we walked up to the reception desk and handed over the precious cargo.

A female lab assistant, who looked about my age, took the pot out of the bag and held it up to the light as she checked the details on a white sticker pasted to the container. She slowly confirmed the correct name, date and time of sample while I sensed Chris inwardly squirming beside me. He kept glancing at the doors, clearly dreading that they might open at any minute.

The lab assistant turned and began to walk away. We waited. Was that it?

"You can go now," she confirmed, looking back over her shoulder as she departed. "Your GP will give you the results within five days."

9.18am. Still nineteen minutes to go before the hour was up. Phew. We had made it.

"Thank God for that," said Chris. "I didn't want to tell you, but I didn't sleep at all last night."

Half an hour later we were sitting in a café, pleased to be anywhere but in the hospital.

Chris looked up from his Full English Breakfast. "I didn't know she'd take it out of the bag in front of me."

I knew this was on his mind because he had already indignantly, and repeatedly, mentioned it on the train home.

"Don't worry," I reassured him, for the third or fourth time. "I'm sure she's seen it all before."

"Do you think they've finished testing it now?"

"Let's worry about that tomorrow. I think we've done enough worrying for one day."

In the back of my mind, though, there was already a niggling anxiety. The sperm sample had looked a bit yellow and clumpy to me. Still, what did I know about it? I had spent most of my life trying to avoid contact with this very substance. I suddenly found myself trying to conjure up mental images of any sperm I had ever seen – why hadn't I taken more notice of these things in my twenties? – but it was no good. All we could do was wait.

SEVEN

CHRIS WAS AGITATED. His words flowed down the telephone in a torrent, and I knew without having to see him that he would be in perpetual motion, probably pacing a corridor, but definitely moving, wherever he was. He could never sit still when the pressure was on. I could even tell when he was mentally unpicking an issue while watching TV – his right leg would start up, jiggling, forever jiggling.

"There's a problem with it!" he said. "I knew there'd be a problem with it, she said there were signs of cholesterol in the sample, they want me to take another one, why did I ring them from work? Why? This is not the place to find out this kind of thing."

"Hang on," I cautioned. "Slow down. It doesn't make sense. What do you mean *cholesterol?* I've never heard that before."

"She didn't explain – she just said exactly what I told you and that I'd have to take another sperm test. That's it, isn't it? I'm not fertile, I knew it."

"Hang on," I repeated. "None of that sounds right. They should have given you a count, they should have told you whether the motility and morphology was okay—"

"No," he cut in. "She didn't mention any of that. That's all she said – cholesterol, the test showed up a problem."

I couldn't make any sense of it; surely Chris had misunderstood. But he was adamant – he had heard correctly and there had been no further explanation.

I was both worried and annoyed. How could a doctor leave him hanging like this, not understanding what he had just been told, and leaving the door wide open for the darkest of imaginings?

"I'm making an appointment for you to go back to the doctor," I said. "They should have given you a bit more information than this."

"I'm not fertile," Chris said glumly. "I knew it."

Four days later, he swapped to a day shift then left work early for an appointment with the male doctor at our surgery.

When he returned home afterwards, Chris looked five years younger. "It's okay," he explained with a grin. "He says I've got enough sperm to fertilise the whole of the UK."

"But what about the cholesterol?" I asked, not meaning to burst his bubble. "What was that all about?"

"I don't really know," he answered. "I just told him I was worried that the results showed I couldn't become a father and he said I had no need to worry about that. 'You've got enough sperm to fertilise the UK', that's what he said."

I rolled my eyes in mock frustration. "But are they properly formed? Are they swimming? What was the actual count?"

"He didn't mention any of that. He just said that there are enough there to—"

"Yes, I know," I said with a laugh, "fertilise the UK."

That was it, then – the problem must lie with me.

And there was more. The doctor had said that even if my ultrasound scan, due to be done the following week, came back clear, then the next step for us would be fertility treatment.

I was startled to hear this. "What? You mean there's no middle ground? There isn't anything else we can do?" I paused to think. "But I'm sure there are still several other tests we could have had."

"He didn't talk about that," said Chris. "He just said we would need IVF, but to think really hard before going down that road – he's seen what it does to people. If you value your relationship, as it is now I mean, he said you should be aware that the pressure of it can tear you apart."

Great. Were all the doctors at our surgery on a mission to destroy our confidence before we had even begun? First of all, I had been bluntly reminded that I was about to fall off the fertile spectrum at any minute and now this.

In addition, we still didn't know the full results of Chris's sperm analysis. It continued to nag away at the back of my mind but Chris, still happily calculating how many children he could apparently father throughout the UK, seemed unconcerned. Again, I knew this was because he didn't have enough information – he hadn't researched what I had researched, and I couldn't seem to get through to him that he could have a trillion sperm but it would be pointless if every one of them was in no fit state to swim anywhere.

Nevertheless, I decided to put that aside until after my scan; it might become irrelevant anyway if we uncovered a serious issue.

My ultrasound appointment was at the same hospital where we had dropped off the sperm test. I had been sent an information sheet about what the scan would entail – I now knew that it would be internal – and, added to the nerves about that, there suddenly seemed to be even more cause for concern about what it would find. What if I had undiagnosed endometriosis? Ovarian cysts? Fibroids? No viable eggs? No womb? My thoughts grew more and more irrational.

Our fertility issue was going to lie with me, I knew it.

On the day of my appointment, I fretted about what to wear. What would best preserve my dignity? What would be easiest to quickly change out of if I was required to wear a hospital gown? Could I just have a general anaesthetic and wake up tomorrow? I really did not want to have that scan, which might sound odd coming from someone who has actual childbirth in their sights. However, I had my reasons for the fear that threatened to overwhelm me and, right then, I just felt like running. It was only the prospect of resolving this increasingly painful problem, which had now plagued us for more than two years, that kept me from doing so.

Chris accompanied me on the train to hospital. He knew that I clammed up under stress, that talking was the last thing I wanted to do, so he just held my hand and smiled reassuringly as we wordlessly passed a cup of hot chocolate back and forth between us.

When we finally arrived at the Radiology Department, I was taken aback to see how busy it was. We were lucky to find two vacant chairs. My hands fidgeted and my stomach flipped as, one by one, other patients were called into the side rooms off reception. The next name was called. Not mine. However, no one responded. The nurse – or was she a sonographer, I couldn't tell? – called again, left it a couple of minutes and tried once more. Still nothing.

Another staff member appeared in the corridor; they consulted, loud enough for all of us to hear.

"My 10.15's not here. How long shall I give her?"

"Okay," said the second woman. "Call through your next patient, if your 10.15 does show up, they can swap places."

The first nurse/sonographer called my name. Chris kissed me on the nose – it was one of 'our' things; "I love you", he whispered – and I was halfway across the waiting room when she called back to her colleague.

"Oh, hang on. This one's *trans-vaginal*." She half mouthed it, half stage-whispered it, which just made it even more noticeable. "I'll need the special attachment. Sam's got it in her room."

She turned to me. "Sorry, give us five minutes and we'll bring you through."

I sat back down again, mortified. Now the entire waiting room knew what intimate procedure I was here for. Was it too late to follow my instincts and run after all?

Eventually, I was called a second time and followed the nurse/sonographer to a door that opened right opposite where everyone was sitting. We went inside and she closed the door behind us; if she had left it open, I could have waved to Chris still sitting in the waiting room outside.

I searched the door for a lock. Was it going to be properly secured during this procedure? I instantly started to worry that someone would walk in halfway through, giving the ready-made audience in the waiting room a good look at my cervix, my ovaries and everything else in between.

I could have done with a reassuring chat, even just a warm look, a nod, anything that said, 'I know this is uncomfortable, but don't worry we'll get you through it.' The sonographer – I had worked out by now that she was not a nurse – was not one for small talk, though. She just confirmed my name, and that I would indeed be having a trans-vaginal scan, and told me to take my pants off.

She looked about nineteen or twenty, but I thought she must surely be older if she was already qualified for this job. Whatever the case, she was clearly many years younger than me. I wondered, did she view my age in the same way our doctor did? Was she secretly thinking I'd left it a bit late? Ridiculously, I attempted to look 'together', confident, as young for thirty-six as a person could look. This, I thought, must be what middle-aged men are attempting when they start 'dad-dancing' at weddings. 'Don't count me out, I've still got it. Yep, I'm young and fit, me.' Why was I focusing on such shallow concerns when I was about to have a scan that might confirm whether or not I could ever have children? Perhaps, on top of everything else, that thought was a bit much to process, in the circumstances.

My legs covered with a sheet, I lay down on a reclining seat that was similar to a dentist's chair. The sonographer had prepared a tubular probe that was covered with a lubricated condom. I had forgotten about condoms; I wondered whether all those condoms I used with Jai in my twenties had actually been a huge waste of time. Maybe I had never needed to be on the pill either; that could have saved me a few mood swings and a bit of weight gain. I was possibly about to find out whether my body had its own inbuilt version of birth control, its own way of ensuring I would never be pregnant.

There was a cold sensation as the lubricant made contact with my nether regions and then the probe, bearing an unfortunate resemblance to a vacuum-packed cucumber, was inserted. I looked immediately to the monitor screen flickering in the dimly-lit room. It was facing the sonographer, but if I peered a bit forward and strained my eyeballs to the right, I could see the ghostly black and white images that were being transmitted from my insides; it reminded me of a monochrome lava lamp. She moved the probe further towards my right hip. It felt a little uncomfortable, but not painful. She held it still, made a couple of clicks on the screen and appeared to be noting the dimensions of something.

"Your right ovary," she said as I craned forward.

"Does everything look okay?" I asked, hoping I had waited long enough for the question not to appear too desperate.

"I can't say. The images have to be referred for assessment."

I knew it, there's something wrong.

The scan continued; more moving around, more clicks on the screen. I noticed that my right side felt more uncomfortable with the probing than the left. Was that a sign, should I read anything into it?

Near the end of the scan, I tried a different tack.

"Would you be able to see from the screen if anything was wrong?"

Finally, the young woman briefly smiled.

"Everything looks fine," she said. "But you do need to wait for the assessment."

Later, on the way home, I felt a dull but persistent ache in my right side, the same dull ache I had felt when the probe pressed deeper and deeper in that direction. Was this normal? Would I ever stop this endless worrying, this search for *the thing that must be wrong?*

When we got home, I lay down on the bed and cried into my pillow. We were now marching ever further into territory that I had always hoped to avoid. I thought of my eldest sister, Jane, who had three daughters, and what she had once told me: "I got pregnant on the first month of trying with each of them." The first month of trying. Three times. What was wrong with us? Why did this easy, natural thing have to be so difficult? Somehow, the stakes seemed to be getting higher. Or maybe these medical tests had just made us consider the reality. We had a definite problem. There would be no more 'trying without trying'.

⁂

After another nervous wait, the scan report came back. Everything was within 'normal' ranges, there were no issues uncovered. I was not sent a copy of the report; I learned my fate via another staccato phone conversation with the stern receptionist. I was relieved, of course, by what she told me but these precious moments of relief were always tempered by the fact that we still didn't know what was wrong. The eternal question remained: what did we do now?

Our doctors had not offered any helpful advice, apart from the fact that IVF was stressful and, although it was the next step for us, we should think twice about doing it. I was not ready for it anyway; for one thing I wasn't convinced about the wisdom of filling up my body with fertility drugs when, conception aside, it appeared to be functioning normally throughout the monthly cycle. I had a history of allergic

61

reactions to prescription drugs – on one memorable occasion it had resulted in a hospital stay due to temporary kidney failure. I feared the introduction of medication at this point would throw my body off course, right at the time I needed it to keep doing exactly what it had always done.

And weren't there other tests? Why hadn't they offered further tests to help pinpoint a cause? It was confusing, not having a name for the thing that was wrong with us. I was unsure which way to turn; I needed more specific directions. However, beyond all of this, there was something else holding us back from moving on to IVF; it wasn't just our doctor's warning about the pressure it might put on our relationship, it wasn't even the drugs. There was something else going on, something that muddied the waters, and so far, we hadn't mentioned it to anyone.

EIGHT

WHEN I WAS YOUNGER, people used to joke that the most frightening thing you could say to a man was: "I love you." However, anyone who has been trying to conceive for any amount of time categorically knows that this is not true. The most terrifying thing you can say to a man is: "Honey, I'm ovulating."

It becomes just another way in which infertility shakes up everything you think you know. Like a lot of women, I spent my late teens and early twenties fending men off. It seemed that they all wanted one thing, and they wanted it now. I even went out with a photographer once, purely on the basis that he was religious and did not believe in sex before marriage, under any circumstances. Excellent, I thought, someone who might actually want to spend time talking to me. I was a little surprised, therefore, to find our first date taking place inside his flat; I had thought we were going out to dinner. The pestering started within the hour. "Stay," he pleaded, his eyes doing that slight upwards roll that some men exhibit when they're feeling amorous. "Stay the night."

It took until nearly midnight to disentangle myself. I would not be staying. Admittedly it was largely because I did not want to fall pregnant to someone I had only just met, but also I wanted to feel a bit more 'special' than that. I was eighteen; I still believed in romance. I also still believed pregnancy was such a supreme force of nature that the only way to thwart it was to place as many deadly barriers in its way as possible. And even then you might not be safe.

The next day, the photographer telephoned and said he needed to see me urgently. I suggested we meet in a café; he

63

couldn't try anything there surely. When I arrived, he looked so anxious that he was all but wringing his hands. The guilt had set in.

"I'm really sorry," he said. "Last night. I mean, I've never done anything like that before. I don't know what came over me. It's not who I am at all."

We agreed to start again. And for the entire eighteen months of our ensuing relationship he would press the issue of sex then disappear into guilty confusion if he ever actually got it.

He was a prime example as to why, right until I was ready to start a family, I thought this of men: even the ones with the best of intentions have their minds on one thing.

So, when it came to timing sex to catch ovulation – actually scheduling it into your week – I assumed that would be about the best news a man could get.

No. Sometimes it is the worst news a man can get. Sometimes he would rather be asked to do anything – anything – than turn up at ovulation and play his part.

❧ ❧ ❧

The first night I spent with Chris was different to any other 'first night', not that I had that many to compare it to. We had travelled back to my flat together on the tube after work; it was the first time we had seen each other in person since the three seven-hour phone conversations that started our relationship. That night, he had put an arm around me as we sat watching the lights on Tower Bridge and, when I leaned into his chest, it felt so natural, so instantly comfortable.

Later, as we rattled along the Northern Line, he stroked my hair – this had been on my secret wish-list of things I wanted in a partner (the men I had been involved with before had each considered themselves too 'tough' to get involved in hair stroking, let alone in a place where other people could actually *see* you doing it) – so I took it as another little sign that we were meant to be together.

When we got back to my flat and ended up sprawled across the bed, I thought I knew what would happen next. However, it turned out I was wrong.

I had recently been so ill with a virus that I had spent two weeks in hospital; I was still often exhausted and still recuperating. So, Chris looked down at me, again resting naturally on his chest.

"I'm just going to hold you tonight," he whispered. "I won't always just hold you but you've been ill, you need time to get better."

I thought that was one of the most romantic things I had ever heard. *I won't always just hold you.*

We awoke the next morning still entwined together. "Hello," Chris said softly when I opened my eyes. I was struck again by how gentle he was, how different, how sophisticated he seemed compared to the men I had known.

Ten years later, I see that night differently because I know what came next but, whatever the reason it unfolded that way, it remains a night to treasure.

As for what did come next, I don't know how to explain it, how to even mention it, because I have largely kept it hidden for ten years. It's as if my job has been to 'protect' Chris and prevent people from knowing about it. It is almost instinctive to keep it close, not to let it out into the light.

The truth is, when I said in the opening to this book that we had spent 120 cycles trying to conceive, that is not technically correct. One hundred and twenty cycles have passed – even more now – but we have not tried to conceive in all of them. There have been some cycles when we have done the exact opposite of trying to conceive. We have, in fact, practiced the most effective type of natural family planning there is – we have not had sex at all.

65

The issue behind this was already sending fault lines through our relationship before we decided we wanted a family; once we began actually trying to have one, the effect was like that of a fully-fledged earthquake. The ructions were so widespread that it seemed impossible to ever recover.

⅔ ⅔ ⅔

It took a long time for the penny to drop that something was wrong. This gap, this time-warp between instinctively knowing and rationally knowing, seems to be a theme with me. I have learnt through infertility that perhaps I give away the benefit of the doubt too easily. Perhaps I have been too eager to keep the peace, keep everyone happy. Perhaps I have been a people pleaser – no, not perhaps; the pre-infertility me *was* a people pleaser. But if your brain is just not registering a problem, what can you do? Instantly, the answer comes. *Listen to your instincts, listen to your instincts.*

If I had paid more attention to my instincts, I would have known that I should have withdrawn from this relationship pretty near the beginning. I should have said to Chris, "You've got some issues to sort out, let's try again when you've dealt with them." The silly thing is that I probably would have done that at twenty. However, I was thirty-three. I felt – and I am embarrassed to admit it now – that I didn't have the luxury of throwing away an otherwise-decent relationship and starting again. Not if I ever wanted to have a family. I know it doesn't make any sense, not a lot about the drive to have children does have an easily-ordered, rational explanation. All I know is that something that had been lying dormant within me had woken up in my early thirties. At first it wasn't even so much that I yearned for children; if I'm honest, it was more that I knew there was now a 'deadline', a timescale in which this had to be achieved – or forever not achieved if you didn't act.

I couldn't have explained it then; it was more a subconscious drive that changed the way I made decisions.

Also, Chris was generally a sensitive, funny, intelligent man. Having never really had a father, I sometimes mused that I would have loved to have grown up with a father like Chris. That was really all I needed to know – would he be a good dad? Because the answer was yes, I perhaps tolerated issues I never should have tolerated. And that mistake at the outset led to a lot of trouble later, when the pain of infertility really started to bite.

The other thing that is embarrassing to admit is that, early in our relationship, when we sat in Pizza Express and chose names for our children, we had not actually had sex. We had more than gotten a little ahead of ourselves.

At first, Chris appeared very gentlemanly in that regard. It had seemed sweet at the beginning but, as time ticked by, it began to dawn on me that there might be more to it. After several months, there had been many false starts – it would seem that we were about to consummate the relationship then Chris would suddenly back off. Finally, I made a stumbling, tentative attempt to raise the issue and he became spiky and angry. I let it drop. There were more false starts; each time the feeling grew that he was actually *terrified* of me, or at least of being with me in that way. I thought there was something wrong with me, something that repelled him. I was close to tears, sometimes, with the rejection.

It didn't matter that I had quickly learned not to say anything about it; my very silence, or even my brimming tears, made him agitated and uptight. He'd tut and sigh and say things like, "I know where this is going, I've been here before" or, "I don't need this." I couldn't understand what I'd done wrong, what had caused him to go an entire day without speaking to me or to turn on me, accusing me of being overly critical, of making something out of nothing.

Once, after a failed attempt at sex the night before, I walked past Chris while he was chatting to a colleague in the office that we still shared at weekends; our workmate greeted me with a warm hello but Chris only sneered, his expression seething with contempt, as if I was barely worth looking at. It felt as if I had been rejected twice, first in the bedroom, then in everyday life. I instantly began to pine for the straightforward men I had always known. I felt homesick, I wanted to go home; I was on the wrong side of the world with a man who despised me.

In the end, it became so obvious that we could no longer avoid facing it. At least, I could no longer avoid facing it. Chris remained in denial, as defensive and tightly wound as ever. There wasn't a problem, he wasn't a machine, it would be okay if I stopped putting such pressure on him.

"I can't handle this," I announced one night, after quietly trying to discuss the issue, only to find Chris had swung straight on to the offensive, turning the conversation into an attack, and one aimed at me.

"Fine," he said. "Leave then."

I started to pack my things; finally my own temper had flared. "I'm not going to put up with you being so angry with me for no reason," I snapped. "It's not right. You can't treat people like this."

I saw it register on his face – I really was leaving.

"Okay," he said. "Okay."

He couldn't look at me as he spoke. Eventually, haltingly, it came out. "There have been problems," he admitted, "with intimacy. Since my divorce. I don't know if I've just lost my confidence or what it is. It's like I've got stage fright."

I nudged aside my half-packed weekend bag and sat down on the bed. "Why didn't you tell me?"

"I thought you'd leave me." He dropped his head into his hands. "Who wants to go out with a sexual cripple?"

"Don't call yourself that! It's not going to help."

"Well, it's what I am," he said. "Let's face it."

I was taken aback by how quickly he could swing from plain hostility to the depths of self-loathing.

"If you knew me at all," I said, "you'd know I'd never judge you for this." I tried to lighten the mood. "For one thing, do you have any idea what a relief it is to meet a man who is not actually fixated on sex?"

I reassured him that plenty of men must experience this type of thing from time to time, that it would pass, that it was natural to lose your confidence after a marriage break-up. In short, I said I understood and would try to help.

That sounds a vastly more secure response than it was; I also asked, was he sure it wasn't me? Was I too heavy, too unattractive, was I the wrong person, was there someone else he secretly wished he was with ...?

"Don't be silly," he answered. "How can you not see that I fancy you more than anyone on this earth?"

I didn't reply; instead I tried to help by taking Chris to the bookshop, where we bought *The Joy of Sex* and *Hot Sex* and the *Barefoot Doctor's Handbook for Modern Lovers*. One day while getting my hair cut, I covertly read a magazine article about what to do 'When Your Man Loses His Mojo'. Apparently, I was supposed to take any sexual pressure off him while simultaneously greeting him at the door dressed in a maid's uniform. How exactly did I do both of those things at once? "No, I'm not bothered about sex, darling, I just thought it would be quite fashion-forward to start dressing as a domestic servant. Do you like my duster?" It wasn't the type of advice I needed.

I tried to keep things light-hearted, to laugh and joke and play-fight in bed; other times we lounged on the pillows at midnight, sharing a spoon as we ate ice cream from the tub or chortling at the words he misread when he tried to quote poetry from a battered book by candlelight. Then we might attempt to have sex and my adored companion would disappear.

The worst thing was that, when it happened, Chris remained as spiky as ever. He would take any silence on my part, or any sign of upset, as a direct attack on him; he responded by stalking off or launching in with a verbal bombardment about how unreasonable I was being. I didn't know what was happening, lying there in lonely confusion afterwards.

Still, he would lure me to bed next time, saying he was absolutely certain everything would be fine, then when the crucial moment arrived he would suddenly become the equivalent of an extremely nervous air traveller on the world's most turbulent flight. His upper lip would bead with sweat and, within moments, it would be dripping off his forehead, too. He would fling the bed clothes away, blaming them for the problem – they were making him too hot, he was being stifled. The thing I found most difficult was that he would actually start to shake. Was I really that repellent? I knew, rationally, that I had very little to do with it – a supermodel could have been lying there and the end result would have been the same. But try telling your feelings that, try walking down the street and feeling in any way attractive when, several times a week, you have taken off your clothes and turned a man into a seemingly repulsed bundle of shivering sweat. I felt bad about myself – and then I felt bad for feeling bad about myself.

We spoke about the other, short-lived, relationship he had had since divorcing. Why hadn't he done something about this issue then? "I thought it would be okay when I met the right person," he said. I shrank a little more inside.

After another couple of months we had failed to have sex at home, in hotel rooms, in a garden shed, on a beach and in a deserted field next to a river. I had never felt so alone – not so much because of the problem itself but because of the lengths Chris went to to avoid accepting that it existed.

I didn't understand, then, the extent of his denial, not really. I just knew that he was like a tiger defending its territory, constantly primed for attack – he was volatile at work, bolshie when walking the streets of London and would become agitated about the simplest things. Even queuing for train tickets became a stressful experience, way out of proportion to the level of inconvenience suffered. He would step in and out of the queue, pointedly craning his head towards the front, while tutting, sighing, swearing and generally acting like a person whose very life depended on that line moving forwards.

Conversely, Chris was still known at work as the man who could flirt for England, people still commented on the number of women who seemed charmed by him. Shortly after we had become a couple, we were talking at his desk when a veteran colleague from another department walked by. "Oh Lord," he said, winking at me, "I see Don Juan's at it again."

I wondered if the pressure to be this 'Don Juan' character, this great seducer of women, was what had knocked Chris off course. Maybe the burden of expectation was a bit much to live up to.

Whatever the reason, the issue, and all the fallout from it, was becoming increasingly damaging. Eventually – nearly six months into the relationship and way beyond the time when I first should have done so – I made it clear that we couldn't stay together unless he stopped lashing out and started seeking help. It had the desired effect; Chris made an appointment with his GP.

On the day of his consultation, we sat in the waiting room holding hands. Both of his legs were jiggling endlessly up and down and, throat dry with nerves, he walked back and forth to the water cooler, knocking back cup after cup. When he was called down the corridor to the doctor's office, I walked outside and paced the pavement. Then, finally, he emerged, looking transformed with relief.

"Well done," I said, giving him a hug. "You did it. How did it go?"

"It was much better than I thought. He's very nice, the old and wise type – we talked about rugby for most of the time actually; he really put me at ease."

"Thank goodness."

"I know," said Chris. "He was great. He asked a few questions and said it's definitely not anything physical. He put it down to performance anxiety, apparently plenty of men get it from time to time, it's really nothing to get het up about."

"That's fantastic!" My hand flew to my mouth as we both began to laugh. "Sorry. I just meant it's good that you're not physically ill. I mean, I'm glad you're fit and well. Anyway … did he give you any advice about dealing with it?"

"Not really. He just said, 'You don't have a physical problem, now go away, enjoy your new relationship and relax.'"

Chris looked a bit pained. "There was one other thing. He thought it might help me to talk to a sex therapist he knows, he says she's very good and he's given me a referral."

"She?"

"I know. I hoped it would be a man too. I don't know if I can talk to a woman about this."

I tried to hide my initial reaction. *Another woman is going to teach my man how to have sex.* I felt like *I* should have been enough, that if I wasn't somehow lacking then it would never have come to this. I knew that was wrong thinking, but the issue was bringing up every insecurity I had. I battled to hide the tears I felt coming and, again, felt bad for feeling bad. If I was a better person, I thought, I would just be pleased for Chris that some progress had been made.

As it turned out, it was a step in the right direction – it seemed to have helped him come to terms with the existence of the problem – but it didn't ultimately solve it.

Chris didn't make an appointment with the therapist. He was only just managing to discuss the problem with me; he was suffering paroxysms of embarrassment and anxiety about sharing this most intimate thing with a woman he had never met. I understood, I would have felt the same, particularly since where I came from, you did not go around spilling your guts to a stranger.

So, we moved on to Plan C, or was it Plan D by now? How to say it? I let him 'practise' with me, with no expectation that full sex would ensue. I thought it made sense because he was suffering from a fear of failure and you can't 'fail' when there's no end goal to reach.

At the beginning, he seemed so out of his comfort zone, so tangibly relieved to physically part from me again, that I suffered all manner of insecurities about what that could mean – was it something off-putting about me in particular, was it women in general, was he in denial about his sexual orientation or was he just plain scared? Only he had the answers and I suspected he wasn't sure what they were himself.

Ten years later, this is painful to write. I want to pick up a loud-hailer and shout back down the years at myself. I want to tell the thirty-three-year-old me: other people's issues are not yours to solve; you don't have to feel responsible for them; you don't have to care quite so much about how other people feel – they are their feelings, not yours. But those lessons were years from sinking in. Unexpectedly, I would have infertility to thank for forcing me to understand these things.

However, in 2002, I continued blindly on. And, hey presto, after months of anguish, the breakthrough finally arrived – one October day, nearly seven months after our relationship began, we finally, elatedly, had sex. The hoodoo was broken. We both cried with relief and happiness. Everything was okay, those strained days and nights were behind us now; it was all over. Over the moon didn't cover it, especially for Chris.

A month later, my contraceptive prescription ran out and we agreed that I wouldn't renew it. We weren't 'officially' trying for a baby – it was far too soon for that, especially given the circumstances – but we both felt it was the right time to get the medication out of my system before letting nature take its course. Anyway, we figured it would probably take a while to conceive, maybe as long as six or eight months.

The 'trying without trying' phase of our attempt to have a family really gathered pace in 2003. And before the end of the summer, we realised that the hoodoo was not broken, everything was not okay and the strained days and nights were very much in front of us. I did not know it yet – I would find out when it was far too late to do much about it – but Chris had vastly downplayed the extent of the problem. What I knew at that stage was just the tip of the iceberg, so I ploughed on, unaware of the struggle that lay ahead.

This hidden factor explains the main reason why we left it for two years before consulting a doctor about our fertility problems: two years wasn't really two years. That amount of time had passed, but it included months when we didn't have sex at all. We had tried each month, but some months had ended in failure. Those months always hurt, but not as much then as they would later, when the very absence of hope during a precious cycle would prove more than I could bear.

NINE

WE HAVE MADE MANY mistakes during our time in the Ten-Year Club, but the worst ones can each be traced back to one thing – the lack of information and support we received on those first visits to our doctors. We didn't realise at the time that, between them, our GPs had effectively turned us around and pointed us in exactly the opposite direction to the one we should have been facing. Right from the outset, we were travelling the wrong way.

We were not told that, up until the age of thirty-nine, I could qualify for a maximum of three cycles of IVF, courtesy of the NHS. We were not told that there was a long waiting list and, before any more time passed, we should add our names to it while we continued to consider the implications. In short, we were not really told anything – except that IVF was stressful and might fatally damage our relationship. I'm not sure how but our doctor also left us with the impression that we would have to pay for any fertility treatment we received. We didn't have that type of lump sum available to spend and we both worried about the pressure it would place on just one cycle if we raised enough for a sole attempt. If that failed, we would still be childless, but also in debt and unable to afford to try again. The fertility drugs were still playing on my mind, too – was there not a way of undergoing treatment without having to resort to ingesting a potent cocktail of hormones and who knew what else?

We should have gone back to our GP and pushed for advice, but the problem is that if you don't know something exists, then you can't ask about it. I could rarely even turn to the internet for help since, in 2004 and 2005, we did not have a connection at home. The best I could do was surreptitiously Google fertility-related information while in the office – but I had to use coded terms to try to make each enquiry appear work-associated, in case anyone realised what I was up to.

Sometimes I would visit an internet café and research fertility problems, trying to touch as few as possible of the filthy, slimy keys on the wonky keyboard, while all around me students and tourists sent their e-mails and loudly debated their holiday plans. It was not an ideal way of operating. Still, we should have found a more informative source, we should have pushed the issue further. We didn't – I suspect this was largely because we continued to live in a dream world where each month we still thought we might be pregnant, each month I mentally calculated another due date when our long-awaited baby would now be arriving. Sometimes, at the internet café, I even keyed my cycle dates into a Pregnancy Calculator. "Congratulations!" it would inform me, "you are three weeks pregnant." It has been a very long time now since I bothered to key my cycle dates into a Pregnancy Calculator; it could only respond: "LOL. Who do you think you're kidding?"

So, seven or eight years ago we made a major mistake and, as is the way when things go wrong, it had a domino effect that led to many other mistakes, many other errors of judgment. However, it does mean that we have explored alternatives to conventional treatment that we might not otherwise have considered. And, really, who can categorically say we've been going in the wrong direction? Maybe there were dead ends awaiting us either way; at least down this road I've sometimes enjoyed the scenery en route. Even if I didn't end up quite where I expected.

It was Chris's mum who encouraged us to try acupuncture. She was one of the few people who knew about our struggle to have a baby – she knew because Chris told her everything. He is the type who tends to share his problems while I am vastly more likely to keep them to myself. I had not told my family about our fertility issues and I didn't intend to, not yet anyway. I didn't mind Rose knowing, though; almost from the day I met her, she became one of my favourite people.

She was in her mid-eighties when I got to know her and, following the recent death of Chris's father, was living on her own for the first time in her life. The first thing I noticed about her was that, when she spoke, her voice could almost match that of the Queen delivering her Christmas message. It was clear she had moved in lofty circles and, on first impression, you might have been forgiven for expecting to find a slightly haughty, cold person sheltered behind that grand voice. However, Rose was one of the most welcoming, open and hilarious characters I have met. She might well have come from another place and time but she could talk to anyone about anything. Rose took great interest in modern life and wanted to know all about everything from mobile phones and eBay (or e*Boy*, as she called it) to fashion, hair and make-up brands. When it came to conversation, nothing was off limits and she swerved without warning from topic to topic.

"Of course," she announced during dinner one night, "we didn't really have decent French Letters in our day. The men didn't like them one bit. Too baggy, I expect. What do you think, Chris? Have you used French Letters? I imagine you must have."

Even Chris, accustomed to her as he was, did not have an answer to that.

Apart from the fact that she was an easy confidante, there was another reason for him to discuss our issues with Rose: it had taken nine years for Chris, her first child, to arrive.

"Charles and I had assumed it would not happen," she said. "I suppose it must have been discussed within the family – after all, there we were, married for nine years and no children."

However, Rose often recounted the tale of the night Chris was finally conceived. "We had been to a fancy-dress ball," she explained, "and got roaring drunk. I think that's what did it – we were so relaxed and having such fun. Anyway, that's how we made Chris after all that time."

By the time Chris was born, Rose was thirty-eight years old and something of a novelty on the labour ward, where she was the oldest first-time mother the staff could remember. She returned two years later to give birth to Chris's sister. I hoped that, somehow, something would eventually click for us – preferably before nine years went by – and we would have a similar tale to tell.

In the meantime, Rose, who always loved a drink, was nonplussed that I had given up alcohol while trying to conceive. She never gave up trying to tempt me; the minute the clock ticked past midday, she would say, "Time for a drink chaps. You will join me, won't you?" And out would come the gin. I had made the mistake of accepting one of Rose's drinks on my first visit to her apartment – it was a weighty tumbler, half gin, half Dubonnet, and it has the honour of being the only drink that has ever choked me. The ferocity of the alcoholic content was mind-boggling, yet Rose would happily knock back three in a row.

In the early days of our struggle to conceive, she would often advocate a shambolic drunken fumble as the best way to achieve success. However, she clearly wanted to help because one day a newspaper clipping arrived in the post. Headlined something like 'Needles gave me my family' it had been ripped out of the *Daily Mail* and was accompanied by a note that just said, "Love Mum." Beneath the headline was a profile of an acupuncturist who was apparently achieving great success with previously infertile couples; some of them were pictured holding the healthy babies they had conceived after undergoing treatment at his clinic. I so badly wanted what those women had.

It was late 2005 and, after discovering the outcome of our initial tests, we were lost. By now, I was spending nearly all of my spare time reading fertility books, looking for that one missing link that would change everything. My study material included *Taking Charge of Your Fertility (The Definitive Guide to Pregnancy Achievement, Natural Birth Control and Reproductive Health)* and *The Infertility Cure (The Ancient Chinese Wellness Program for Getting Pregnant and Having Healthy Babies)*. Each of these was more enlightening than anything I had been told by our doctors and I instantly found that a more natural philosophy felt like a perfect fit for me. I was eager to explore these so-called alternative avenues.

Inspired by *Taking Charge of Your Fertility*, I began 'charting', which involved noting crucial changes in my body throughout the monthly cycle, from day one until the onset of menstruation. I took my temperature every morning and recorded it on a monthly chart, alongside other observations, ranging from any exercise taken to the quality of my cervical mucus (which was not a topic I had ever considered, let alone expected to encounter on a spreadsheet). Ideally, my temperature graph would reveal a 'thermal shift', or the rise in temperature that happens after ovulation. The graph would head downwards again when my next period was due – or if the moment of all moments had finally arrived and I was pregnant, I would clearly see the evidence on my spreadsheet (if temperatures remain higher for eighteen or more consecutive days after ovulation, with no sign of a period, it almost always indicates pregnancy). The use of this simple cycle tracker could also highlight a range of issues that might otherwise have remained hidden. I was fascinated to see what my body had been up to all these years, with absolutely no help or understanding from me.

Unfortunately, as with many of my fertility adventures, there was already a bump in the road. My temperature chart had given me a new thing to worry about; it had become immediately apparent that I did not fit the 'norm'. The chart provided with the book listed a temperature range, travelling upwards 0.1 of a degree at a time, from 97 to 99 degrees Fahrenheit. Much of the time, my temperature was lower than 97, which meant I didn't even register on the chart. I got around that by photocopying it and customising the grid, to start at 96 degrees instead. It was official: I was a cold-blooded reptile. The book suggested that this could be due to my old friend, the thyroid. Tests repeatedly showed it was functioning normally, but was it actually still sluggish? On the other hand, I knew that Mum and Vanda also had the same low-level temperatures as me – they each barely hit 97 degrees, yet they had eight biological children between them (plus me, the non-biological one). Trying to unravel all of this was starting to give me a headache to match the heartache.

I had reached this very point when Rose's newspaper article arrived. Typically, she had sent her beacon of hope through the post at just the right moment. I read the article several times and instinctively felt I would respond to the type of therapy it described, certainly more positively than I would to invasive fertility treatment. And so, for the second time, I set off down the path of private healthcare. Hope sprung anew. *This* would be the key. This would be the vital piece of information that led to me getting pregnant!

I wasted no time in digging out the acupuncturist's contact details and making an appointment to see him. Once again, I would be heading to Harley Street for help.

On the day of my appointment, I entered another grand old building, similar to the one that had housed the thyroid specialist, but at the opposite end of the famous street. As I sat down in the reception area to complete my introductory questionnaire, I looked around at the other women waiting there and wondered, 'Are they going through what I'm going through? Do they feel it too?' I sank back into one of the plump couches that bordered the room; it was like being in the lounge of a period country house, I think *Country Living* magazine was even displayed among a raft of glossy titles on an ornate central table. Unexpectedly, I felt comfortable in all senses. *Please let that be a good sign.* Before long, a man who I recognised appeared – the photo in the newspaper article had captured him exactly. I thought he might be about my age, or perhaps a bit younger; maybe he was actually older but had been using his acupuncture needles and herbal potions to hold back time. Why did I think these random thoughts whenever I was about to front up – again – to this fertility problem, this thing that might overwhelm me before I knew it? Maybe I wanted to put off the face-to-face 'confrontation' with this damn issue for as long as possible.

David Taylor led me down the hall to another high-ceilinged room with sash windows framed by heavy drapes. An old-fashioned desk in dark wood stood near the centre of the room, with a treatment table along one wall. We both sat down on the same side of the desk as I prepared to tell him my tale. As always when discussing it, I steeled myself to appear matter of fact. I did not want to find tears creeping into the corners of my eyes when I said, "My partner and I have been trying to conceive for nearly three years." Sometimes when you said it, it could take you by surprise and a wall of emotion would surge up, unbidden and unexpected. I got the opening line out, hoping I sounded just casual enough but not *too* casual.

We went through the questionnaire, about my health, menstrual history and lifestyle. Did I get menstrual cramps, what colour was the blood, was there any clotting? Poor man, I thought, having to discuss this all day. Luckily, he didn't appear to share my thoughts; he was interested, empathetic and, the thing I welcomed most of all, down to earth. He took my pulse at several different points on my wrists, observed my tongue and scrawled many notes on a pad. I had never been so comprehensively questioned about anything health-related; I was intrigued and encouraged by this holistic approach.

David then asked how much I knew about Traditional Chinese Medicine and whether I had experienced this type of treatment before. "I've read one book about it," I offered, "but that's pretty much it."

My education began instantly. He explained thoroughly but simply the principles of TCM, even drawing a diagram to illustrate the core concept of yin and yang, the two opposite halves that, when in balance, contribute to a perfect whole. Yin, he explained, was associated with female energies and its basic qualities included coldness, darkness and stillness. Yang represented the opposite – male energy, heat, activity, brightness. In fertility terms, yin energies governed the first half of a woman's monthly cycle before converting into yang at ovulation.

I wish I had written all this down at the time; the fact that I didn't reminds me that, even then, I had still not reached the point of obsessing about fertility. I didn't need to bombard him with questions or painstakingly document every word he said for future reference; I was still content to go with the flow, to keep things low-key.

In my case, I was being affected, said David, by an over-abundance of yin energy. Great, I thought, I'm cold and dark; why can't I be bright and hot for once? However, it was not all bad; David was actually very positive about my overall situation. Apparently it was good news that the first half of my cycle – the one governed by all this yin I had – appeared to be functioning smoothly. Tests had confirmed that I was ovulating and, from what I was able to observe through charting and checking my body's changes throughout the month, I was as sure as I could be that this was correct. His diagnosis chimed with this; it was yang energies that were lacking, the ones that governed the other end of my cycle.

David explained that I would need "just a few tweaks" to improve the situation. Treatment would involve regular acupuncture and I would also take Chinese herbs daily.

"We need to heat you up a bit," he said, "and get any stagnant blood moving."

The required treatment was relatively straightforward, and results could be achieved more quickly than with other, more complicated, issues. And there was more encouraging news. "You'll find your menstrual cramps will disappear after this treatment," he said. "You won't have any need for those pain-killers you're taking at the moment." As far as I was concerned that, on its own, would make this experience worthwhile. I was eager to get started.

What I remember most about my first acupuncture treatment with David is the feeling of surprise that he had inserted needles into my body yet I remained completely unaware that he had done it. I was lying on the treatment couch with my shoes off and trousers unzipped as David showed me the ultra-fine acupuncture needles he imported from Asia; they were like long slivers of frozen spider web, each sealed in a separate paper packet. He was moving around the bed, chatting about the workings of this type of acupuncture when he explained why he had placed needles in my toes, feet and calves.

What? There were needles in my legs? I glanced down; sticking out at right angles from my little toes, I could see the silver needles, with more protruding from various points of my feet.

"How did you do that?" I exclaimed. "I didn't even realise."

"Years of practise," he smiled, while carefully and painlessly inserting more needles into my lower abdomen and then into each hand.

Finally, he wheeled over a tall heat lamp, which he angled over my stomach. "Now," he said, "I'm going to leave you to cook for half an hour. I'll be just out there if you need me," and he gestured to an ante-room on the other side of the door.

At first, I was afraid to completely relax in case I dislodged any of the needles or, even worse, managed to poke one further in. I hazarded a glance around the room, taking in the prints on the walls and the books on the shelves. One of the faded curtains at the window was crooked, it needed hauling back up at one end. I wondered if anyone used the courtyard that I could see beyond it. The thirty-minute finish point felt a long time away. However, the sensation of heat over my stomach felt so soothing; I wished I could carry that warmth around with me all the time. I closed my eyes and felt my body sink further into the bed.

Then I heard the door softly open and realised David was quietly moving the heat lamp away. I half-opened an eye.

"How did you find it?" he asked. "You were looking very relaxed there."

"Oh my goodness," I said, drowsy and perplexed, "I think I must have dropped off for a minute or two."

"Excellent. That's what we want – some nice, restful time for you."

He quickly and efficiently removed all of the needles; they would not be used again, it would be a fresh set each time. When I stood up, I felt like a cat who had been dozing in the sun and needed a good stretch to fully wake up.

Sitting at the desk again, David showed me the bottle of Chinese herbal capsules that he had brought back in with him, explaining how many to take and how often.

I left full of confidence that this new treatment would work, that I would join the ranks of those women – those mothers – featured in Rose's newspaper article. At reception, I instantly made an appointment for my second acupuncture session.

So, acupuncture (£35 per half-hour session) and Chinese herbs (£20 a bottle): entries five and six for my notional fertility accounts book. Unaware that the 'book' would remain active for another seven years, I had my first three treatments only a week apart, then moved my appointments out to once a fortnight. It felt good to be doing something positive; even better, I enjoyed acupuncture so much that I felt it was something I would want to continue even if I wasn't attempting to have a baby.

Meanwhile, David suggested that I bring in the charts I had been keeping to track my cycle. I instantly felt a shot of alarm at the suggestion; I couldn't let him see the truth! So I did two sets, one for him and one for me. On David's charts, I filled in only my daily temperatures and the days when my period fell, along with any other menstrual symptoms that arose. "Things are a bit hectic," I said, trying to explain away the swathes of white space on the chart. "I think it takes a more organised person than me to keep it up to date."

But that wasn't true. I had purposely left gaps on the pages I showed David because I was too embarrassed to show him my 'real' charts. For him, I always left out 'cervical mucus signs' and 'breast symptoms', but those omissions were just smokescreens – what I really didn't want David to see was the part of the chart where you are supposed to colour in a square on each day you've had sex. On some months, on my 'real' chart, there were no squares coloured in at all. I was nearly three years in to trying to conceive and I was still uncertain whether I could ever rely on 'catching' ovulation (or any other stage of the cycle for that matter), whether Chris would manage to turn up and do his bit. How could I tell David, "Yes, I'm expecting acupuncture to give me a baby, but I don't think I'll bother much with actually having sex?" I knew already that acupuncture was a powerful force but nothing, short of divine intervention, was *that* powerful. Deep down,

I felt stupid for even pursuing treatment, but I also believed that acupuncture could help me cope with the stress of sometimes *not* being able to have sex. Of knowing that you're about to turn thirty-seven and, for some months of the year – as if your 'youth' will last forever – you are wasting the precious gift of a body that still ovulates.

I also noticed a shift in my mind-set once I started having treatment to improve my fertility. I had already been noting in shorthand at the top of my diary pages the days when we had managed to have sex; I wanted to know what was happening on the day my baby was conceived and, also, it was necessary information on the charts I did 'for my eyes only'. However, now I started noting something else in my diary. Every so often, the words 'failed attempt' would appear at the top of a page. This was new; unconsciously I had now started counting the cost.

Back at the acupuncture clinic, though, the signs were more encouraging. After a couple of months of treatment, my temperature chart had changed markedly. To begin with, it had looked like the graph of a particularly violent earthquake; the lines drawn between each temperature raced erratically up and down. *Taking Charge of Your Fertility* described this as a 'sawtooth pattern'. It was probably partly caused by the fact that I worked nights – I would get home from work around midnight, and by the time I wound down, I might fall asleep anywhere between 1.30 and 3am. That impacted on the time I awoke the next day so my first temperature of the 'morning' was not always taken at exactly the same time.

However, once I was having acupuncture, the sawtooth pattern began to even out. A couple of months in, I was thrilled to see my chart had taken on a new, streamlined look – my temperatures were much more consistent. That was not the only thing to have improved. I had never particularly considered the colour of menstrual blood before, but at the start of my cycle it was suddenly transformed from a gloomy, muddy brown to a clear pink. I also stopped spotting before my period and – for the first time in my life – felt hardly anything in the way of menstrual cramps.

David had also helped with more prosaic matters. For one thing, he confirmed that the niggling worries I was still having about the results of Chris's sperm analysis should not be ignored. He had asked for the test details at the outset as he tried to build as accurate a picture as possible of our combined fertility. When I explained what our GP had said, and that we hadn't received specific results, he suggested that Chris take another test. There was certainly much more that we should have been told about, including sample volume and count, morphology (which would show any structural defects) and motility (the percentage and progression of forward moving sperm).

At one of our treatment sessions, David wrote neatly on a piece of paper the details of a private laboratory nearby, where we could have another sample tested and receive the results within two to three working days. It would mean paying to have it done – I think it was just under £100 – but it was preferable to trying to explain to our doctors the very things that they should, in fact, have been explaining to us. Also, the private lab accepted credit cards, something that we were relying on more and more as we – literally – began paying for our lack of fertility.

When I got home, I told Chris about David's suggestion and handed over the piece of paper.

"Mm." He glanced at the name of the laboratory before discarding the paper on the kitchen bench.

"I think it would be a good idea to do it," I persisted. "We don't really know where we are otherwise."

"The first one must have been okay, though," Chris countered. "Otherwise, why would he say I've got enough sperm to fertilise the whole of the UK?"

"I don't know," I said, privately thinking I would happily strangle our doctor for making this ridiculous, subjective comment when what we really needed was facts. "But wouldn't it be nice to have the details to back up the theory? And they did say you'd need to take another one."

"He seemed pretty positive about it," Chris said doubtfully. "But okay, yes, I'll do it."

It was late 2005. I was turning thirty-seven years old, a number I had dreaded for some time. *Surely our problems would be resolved before I turned thirty-seven.* Everything I read, everywhere I turned, there seemed to be someone pointing out that women's fertility levels fell "even further" from the age of thirty-seven; there was also said to be an increased risk of miscarriage and foetal abnormalities. I remember thinking, 'We can't all be the same. Someone must buck the trend.' But I was still afraid. I had started 'trying without trying' for a baby at the age of thirty-four precisely because I wanted to avoid this; I could take two years on the slow road to conception and still have time to play with before I turned thirty-seven. Clearly, it hadn't worked out that way – I was not so much on a slow road as stalled in a cul-de-sac. I felt a ratcheting up of pressure as I marked my thirty-seventh birthday. However, I reminded myself that I was still in my thirties and plenty of women conceived in their late thirties – didn't they?

As it happened, plenty of people certainly did and – as I was soon to find out – I even knew some of them.

TEN

I WAS WALKING ALONG the banks of the Thames with my friend Suzanne in the early autumn of 2005. We met every so often in west London and strolled down the tree-lined path while catching up on each other's news. Usually, there would be three of us on this walk – Suzanne, myself and Lisa, all of us from the southern hemisphere, all of us born in the same year. But that day Lisa was missing.

"I haven't seen her for ages," I said. "I was hoping to catch up with her today."

"Hmm," said Suzanne, uncharacteristically short of words.

We followed the dirt and gravel track west, falling obediently into single file whenever a suburban cyclist, as they were wont to do, tore past as if competing in the Tour de France.

"So," said Suzanne eventually, "what's happening with the baby thing?"

I told her about acupuncture, how much I enjoyed it and how I thought it might be able to help with the asthma she suffered.

"Yeah, but how much does it cost? I mean Harley Street, trust you to have acupuncture in *Harley* Street."

"That's what credit cards are for," I joked.

"Oh Lord," she said with a groan, "please tell me you're not back to paying your rent with a credit card."

"No I am not." I gave a wry laugh. "I'm still paying that off as it happens. I can't believe I was so stupid."

"Well. You thought that bloody husband of yours was going to come back, didn't you? Although we did think you were mad to keep a two-person flat going – and in one of the poshest parts of London, of *course*."

"Oh, don't," I said. "He was already involved with *her* when all that was happening."

"We're not going to talk about her again, are we?" Suzanne decisively kicked aside a stray stone. "She was a crappy, crapola, crapshit friend. Let's talk about *me* instead. Anyway," she added, "you're much better off with Chris."

"Do you think so?"

"Well, he's a much better conversationalist. I know Jai was a big, buff, muscly hunk of a man—"

"You noticed then?"

"Hello Louise? I did spend some time with men before deciding I preferred women. I even lived with one once ... poor man. Anyway, the point is, I just think you'll have more intelligent children with Chris."

I burst into laughter; Suzanne had an amusing tendency of coming right out and saying what other people were thinking but wouldn't dream of sharing publicly.

"And it's not as if he's been hit with the ugly stick either," she continued. "Even I can see he's a good-looking man."

"Well, I'm pleased to hear we've got your blessing."

"Yeah, well just don't think I'm changing any nappies or dealing with any sick-ups – I'm sure you'll think your kid's cute even if it's covered in snot, but I won't. Please remember this and don't ever make me hold it, touch it or talk to it in funny voices when it's in that state."

"Noted," I said. "It's not as if I'm exactly keen on any of those things either."

"I know." She chortled, waving a sunset-coloured leaf in my direction. "I can't believe you want to have children. How are you going to afford all your glam lotions and potions when you're running around the house cleaning up sick all day?"

Twenty minutes later, we had reached the end of our walk and were happily resting in the beer garden of a riverside pub, Suzanne enjoying an oversized glass of red wine and saying, almost loud enough for every other punter to hear, "Get you with your lemonade. You're really serious about this aren't you? Who knew two years ago that you'd give up drinking for sprogs?"

We were on the second glass when the conversation returned to Lisa, our missing friend.

"Do you think she's all right?" I asked. "It's not like her to miss out on a drink."

"Mmm," said Suzanne.

"I've texted her a bit but I can't think when I last spoke to her. Oh no! You don't think I've upset her and not even realised?" I ploughed on, answering my own question. "No ... no, that can't be it, she's not like that is she?"

"Ach," said Suzanne, "this is stupid. I'm just going to tell you."

"What? Tell me what? Is she okay? Has something happened with her and Pete?"

"The thing is," Suzanne began, "she's pregnant. She didn't know how to tell you."

I was stunned; apart from Suzanne, Lisa was one of the most unlikely candidates for pregnancy that I knew. But *pregnant*. Lisa was pregnant.

"Wow," I exclaimed. "Lisa?"

"Yep."

"But why would she think I'd mind? Why didn't she tell me?"

"Well. It's been a bit tricky," Suzanne explained slowly, looking as if she was, unusually for her, weighing up what to say before she said it.

"How far along is she?" I asked before she could get any further with her deliberations. "When did she find out?"

"Um. Twenty weeks."

"Twenty weeks! She's twenty weeks pregnant?"

Suzanne nodded.

"But that's ... that's ... bloody hell, isn't that about five months?

"Yeah, I think it was a bit …" She tried again. "Well, she had to think about whether—"

"I didn't even know she wanted children," I interrupted again as the news slowly filtered through my brain.

"Me neither," said Suzanne. "She was on the pill. She didn't find out until quite late, she didn't think it was possible. Then she had to think about what to do, you know …" and she trailed off, unable to find a suitably discreet way of saying 'whether to continue with the pregnancy'.

"Wow. She's nine months older than me and she's managed to get herself up the duff even on the pill."

"Um," said Suzanne, "I think they used condoms too – I know she was really careful, she didn't want anything like this cramping her style."

"Amazing. She must be fertile as all hell. And when you think how much she drinks in a week. So much for the theory that we're all past our use-by date at thirty-five."

I paused.

"But why didn't she tell me?"

"Ach, I don't know," said Suzanne. "I think she was a bit embarrassed and she was worried it might upset you, with the way it happened and everything. Silly really. I thought she should have just told you, like everyone else."

Despite trying to conceive for nearly three years, this was the first time anyone really close to me had announced a pregnancy. My brothers and sisters were all so much older than me that I was still at secondary school when most of them had had their families. In London, my friends were all women much like myself, either travelling or building careers before finally 'settling down' – or not planning to 'settle down' at all. It was the first time I realised that, while my life was stuck, other people's lives were moving on.

That night I told Chris the news. "Guess what?" I said. "Lisa's five months pregnant."

"*Lisa?*"

"Yeah, I know."

"I didn't realise they wanted children."

"She was on the pill. I think it was more than a bit of a surprise. Can you believe it? We've been trying to do the deed – at the right time – for months and months and I haven't had so much as one drink. And she's nine months older than me, she's nearly thirty-eight. I didn't even know you could get pregnant by accident at thirty-eight."

"Well, that's exactly why people should shut up about your age," said Chris. "They're just trying to scare you with their statistics. It's not what you need to hear. And look at you – you're the picture of health."

"Yes," I said. "But I'm not pregnant."

"I'm sorry sweetheart." Chris reached out and pulled me close. "Your turn will come one day, I know it will. It would be a travesty if you never got to be a mother."

"Well, anyway, that's not why I'm upset," I said. "Lisa's lovely, that baby is so lucky she'll be its mum. But," I added, pulling away to launch into a full explanation of my grievance, "she's told everyone else except me. I heard it from Suzanne. She said Lisa didn't know how to tell me. Why didn't she tell me? I feel like a freak."

"Lou," Chris said patiently. "You are not a freak."

"Well, I feel like one. Why would you leave me out? I feel weird enough as it is, not being able to get pregnant. And now everyone's going all strange around me. Why, oh why did I have to tell them we were trying for a family?"

"I'm sorry," Chris repeated. "She should have just told you. But I'm sure she was genuinely trying not to upset you. And she probably felt embarrassed."

"That's what Suzanne said. But why did she have to leave me out? Why do I have to be the weird one who can't be told about it?"

"Look," said Chris. "You are *not* weird. You are generous and kind and strong and one day it will be *you* telling them *your* news. Now you just go out there and show them you're not bothered by any of this."

I smiled. Chris took his pep talks very seriously and he often reminded me of a father figure when he delivered them.

Later in bed, I was still mulling it over, going through all the reasons I could muster as to why Lisa had not told me she was expecting a baby.

"And another thing," I said into the darkness.

"Huh?" Chris was clearly already drifting in and out of sleep.

"Do people think there are a limited number of babies given out each year – and if they've got one, I'm less likely to have one of my own?"

"Hmm."

"Well, why is their conception such bad news for me? Surely it gives me hope that it can actually happen. It's not like they've scooped up the last of the available babies this year and now I'll have to wait for the new allocation to be given out."

"Come over here," ordered Chris, now fully awake. "Why don't you put your head on my chest and see if you can go to sleep? Just let the warmth draw you off ..."

ᘔ ᘔ ᘔ

It turned out that, in late 2005, Lisa was not the only one with news to impart.

In mid-October, I received an e-mail from Jai, once again while I was at work. 'That's odd,' I thought, 'it's not my birthday. Maybe he's writing to tell me he's finally realised what a pain in the butt the praying mantis is.'

Our new name for Dana: *Praying mantis,* an exclusively predatory creature, largely of the ambush variety. (You might also like to know that the praying mantis has grasping spiked forelegs in which prey is caught and held securely; it is also closely related to the cockroach). Optimistically, I thought Jai might finally have recognised this description for himself. However, as so often, that was nothing but wishful thinking. Back in the real world, another shock lay in store, and this one hit right where it hurt. It turned out Jai had not escaped the grasp of the praying mantis – far from it. He had actually gone and *bred* with her. He was, he casually informed me, about to become a father.

"Hi," he opened before managing an innocent-enough line of chat about the northern hemisphere summer.

Then, in line three: the grenade.

"I'm e-mailing you to let you know of some big news, I'm gonna be a dad. I know you probably don't care less and wonder why I'd bother telling you, but I felt I needed to for obvious reasons. I haven't told anyone yet other than my flatmate as I'd rather you heard it first from me … When I found out you were the first person I thought of."

When I found out. Another accidental pregnancy? Was someone, somewhere playing some sort of bad-taste cosmic joke on me? *Yep, you try all you like to get pregnant, everyone else will just do it without even noticing. That's how easy it is. That's how deeply flawed and useless you are.*

Jai offered a few more thoughts about how he had become more of a free spirit – like me, apparently – and wasn't sure whether settling down was really for him. Little did he know, we had strangely swapped roles since parting – the man who had wanted to live in one small place for his entire life had become the man who wanted to travel the world and the woman who had never looked like settling down now wanted to do exactly that.

He signed off with, "Anyway that's the news … I ain't told anyone else yet, will do over the next week.

Me."

There were tears rolling down my face before I reached the end. I left the e-mail open on my computer screen and, head firmly fixed to the floor, rushed for the sanctuary of a toilet cubicle, glad that my long hair was flopping forwards to camouflage my distress on this desperate surge through the room. I had no thoughts and hundreds of thoughts; all I knew was that every bit of me seemed to be hurting and I couldn't control it. Somehow I reached the toilets without anyone noticing and – one small mercy – no one else was in there. I flung open a cubicle door, kicked the seat down with my foot and slumped there with my head in my hands. Mascara-stained splashes coloured my palms and spilled onto the front of my skirt. The childish mantra, 'It's not fair, it's not fair, it's not fair' danced in my head. Everyone – even so-called best friends who went round stealing other people's husbands – got to be a mother. Everyone except me. I had tried and tried and tried but motherhood instead chose to bestow her gifts on people who had not tried at all, people who didn't even know if they were ready to be parents. What was wrong with me that it should happen this way? Was someone, somewhere trying to tell me that I would be a *really bad* mother, that I didn't make the grade, I didn't cut it?

That was one wave of pain: I'll never be a mother. I'm not *meant* to be a mother. It will happen for everyone else but never for me. Yet, simultaneously, a second wave was wreaking its own havoc. It tore through my defences and exposed all that I had concealed, even from myself. But there it was, sitting jagged on the surface: I would have done anything to be the one announcing a pregnancy with Jai. It came as a jolt to consciously think it. However, he had said – not so long ago, as it happened – that he felt 'some kind of bond' with me and knew it would be there for life. Similarly, since failing to conceive, I had increasingly wondered if Jai and I hadn't been knocked off the path we should have been living together.

Maybe I was living the wrong life! Maybe that was why I had been unable to have children with Chris. Or was it just that I wanted to go back, now that going forward had become so painful?

It didn't help that infertility was causing me to question everything. Just as I sat in a toilet cubicle and wondered whether I was ever 'meant' to be a mother, so I wondered whether I was ever 'meant' to be with Chris. Maybe I was wrong, maybe the relationship was wrong, maybe we were both wrong. Round and round in my head charged this unstoppable tumult of thoughts, all converging every so often at the same point: *Jai is going to be a dad.*

I remembered his last line to me. *I ain't told anyone else yet, will do over the next week.*

By this time next week, everyone would know. It would be clear to all that retracing my steps back to the safety of Jai could never be an option. In fact, it never had been; I had just held on to the thought as a method of keeping afloat, pretending there was another choice because if I knew that, then I might not sink completely. So Jai was going to be a dad with someone younger, blonder, slimmer and, very obviously, more fertile than me. Meanwhile, I had been trying for nearly three years to have a family with a man who could sometimes bring himself to make love to me and sometimes not. In all of that time, despite all of the trying, there had not been one positive pregnancy test, not even a faint line on a pee stick that made you catch your breath, made you think, 'Ooh, is it or isn't it?' Sitting there in the toilet cubicle, covered in mascara blobs and runny snot, I thought, 'Look at me, no wonder Jai prefers *her*, no wonder Chris can't touch me … who the hell in their right mind would want me to be their mother?'

I think that is when I first lost my grip on whatever it was that had been keeping me from falling. That's when infertility, the adversary I had fended off for nearly three years, really started to get the better of me. In an unguarded moment, it had just punched me in the face, knocked out a few teeth and walked off laughing.

⅔ ⅔ ⅔

That night, as usual, Chris met me at the tube station. Again, I had sent a text ahead with the painful news. He was at the exit barriers as I came through, his arm around me immediately. "Oh Lou, I'm sorry," he whispered. Outside, he hugged me close, kissed the top of my head then handed over a bar of dark chocolate and a single blue flower, an Iris. "A little present," he said. "To cheer you up."

The blue flower was one of 'our' things, a joke that only we understood. It had started not long after our relationship began when Chris had presented me with a bunch of plastic flowers, in the same shade of artificial blue that elderly ladies chose to dye their hair. There were 'dew-drops', like oversized globs of mucus, on the 'leaves', which were connected to fuzzy, Kermit-green stems; I had never seen anything that looked less like an actual bunch of flowers.

It was several hours later, when Chris enquired as to why I hadn't put the bouquet into water, that he finally realised they were not 'real'. "What?" He looked stricken. "Plastic? They're plastic?"

"Well. Yeah. But they almost look real," I lied.

"Oh no! It was dark, I couldn't see properly, they were just outside the service station and I thought ..."

I started to laugh. Chris shook his head. "What must you think of me? I've given you cemetery flowers."

"From a service station." I giggled. "At nearly midnight. What did you expect?"

He picked up the offending bunch and studied them under the light. "These really are the most appalling flowers I've ever seen." We stared at the flowers, stared at each other, then rolled around the couch in fits of laughter.

"Please," he managed eventually. "Please throw the bloody things out. No one is to mention these Frankenstein flowers ever again."

But, of course, we did, often. And secretly I was relieved; I did not want to be with someone *too* serious and sophisticated – I was glad to know Chris did these haphazard things, because I did them too. I could boast a lengthy back-catalogue of dorky moments of my own; it was nice to know the two of us could bungle along together and laugh about it afterwards. I kept the flowers.

And now, on this night when I was overcome by nearly every miserable emotion you could name, Chris had thought to produce a blue flower, not just to cheer me up with the shared memory, but to say *I know you and I'm still here*. It somehow reminded me of who we both were, infertility or no infertility.

Later as I snuffled into my pillow, not quite managing to cry myself to sleep, he soothed and consoled me. "I love you," he said over and over. "You *will* have children, you will be a mother. Your time will come, I promise you."

Sheltered in his embrace, I felt guilty for the disloyal thoughts I had harboured while having a meltdown in a toilet cubicle. *Forward, I have to look forward.*

My mind, though, had no intention of being corralled into laying out its thoughts in a nice, clean straight line all the way into the future. At sickening speed, my thoughts raced back and forth across the world. *Jai is going to be a dad.* So easily, so casually. Why? I asked again, that futile question. Why does it work this way?

I pictured all the people who would be hearing the news over the next week. Most of them had been guests at our wedding, when I wore white and Dana followed me down the aisle in a blue bridesmaid's dress. *Don't think it, don't think it, don't think it.*

I thought of our old friend Dean, one of the few people who knew I had been trying to have children. Dean, who would soon know that I wasn't pregnant, but that Dana was. Again, I admonished myself: why had I told people? Why had I blurted it out? Why had I not just waited to see what happened? I understood, too late, that it would be so much easier if I had just let old perceptions lie; I wanted travel, I wanted a career, I did not want children. Now, thanks to my naive announcement – '*We're trying to have a family*' – I had to face friends like Dean, who would at least approach the delicate situation head-on, and friends like Lisa, who would try to avoid it, avoid me, altogether.

This was getting a lot more complicated than I had ever expected. As I lay there, tossing, turning and dripping tears into the dark, I wondered whether it was time to just take the hint: it appeared I was not meant to be a mother. What other message could I take from it when conception happened so easily for everyone else? For the first time, I felt my intentions wobble. Maybe the path to motherhood had already ended for me.

ELEVEN

IT WAS A NEW year – for the fourth time since we had set out to have a family, this date that was supposed to mark new beginnings had rolled on by. It is now more than seven years since January 2006, but I don't need to trawl through my memory banks or to check diaries or appointment books to know how I was feeling. I know I was feeling desperate because I did something that would normally be quite out of character: I visited a psychic. I had officially become a walking infertility cliché, endlessly searching in increasingly futile places for anything that would take away this pain, any glimmer of hope that one day it might happen – I might have a child.

The darkness that had started to fall after Jai's announcement had not lifted. Christmas, once my favourite time of the year because it meant 'family', was now my least favourite time of the year for precisely the same reason. I had wanted it over with quickly while, paradoxically, not wanting any more time to pass. Either time had to stop or I had to get pregnant because, if neither of those things happened by January 1, 2006, then I would be at least thirty-eight years old before I had my first child. Thirty-eight. Perilously close to forty and definitely not close enough to thirty. With these thoughts weighing on me, I felt constantly 'heavy', as if everything was an effort. And yet, somewhere inside, there was still that little voice, piping up to pierce the January gloom: *this* could be your year. *This* could be the year it happens. It was like simultaneously juggling balls of despair and hope, one low and heavy, the other high and light – it was impossible to keep both in the air at the same time without contorting body and mind into an unlimited range of tortuous states.

This was the tangle of contradictions that was me when Chris and I took a trip to Brighton on a dull winter day that January. We first visited the seafront, its contrast to a southern hemisphere beach never more obvious than at this darkest month of the year. "I don't get the fuss about this beach," I muttered from beneath the hood of my coat. "It's all stones. There's not even any sand."

"Well, nothing looks the same when you've been to Bondi, does it?" said Chris.

"And that's not even the best beach in Australia," I harrumphed, casting a scornful eye out over the ocean. "Have you noticed," I continued, "that there is no actual horizon? It's just grey rocks ..."

"Stones," said Chris.

"Okay, stones. Grey stones, grey sea, grey sky. Grey, grey and more grey."

This was not like me at all; normally I could find beauty in any place, normally I was excited to see a different way of doing things, normally I loved the northern hemisphere with a passion that other people couldn't always fathom.

"C'mon," said Chris. "I think it's just too cold for you down here. Let's go to The Lanes, it's more sheltered there." He was looking at me with an expression I had seen more often lately, worried and a little perplexed, as if he was thinking, 'Where have you gone? I'm not quite sure that I recognise you.'

I perked up a bit as we disappeared into The Lanes, the labyrinth of pedestrian passages that weaved in and out between Dickensian buildings bursting with character, the independent shops and restaurants within still twinkling with seasonal lights. Chris had walked these Lanes since he was a child and always knew where we were going and what we would see next, but I never failed to be surprised by wherever we ended up; no matter how often we walked through, the layout seemed to have changed since last time.

So I had no clue as to our precise whereabouts when we suddenly rounded a corner and found ourselves at the end of a Lane, facing a new-age shop and spiritual centre. I knew this place; we had passed it many times before but that was not why I remembered it. The reason it had always stuck in my mind was that, after a scathing argument early in our relationship, Chris had come to this very place to see a psychic and tarot card reader. This was not a particularly unusual thing for him to do. Although you wouldn't credit it from first appearances, Chris came from a family where the dreaming of events before they happened was fairly commonplace. His grandmother had dreamed, in full detail, of a zeppelin crash and had been desperate to warn someone of the impending disaster; her fears were borne out when her dream tragically morphed into reality a fortnight later. His mother, on a less distressing note, had a childhood dream in which the Grand National steeplechase played out before her eyes and she clearly saw the winner. However, no one took her seriously – until the horse in question romped home at the front of the field. Chris himself had often experienced disturbing premonitions and was left particularly shaken by a precognitive dream that showed, in the exact manner it would later happen, the death of a young celebrity during the 1990s.

In addition to all of this, he seemed to have the knack for randomly attracting people who described themselves as fortune tellers or 'seers' – one of them, a Romany Gypsy who stopped him in a car park had, allegedly, predicted my arrival in his life. "You won't be alone much longer," the old woman had told him, "there's someone coming from the other side of the world. She has had a challenging life and travelled a long way. You will know her when you see her."

Because this part of the prediction appeared to have actually happened, he set a lot of store by the other things she had to say. Unfortunately, she had also reported that he would have a daughter within eighteen months and that, in twelve years' time, he and his three children would meet her again in Cardiff. "You will have a little problem with making babies," she had whispered, patting him on the arm, "but it is not major, it is something that will be easily fixed."

I often wondered whether the faith he had placed in this random prediction was the reason he took such a *laissez-faire* attitude towards our fertility problems. As far as he was concerned, it was all destined to work out just fine and, by 2012, we – or at least he – would be sightseeing in Wales with not just one but three children.

I worried that he gave away too much during these encounters of his, that he was unable to keep information back. However, I had to rethink that belief right after his reading with the psychic at the little shop that we now stood outside in Brighton. This was because the psychic had revealed one of *my* secrets, something that Chris knew nothing about. Apparently the Libra card had come up repeatedly during the reading and I am indeed a Libra. But that was not the interesting bit; that was still to come: "Don't get too attached to the Libra in your life," the psychic told him. "I'm really sorry, but she's got another agenda. Whether she stays here or not could go either way."

What Chris didn't know at the time was that I was feeling increasingly uneasy about the sheer force of his defensiveness whenever I tried to discuss our issues with intimacy – so much so that I had discreetly packed some of my things into boxes and hidden them under the stairs. I wanted to be ready for a quick getaway if needs be. I didn't know how the psychic had managed to hit pay-dirt with this, but it did pique my interest. So when, in my devil-may-care mood of January 2006, I came upon the spiritual centre again, you didn't exactly need to consult an oracle to see what would happen next.

"Stuff it," I announced. "I'm going in."

Ten minutes later I was perched on a chair on an upstairs landing, about to see the same psychic who had earlier divulged my secrets to Chris.

"You're in luck," the young woman at the front desk had said, "he's normally booked out for weeks in advance. People travel from all over the UK and Europe to see him."

As I sat there on the landing – a little more energised at the thought of trying something different, but still in the funk that wouldn't lift – a smiling woman of about sixty emerged from a room further down the corridor.

She sat on the chair next to me, apparently gathering her thoughts. "Are you waiting to see Sebastian?" she asked.

"Yes." I nervously returned her smile.

"Been before?"

"No, it's my first time, just a spur of the moment thing really ..."

"Well, don't worry," she said warmly. "He's good. He really is fantastic. You'll get a lot out of it."

All I seemed to be doing since failing to have children was sitting outside doors like this, hoping that they would open and the person within would emerge to say, "Here's the solution! We'll fix it. Problem resolved." But was I really so lost that I needed a psychic to point me in the right direction?

A slim, dark-haired man, probably slightly younger than me and definitely trendier, emerged from the door down the corridor and welcomed me in. He was softly-spoken and friendly. Definitely not a show-off, I noted, relieved.

When the reading began, he handed me a deck of tarot cards to shuffle, then laid them out in a horseshoe shape on the table. He asked me to choose nine of them and I went for the symmetrical look, plucking cards from the centre-left, centre-bottom and centre-right; even when divining my future, I like the aesthetics to be evenly balanced.

"Oh," said Sebastian on viewing the first set, "I thought so."

He sounded genuinely sorry. "There's a relationship that has meant a lot to you. There's been a betrayal but it seems like the feelings on both sides have still been there, they haven't gone away. Something is going to happen, though, in the next two months, an event that will mean it's over for good, there's no going back. I'm sorry." He gave an apologetic grimace. "I didn't want this to come up for you either."

Crikey. Jai's baby was due in two months. Was it just a fluke that this scenario fitted perfectly? Or was the description general enough that anyone sitting here could have taken any situation and made the two halves match?

I kept my gaze down on the table; I didn't want to give anything away and furthermore Sebastian, I had noticed, had the most unusual, piercing blue eyes I had seen. I did not want him using them to x-ray my soul. Still, I thought, it must be a handy asset for a psychic, the requisite set of eyes that appear to bore right through you.

"Tied up with this situation," he continued, "there's a female who was in your life and I'd describe her as … a human leech."

I laughed, a bit more loudly than I meant to and, seeing that I was not upset, he joined in. "Sorry, it was the only way I could think of saying it!" From now on, I thought, I must remember to interchange praying mantis with leech.

"Why am I getting so many Pisces cues?" asked Sebastian. "You seem to be surrounded by Pisces energy."

Oh. That was good. Both Chris and Jai were Pisceans, though the vast differences in their characters, their opposite, almost *opposing* personalities, did little to reassure anyone that there was anything in this star sign lark.

Sebastian was off and swimming in the Pisces pool, though. "The Pisces you're with now," he said, "for some reason I link him with children, as if children are important to him, I get a real feeling of 'family' around him. Having a family is important to him."

Well, that was just typical. I was the one who did all the legwork, all the research, all the *attempting* to get pregnant, yet Chris was the one who the cards recognised as the wannabe parent.

I gave in and offered the information that we wanted to have a family, but it hadn't happened for us so far. As always, I tried to do this lightly, casually.

"Hmm," said Sebastian. "Let me see your palm."

I held out a hand, trying to look nonchalant.

"This is unusual," he said. "I'm getting two children from your palm, but psychically I can only see one pregnancy, a little boy. I think you will have a little boy, around thirty-eight, thirty-nine, that stage of your life. But it seems as if there is another child there as well."

He studied my palm again. "Yes, definitely two children. I don't know why I'm only seeing one psychically but that's what I'm seeing. I suppose it could always mean one pregnancy but two children. Maybe there's a twin hiding in there. Or maybe you will adopt a child. It's a bit odd. But there's definitely one here – I can see him, a little boy."

Naturally, my spirits leapt when he described all of this, however, I was not prepared to unleash my hopes on the strength of a prediction plucked out of the air by someone I had only just met.

Then he said something so specific that it stopped me in my tracks. "I can see two people who will help you with this," Sebastian informed me. "Someone called David will play a role and there's another who will help, called Sam. Those are the names I'm getting, but I don't know whether they mean anything to you yet or whether they will help you in the future."

I couldn't help myself. "Wow. David is the name of my acupuncturist. And Sam works at the same clinic – I see her sometimes when David is away."

"Oh," Sebastian said with a smile and a shrug. "There you are then. Although," he added, "the Sam I'm seeing is a man. Perhaps you are still to meet him."

There were other comments that could be described as 'hits' throughout the reading, although I didn't know that at the time. Sebastian predicted that I would become self-employed and also that I would live overseas – "I know you're already living overseas," he said, "but I mean somewhere else, another country, not this one and not your home country." As it transpired, he was right on both counts. Each of those things happened.

Near the end of the reading, he stopped and said: "I feel like I need to tell you again to leave that old situation behind. Sorry to go back to the first cards again, but the first Pisces, he wasn't who you thought he was. I sense you might have … sort of put him on a pedestal. But this Pisces, the one you're with now, give him a chance – he's genuine. And remember, the cards that have come up later, they're all really promising. There's a lot for you to look forward to."

When the reading came to an end and I got up to leave, Sebastian looked at me kindly. "There's a real sadness coming off you," he said. "I can feel it so strongly. But it will get better, it won't always be like this."

Whether he really knew that or not, I didn't care – at least he was displaying empathy and that was more than could be said for some of the medical professionals I had already met, and would go on to meet in the future.

I liked Sebastian, his gentle manner, his sense of humour and the modest, low-key way he responded whenever I couldn't help but say 'that's *exactly* right'. If he did have a gift, he wore it lightly, clearly regarding it in the same way the rest of us would regard breathing. It was just there. There was no point making a fuss about it, trying to build it up into something bigger than it was.

When I left the shop after the reading and crossed the street to meet Chris, I caught a glimpse of Sebastian looking out on us from an upstairs window.

I still had the feeling of 'heaviness' that was now starting to feel like normality to me, but I was eager to tell Chris about my brief trip to the spiritual side. I explained what Sebastian had said about children, trying to remember word-for-word what he had told me.

"We can play it back on tape when we get home," I added, "he gave me a recording of the whole thing."

When I mentioned his prediction about me having a little boy in the next year or two, Chris grinned and said, "See, I told you everything would be all right. I knew it would all work out okay in the end."

I still have the tape of that reading and, when I play it back now, I'm surprised by how many of Sebastian's predictions later appeared to have been borne out – from descriptions of buildings, which included correct street numbers, to the names of people I would encounter and places I would live. As it turned out, I did go on to seek help for infertility from a male practitioner called Sam, but that was still a good six months away at the time; I didn't yet know he existed.

The only thing that drew a complete blank was the little boy. He did not appear when I was thirty-eight or thirty-nine – he has never appeared and, of course, it now seems he never will. When I point this out to Chris today, he says, "Well, they get their timings wrong sometimes, it's quite hard for them to pinpoint actual times. An Irish palmist I met once told me that – these things can be very fluid. Don't give up yet."

I think about Sebastian sometimes when I'm looking back over the past ten years, beating myself up for the decisions I took and the decisions I didn't take, and the one thing I come back to is that old mantra of regret: 'What if?' What if, I think, we had managed to make love every single month during my thirties? Would the little boy have appeared then? Was he all ready to appear one August, say, but we shut the door, closed him out because we didn't provide any opportunity for sperm to meet egg? It is amazing that, even after an entire decade, these ridiculous thoughts will make their way into your mind. And yet, putting esoteric predictions aside, what is so illogical about 'what if?' It would take more than a psychic to answer these questions. Sometimes it's easier just not to ask them.

Over the past decade, Sebastian was not the only psychic who told us we would go on to have children. A young Irish clairvoyant who was getting rave reviews in *Time Out* told Chris I would fall pregnant in autumn, at the same time as he received a fantastic career offer. Six autumns have passed since then and I have not fallen pregnant in any of them. Chris is also still waiting for his big offer.

"These things are fluid," he repeats, "time is a very difficult thing to quantify if you think about it."

Although I remain sceptical, there was one woman who I encountered while traversing this fertility no-man's-land who did give me pause for thought. She was a psychic astrologer who I had read about in *The Times* newspaper, of all places. I liked her because everything about her was so unexpected, from her Oxford education to the earthy, direct manner in which she delivered her thoughts. She was renowned for her prescient advice on property purchases so, in another devil-may-care moment, I consulted her about a house move we were considering. I soon realised she was happy to discuss other matters and inevitably I questioned her about Chris and about having a family.

On whether Chris was the right man for me, she said something along the lines of, "He's okay, no better or worse than any of the rest of them."

I enjoyed this no-nonsense approach; it was a lot more fun than hearing about perfectly tall, dark strangers who could never exist.

She also reported that she would rather I achieved more for myself before having children. "There are a few other things that I want to see you accomplish first," she said.

Recently, I have gone back through the notes I took during our session because I was saddened to stumble across her obituary in a national newspaper. It turned out she had been the trusted advisor to a cast of stars, from big-name writers and publishers to barristers and investors.

There was one thing she said about pregnancy, which is written clearly in my notes: "It will happen, but it will happen in a month when you think it's well-nigh impossible."

I know. I know. Anyone could say that about anything, famous astrologer or not. But sometimes, when I'm worrying about what will happen next, I hear those words and a little bit of me still thinks, as futile as it might seem, 'Keep going, just keep going.'

TWELVE

WHERE IS THE ADDRESS card David gave us?" I was trying to get Chris organised. That's the positive way of saying it but, really, by this time it had come down to good old-fashioned nagging.

It was early 2006, not long after my visit to Sebastian the psychic, and Chris still had not taken his repeat sperm test. The details of a clinic where this could be done were on the back of a card that David, my acupuncturist, had provided more than three months earlier.

"Did you put it in your wallet?" I asked.

"Don't worry," Chris replied. "I've still got it. I'll look it out and contact them. I'll get onto it this week if you like."

"I can't see it here," I said, riffling through a pile of business cards and receipts in his wallet.

"It's probably in my desk."

"Probably? So you don't know where it is. Why didn't you just say so?"

"Well, it's around here somewhere. I mean, I haven't lost it. I've just got to remember where I put it."

I sighed. "Don't worry. It could be anywhere by the sounds of it. I'll just ask David for the details again."

"No, no," said Chris, "no need to do that. I'll get onto it, I give you my word."

I wondered if I should let it drop, hoping that, as with most things, he would get there eventually in his own vague and shambolic way. I didn't think he was stalling exactly, but I still wasn't convinced that he understood the importance of a detailed test. I had tried to explain it many times but something wasn't right – it just didn't seem to be sinking in.

"There's no point in us having any further tests until we know the outcome of this," I told him. "If it uncovers any severe problems we'd have to go straight on to IVF anyway."

He nodded and I knew he was still thinking – *but I've got enough sperm to fertilise the whole of the UK, the doctor said so.*

I tried another tack, albeit one I had used before. "The thing is, a sperm test comes right at the top of the list partly because it's quick and non-invasive. Also the results can shed a lot of light on what's happening all-round. If you're okay, it probably just confirms that we need to focus all our efforts on me."

"I'll get it arranged," Chris promised. "Don't worry."

Not long after that discussion, we were visiting Rose, Chris's elderly mother. Over tea and fruit cake, the conversation ranged, as always, across vast expanses of territory.

"Patrick has started a business," Rose said, discussing one of Chris's cousins. "He's very clever, he's done it all on the Circle Line you know. You can do that these days of course, but I must say it does sound very complicated."

"The Circle Line?" queried Chris.

"Yes, you know, it's on the Circle Line. Everyone's doing it now apparently. Of course, I haven't got a hope of getting on to visit it. I expect I'd have to get a computer for that." She laughed. "Can you imagine?"

Chris cast me a perplexed look, obviously wondering whether I had any idea what Rose had just said.

"Do you mean he's got an online business?" I ventured.

"Yes," she said, "that's it. You can do it all on the line. Quite extraordinary. But I expect you know all about that. After all, you were the one who finally taught Chris to do texting. I never thought you'd do it." We shared a conspiratorial giggle.

"Hey," Chris protested. "I'm actually pretty good at it now. It's quite straightforward. I don't know what all the fuss was about."

"Exactly," I said, laughing at the memory of him scrawling the most basic of instructions on torn pieces of paper, only to lose them again before his next attempt at sending a text. The same thing had happened with online banking. I had shown him how it worked and provided him with a customer number, password and pin – which he had subsequently noted down in too many random places to remember. I had grown so tired of him saying, "Just remind me, Lou, what is my customer number?" that I had ended up doing his online banking myself; it was quicker that way.

I was jolted from my ruminations on this by the realisation that, somehow, Rose and Chris were now discussing sperm tests. If there was a link between that and mobile phones, I couldn't see it. Still, it was time to catch up with the galloping conversation.

"Really?" Rose was saying, clearly sceptical about something. "We didn't have that sort of thing in our day you know. No one even mentioned it. It was always a women's domain, not something men were brought into at all. I suppose it's one of these modern things they feel they have to do."

Chris broadly explained the type of things such tests could show and why they were important. So, some of it had sunk in after all.

"I have to do another one," he told her, "to see what sort of state my sperm's in."

"Well, I'm sorry," Rose declared with a defiant shake of her head, "but no son of mine is going to have substandard sperm."

Chris laughed; I probably did too. But inside, there was that sick feeling again, the warning sign that I was so very accomplished at ignoring. 'It's me,' I thought immediately. 'She thinks we can't have children because of me.'

No son of mine is going to have substandard sperm.

Later, on the train home, Chris reassured me. "She didn't mean it," he said. "Not like that."

"I *know* it's probably me," I said. "I know that. But she didn't need to say it in front of me. She sounded completely serious."

"I know, I know. I'm sorry."

"Anyway," I added, "we're supposed to be in this together. It doesn't matter what the cause is – we just need to find it so we can move forward at last."

"That's exactly right," said Chris. "We'll do this together. It's not about blaming anyone. It's about the two of us."

He was saying the right things, the right words in the right order, but inside I still had that little warning twinge of uneasiness. Something wasn't right. I felt it, I knew it, but I couldn't yet put it into words.

⁂

By this stage, I had spent well over £500 on acupuncture and Chinese herbs. The investment had paid off in terms of my menstrual cycle, which seemed to be running more smoothly than ever, and, while lying on the treatment bed, I had several times experienced moments of complete clarity; it was as if a voice was whispering, 'You are right where you're meant to be. This is where you should have been all along.' I hoped that rare sensation related to my quest for pregnancy, but I was increasingly wondering if it wasn't a broader hint: maybe it was time for some more widespread life changes. As I lay there with eyes closed while the needles did their work, I daydreamed about having a family but, more and more, it was the burgeoning idea of a new career that danced to the forefront of my mind. Was I meant to be working in a field like this? It certainly felt like it – it seemed I was right at home there, among the meridian charts and the herbal concoctions that smelt of burnt coffee.

Conversely, I had known since the age of seventeen that I was not suited to the career I had chosen, but typically I ignored that and ploughed on nonetheless through the snake pit that was my profession. There had been many occasions when I had wondered how I would maintain the pretence that I was tough enough to belong there for a full forty-five-year career span. However, as I reached my thirties, I began to formulate a solution: with fifteen to twenty years' career experience behind me, I would take a break to have a family. That was phase one. Phase two was that, once my children had reached a suitable age, I would retrain in a new field. This was now just another plan that was beginning to unravel as infertility took hold. It seemed there was no part of my life that it couldn't shake up and disrupt. And something else was starting to happen; I would imagine bright new opportunities, from travel to study, then find myself putting them on hold 'just in case'.

I would be lying there at acupuncture wondering if I should take the hint about moving into a profession that better suited me, but then another voice would intervene: 'You can't retrain now – what if you get pregnant halfway through the course?' Or, if I was arranging a family reunion in my mind, each hemisphere meeting the other halfway, it would say: 'You can't fly long-haul to Hong Kong – what if the flight ruins your chances of conception?' After more than three years, I was still arranging my life around a pregnancy that had never happened. When would I get my actual life back, the one I recognised?

Then, finally, in March 2006, came the moment, the stab of hope that signalled I was about to get right back on track. My track, the one I had planned, not the alien road that infertility had led me down.

Chris and I were on holiday in the Lake District when, after an untimely storm, we found ourselves snowed in at the cottage we had rented on Lake Windermere. We ate meals in bed, swam together in the indoor pool and read books and magazines in an intertwined heap, joking that we were snuggled up like a pair of hibernating moles.

"*Do* moles hibernate?" I asked. "You don't hear much about moles in the southern hemisphere."

"I've got no idea," Chris replied. "But if I was a creature who hibernated, this would be the way I'd do it."

"Would you take me with you?"

"Of course I would, Lou. You know I'd miss you, even in my sleep."

"Good!" I laughed. "We're pretty companionable for a pair of moles, aren't we?"

"Yes, that's exactly the word. Companionable."

We had retreated into our old familiar bubble – just the two of us, with no care or idea what the rest of the world was doing. Cocooned by gently rising banks of snow, I was nursing a secret hope, almost daring to wonder whether this perfectly-scripted setting would provide the scene for our happy ending – at last.

My period was three to four days late. This had never happened before; my cycle was always twenty-seven or twenty-eight days long and, on the rare occasions when it varied, it would get shorter, never longer.

I didn't *feel* pregnant, not that I could really know what that felt like, but I didn't feel the same as usual either. Had we not been snowed in, I might have dared to buy a home pregnancy test. I didn't have one with me because I no longer kept any on stand-by. We were now in our fourth year of trying to have a family and I knew all too well how demoralising it is to stare at a white stick, willing a vertical line to appear, bringing with it the best news of your life. I had taken plenty of tests, all starkly negative, during the early years of our attempts at parenthood, and before long I had realised that, for me at least, it was best to remove that particular scary dip from the roller-coaster ride. I preferred not to be confronted with the proof that we had failed again; it was just another way that infertility could kick you in the teeth. Better to let my body tell me in its own good time, rather than having such a tangible reminder that, yet again, you've lost the fertility lottery.

So, in the Lake District, I did what I always did – waited to see what happened.

With each day that ticked on past day twenty-eight, I felt an increasing surge of adrenaline. I checked my diary over and over in case I had made a miscalculation, but it was all written there, ready to be transferred at some stage to the cycle chart I was still supposed to be keeping. It was day thirty-one and my period had not arrived.

I was done with getting our hopes up all for nothing, so I had kept my comments vague when I discussed it with Chris.

"I must have got my days muddled up," I said at first, "this seems to be a bit of a long cycle."

He visibly brightened even at that.

"Do you think it means anything? It must be a good sign mustn't it?"

"No." I shook my head. "No, I'm sure I've just miscounted."

Each morning, he would ask casually, "Any sign yet?" and I would say, "No, doesn't seem to be, must be the acupuncture – or maybe I've just written the wrong thing on the wrong day in my diary."

"I doubt it," said Chris, "that wouldn't be like you at all. I'm the one who never knows what day it is."

Now, on day thirty-one, I finally buckled and let him in on my private thoughts.

"This is really strange," I admitted. "I've never had a cycle that went into the thirties in my entire life. I think I've only even had a twenty-nine day one once."

"Just remind me," said Chris, "how many days is it usually?"

"Well, twenty-seven really. But it's twenty-eight sometimes, just depends what's happening."

He smiled. "I think this is a very good sign. I mean, if it's never happened before?"

Never happened before. I suddenly had a terrible thought.

"Oh no," I said. "Maybe I'm starting the menopause, maybe this is what's going to happen now – my cycles are just going to get longer and longer and then they're going to stop completely."

Chris looked momentarily alarmed. "Can you get the menopause at thirty-seven then?"

"Yes. You can start it even earlier than that … but it is quite uncommon."

"Well, there you are then. Anyway, wouldn't the acupuncture people have said something? Surely they'd be able to tell if that was happening. And wouldn't there be other symptoms first?"

"Hmm, I suppose so," I replied. "Maybe it's best if we don't read anything into it for now. It's just hard, you know …"

"I know," finished Chris, "when we've been waiting so long."

By the time we went swimming together on the morning of day thirty-two, I was starting to run out of 'other' explanations; perhaps this really could mean I was pregnant. There was absolutely no sign of my period and, joy of all joys, we had actually had sex three or four times around ovulation. If this was going to be the time when we discovered that the interminable wait was over, then it would all have been worth it. In my mind, I was already cutting free the shackles that had so painfully tied me to infertility. I felt my old energy surging back, as if I had been weighted down but now I was free to fly. For a couple of days, it was as if I was catching a glimpse of both the person I used to be, before this, and the person I would be, afterwards. The rising sense of relief this provided was almost more powerful than the hope and joy I had finally allowed myself to feel.

And then. The next day I woke and, within minutes, I knew that something had changed; whatever it was that I had been feeling had disappeared into the night. Something had shifted physically, something I couldn't even describe. But that 'different to usual' feeling, that 'otherness' had just gone. As we sat down to lunch on day thirty-three, my intuition was confirmed – a cramping pain unlike anything I had experienced was gripping my lower back. I had never felt menstrual pain in that area; any cramps were always centred on my abdomen and those had dissolved completely since having acupuncture. What was this?

The pressure in my back was joined by a growing wave of nausea and, before long, there was nothing for it but to lie down.

"Thank goodness we're on holiday," I groaned as Chris hovered anxiously over the bed. "Can you imagine all those bloody men in the office being confronted with this?"

He ignored my attempt to shift the focus onto something else. His words were short, crisp, hurried, his voice a little too loud. "Sweetheart, I think I should call a doctor! I'm going to phone for a doctor." And he dashed out of the bedroom door.

"No!" I pleaded to his departing back. "No, don't do that. I'm fine, it's just the pain in my back, that's all. Come back. Chris? … Chris?"

He appeared at the door with cellphone in hand.

"Honestly," I reassured him, "don't ring anyone. I'd feel an idiot ringing them up for this."

"But you don't look well," he said. "You've gone very pale. And look. You're shivering."

"Of course I'm shivering. It's snowing outside."

Nonetheless, I furtively glanced down, surprised to notice that my limbs did seem to be involuntarily shaking.

"I just need some paracetamol," I decided. "That'll sort out these cramps."

"Where is it?" asked Chris, still sounding panicked. "Where's the paracetamol? I'll get it. You must take it immediately …"

And he was off out the bedroom door again.

"It's in my handbag over there," I replied to the empty space in the doorway.

A couple of minutes later, he raced back in. "I can't find it! It's not in the kitchen. Or the lounge. Where did you put it? Do you really think it will help? Don't you think I should ring a doctor, just in case?"

"It's in my handbag." I sighed, gesturing to the chair where I had deposited it days ago, when we were last able to leave the house before the snow set in.

He dug around in the bag like a frenzied groom who has lost his wedding ring in the sand during a beachside honeymoon.

"It's in the side pocket – there," I pointed, the intensifying cramps almost taking away the breath I needed for speaking.

After taking two capsules – precipitating another haphazard dash to the kitchen for a glass of water – I sat up in bed and shuffled off to the bathroom. It was instantly clear that I was bleeding much more heavily than usual and, just to underline that fact, a clot of blood, about half the size of my fist, plopped to the floor with a violent splash. There were many reasons why it was best not to pass on this graphic news to Chris.

"Is it your … you know?" he needlessly asked as I crawled back into bed.

"Yes, afraid so."

"Oh. Oh I am sorry."

There was silence, even from the groaning blocks of snow that had begun to slip from the roof in unruly clumps.

"Sweetheart?"

"Mmm."

"I'm worried about you. Shouldn't I call a doctor?"

"I'm fine," I muttered into my pillow. "I'm pretty sure all you need to worry about are fever and sharp pain and I don't have either of those."

"You're still very pale," he said doubtfully. "But at least you've stopped shaking."

"I feel a bit better now," I said truthfully. "I thought I was going to throw up on their nice bath tiles for a minute, but it's just back cramps now. It's okay."

Chris finally stopped hovering and lay down beside me, propped up on one elbow as he stroked my hair.

"Don't worry, I'll keep an eye on you. I'm not going anywhere until I'm sure you're all right. Remember when you had sunstroke and I sat up all night wrapping you in wet towels and trying to cool you down?"

"Yes," I replied. "Just as well you did. I don't think I've ever felt worse."

"I soaked every towel we had in that motel …"

I lifted my head out of the pillow as we both laughed at the memory of our first holiday together, now more than four years ago.

The next morning, much like the sunstroke incident, I awoke feeling drained but almost fully recovered. It took another four paracetamol – I had refused to take anything stronger since we had been trying to conceive – but the cramps had now returned to a mediocre, manageable level.

We don't know what happened in the Lake District; there could have been many differing causes for it. For us, it's just another 'what if?' among ten further years of 'what ifs?' All I know is what *is* – I did not go on to have a child in late 2006 or early 2007, despite my rising hopes that our time might have arrived. Oddly, I don't remember any tears on that holiday. I probably cried them later, when what was happening to me really began to sink in. But at that point in 2006, I just resumed my familiar feeling of heaviness, trudging on as if it had never left me in the first place.

I had kept up my acupuncture treatments, but began booking them further and further apart as I lost heart about achieving a breakthrough. For the past few months, I had been treated by David's colleague, Samantha, purely for the reason that my work schedule did not fit in with the days he was available.

By April, more than six months after I had started treatment, it seemed that Samantha herself was at a loss to explain why I had not fallen pregnant.

I watched as she painstakingly revised my treatment notes and studied my temperature charts.

"Everything appears to be progressing as we would want it to," she said. "And you've noticed improvements with menstrual flow and cramps?"

"Yes, definitely."

"Fresh pink blood, no brown or black? No spotting before your period? No clots?"

"None of that, no. It's all gone. Well, apart from what happened on holiday, but you know about that. And it's a totally different colour, much 'fresher' looking, if you know what I mean."

"And no cramps?"

"None. I can't believe it. I've always had cramps."

"I know." Samantha looked up from the sheaf of papers she was holding. "We all put up with cramps because we think they're normal, that we're supposed to have them. But, actually, when your body's in balance, it's normal *not* to have them. I wish more women knew that."

Samantha returned to my charts again, frowning as she tried to uncover the missing link. "Your temperature graph is much more even and there's an obvious shift at ovulation."

She paused. "I can't see anything else here that we should work on. The only other thing I can wonder about is your lifestyle. Are you still dealing with deadlines at all hours?"

I confirmed it with a grimace.

"About 11.15pm for the last one. It's just the winding down afterwards. I can't shut my brain off for hours. My thoughts start racing – I can't stop them."

She nodded sympathetically. "Yes, it can have that effect. So what time are you getting to sleep generally?"

"Probably 1.30 or 2am. Unless I'm really stressed out, then it's later."

"Mmm. It's obviously not ideal, but you've responded well to treatment and your charts are looking better."

We mulled it over for a bit longer.

"There *is* one other thing," said Samantha. "Has your partner been retested? I'm wondering whether his sperm analysis results might clarify things for us. We really need to get a picture of your joint fertility as a couple."

She looked at me expectantly.

I shook my head. "No. He hasn't done it yet."

"I really would advise it," Samantha said. "I see here that David has given you the details of a lab we often recommend. Have you still got their number?"

"To be honest, I'm not too sure. I gave it to Chris and he may or may not have lost it."

"Oh dear." She reached for a notepad. "Well, here, I'll write it down again. I'd definitely get onto it. There's not much more I can see here that we can do to improve your cycle ..."

That night, I took the newly-provided piece of paper out of my work bag and handed it over to Chris.

"This," I said with a glare, "is that thing you said you'd do months ago."

He looked momentarily confused. "It's the lab details again," I explained. "For your sperm test."

"But Lou, I haven't lost David's card. I've put it away very carefully."

"I don't care what you've done with it," I said.

"Well, that was a very critical tone for someone who doesn't care."

"Oh for goodness' sake. It's not a criticism. It's a *please pull your bloody finger out.* I've been told again today how important it is for you to take this test."

"I know that," Chris snapped. "I'm getting on to it. Honestly, there's no need to row about it. I'll get on to them this week, I give you my word."

Thirteen

I WAS IN THE presence of a God. Well, that was the impression I gathered I was supposed to be taking from the encounter. There I was trying yet another method to get myself pregnant, the most expensive so far as it happened, but then, by this time, the stakes were getting higher in every possible way.

I had not returned to acupuncture after that last appointment with Samantha. It felt like there was nowhere else for us to go, no further improvements to make, almost as if we were both baffled by what was wrong with me. As much as I had enjoyed the treatment sessions, I lost heart and gave up on acupuncture. The stalemate lasted two months. Then, inevitably, I was off again, galloping down the next path that would surely lead me to the family I so desperately wanted. I had found another fertility guru in the feature pages of a national newspaper, but here was the thing: his method of treatment differed from any other, and, through it, he was achieving remarkable success with previously infertile women. Hope sprung anew. *This* would be the key. This would be the vital piece of information that led to me getting pregnant!

Again, acupuncture was involved, but not the common or garden sort apparently. This style of treatment was based around the ancient study of five natural elements (wood, fire, earth, metal and water) and their influence within the body. However, that wasn't the big news as far as I was concerned. I was drawn in because of another beguiling component – practitioners focused on treating the emotions as well as the body. It sounded like a cross between acupuncture and therapy. We hadn't yet found a physical cause for our infertility; perhaps there was something in this theory, perhaps it was an untapped psychological block. Certainly, given my own arrival into the world as an unwanted baby, I had more reason than most to unconsciously fear pregnancy. I had even wondered about it sometimes. Deep down, did I still believe that getting pregnant was the absolute worst thing I could do? Was some unseen part of me fending off conception for all it was worth?

The 'guru' in the newspaper had spoken about how it was important to treat the emotional as well as the physical in order to achieve balance and, ultimately, success. I think he called it the 'whole person approach'. I have not done it justice in describing it – it is more than seven years since I read the newspaper article – but a lot of what I saw resonated with me.

And there was something else: I had not been brought up to ask for help with emotional issues, let alone discuss them with a stranger. I came from a farming family where you just flexed your muscles and got on with things – the type of people I grew up with included an eighty-two-year-old man who was still breaking in volatile young horses, even with one arm in a sling after a previous fall. His daughter eventually confiscated his saddle; even that didn't stop him. These gritty men and women held no truck with sitting around examining the contents of your soul – and my own parents, who had each left school and joined the workforce at the age of fourteen, were among them. While it was obvious that I had always been more highly strung than the average weather-beaten dairy farmer, there was no way I was going to completely break the mould and admit that I needed help, needed propping up from an outside source. Something ingrained in me, some type of pride about standing on my own two feet, had prevented me from doing so, even though there had been many times, even before infertility struck, that a good counselling session might not have gone amiss.

So, the question was, could I now put all this conditioning behind me and try this new treatment?

I actually thought I could. Despite a natural aversion to baring my soul in public, the acupuncture guru's theory seemed less alien to me, purely on the basis that it included a practical component as well. So, this would be different – this would be therapy by stealth. I thought I might just be able to do this foreign thing, to share my worries with a stranger, if I walked in there and called it 'acupuncture'. I still didn't expect it to be a comfortable experience but, by this time, my desire for a family was so overwhelming that I was willing to try anything, even breaching those barriers that had previously seemed impossible to breach.

As ever, there was a waiting list to see the guru himself, but I happily bided my time for the chance to consult with him – I wanted to see the miracle worker who had given the women in the newspaper article their families; I wanted exactly what they had. If he could do it for them, surely he could do it for me too. After three-and-a-half years of trying to conceive, I had found something else, or maybe someone else, to trust with my fragile hopes.

The way it worked was that you had an initial appointment with the guru – a bit like a counselling session where you told him about yourself, discussed your anxieties and spoke about any potential emotional blocks that might be holding you back from conceiving. Then he decided what treatment plan would suit you best and, once again, it would be back to regular acupuncture sessions. So I took a deep breath, booked in, and eventually trooped off to Harley Street again to find the third clinic I had consulted there since struggling to start a family. Another grand building, another reception room where those in crisis signed over their hopes to someone else. Unfortunately, I was getting used to this. When would I graduate from all this waiting and hoping?

I climbed a wide staircase, trailing in the wake of a young woman dressed in white, and was shown into a consulting room where I sat and waited for the guru to appear. I felt unexpectedly excited, relieved even, to have the opportunity to discuss the thoughts and fears that had taken to relentlessly chasing each other around my head. If I had been of a less proud bent, I might even have thrown myself at his feet when he walked in and yelled, "For the love of sanity, please make it stop!" Instead, I smiled and tried to look confident, laid-back. Why did I insist on doing this when all I really wanted was to weep and wail? Oh well, if he was any good at his job, he'd soon realise it was just a farcical front.

There were the usual preliminaries, with the length of time trying to conceive now adjusted upwards, given that nearly a year had passed since I last went through this routine. I think he took my pulse and studied my tongue – only *think* because that wasn't the part of the session that has stuck with me all these years. The bit I remember is the 'talking' segment of the appointment and the way the whole experience made me feel. Maybe it was anxiety, maybe it was my earthy background, but something about the encounter made a small part of me want to giggle. I liked the guru – I did – but there was something about him that made me think of the sleek Burmese cat who lived in an imposing house further down our street; he frequently sauntered into our flat with the air of one who thinks, 'Yes, I am lord of all I survey, you may plump the cushions for me now.' I kept getting the unshakeable feeling that I had been granted an audience with the very God of acupuncture himself. Still, mere mortal that I was, I ploughed on, eager to make the most of this opportunity.

We had an hour in which to unravel the mystery of my failed attempts at motherhood. I decided there was nothing for it but to dive in with both feet. As we sat opposite each other and talked, I told him first of all about my background.

"I'm adopted," I explained. "I don't know who my birth father is …"

I trailed off; how do you explain in a few sentences the complex array of emotions that evokes, not to mention the shadowy feelings that control you like a secret master key, without you even realising?

"How about your birth mother?" he prompted.

"I've mainly had to pretend she doesn't exist," I began, a nervous giggle overtaking my words. "I didn't want to hurt Mum's feelings ... my adoptive mum, I mean, because she's amazing, especially the way she took me in. But it's just nature, you know, that bond you can't help feeling with the woman who carried you." I momentarily broke off, my voice threatening to catch at the thought that I would never know that bond, that I would never carry my own baby, who I would surely love and nurture with all my heart. "It's not like you can do anything about it," I continued, "make it go away."

He nodded. "I can see mothering has been a complex area for you."

Later, the conversation moved on to Jai and Chris.

"The thing is," I said, "I worry sometimes that it doesn't seem like a natural fit with my partner now. We've argued almost since day one and I don't get that because I never argue with anyone." Another nervous laugh. "My ex-husband and I never had any massive bust-ups, we went for years without arguing. We just went together – like salt and pepper. We just matched."

I was too embarrassed to add that the source of most of my arguments with Chris had been the performance anxiety issue, or more aptly his refusal to admit it existed. As much as I knew it would never happen, I still had visions of one of these fertility experts saying, "So let me get this right? You want to have children, but you don't always have sex?"

Even *I* thought I was ridiculous, pursuing all these avenues of inquiry on my quest for answers and yet the most basic of solutions had been writ large right in front of me all along.

I batted aside those thoughts and tried to concentrate on my ruminations about whether relationship concerns were blocking the path to pregnancy, whether some part of me knew this was the wrong road to take.

"Maybe it's because my current partner is a much better conversationalist," I said, by way of rationalising the number of arguments we had had. "He's certainly a big talker. My husband was much quieter. Maybe he and I weren't really communicating properly, maybe we actually *needed* the odd row. I don't know really ..." I shrugged.

Later, when we returned to the topic, via a description of Jai becoming a father while I struggled to become a mother, the guru said, "This is the salt and pepper man?" and I warmed to him because that meant he'd really listened, taken an interest, not only in what I said, but the *way* I had said it.

The guru, I decided, may or may not be the God of acupuncture but he was also a very nice earthling, kind and easy to talk to. I had the impression he was really 'getting' what I was doing my best to explain. So my confidence grew, I began to feel secure and a voice inside me said, 'Tell him! You can do it – tell him.'

This did not relate to Chris and our issues with performance anxiety; I wanted to confide a much darker burden than that. It was something I had never told anyone, except Mum, Jai and Chris, and even they didn't know the full story. But since infertility had come calling, this secret had been playing on my mind. It was like an intruder who had been lurking in the shadows but never quite jumped out to deliver the killer blow. Now, with each day that passed, the lurking figure was becoming more threatening; I feared it could burst into the light and finish me off at any minute, this thing that stalked me.

Was there a psychological block affecting my efforts at conception? You bet there was.

I padded out the conversation with things that didn't matter to me, stalling for time while an inner debate raged about whether it was safe to share this secret. The yeas and the nays were equal, except for one thing: the voice that was arguing, 'Yes! Yes, do it' was backed by the powerful force that was my desire for a family. It had become so strident, so insistent, that it was impossible to silence. It knew, and the rest of me reluctantly agreed, that this secret issue was making me feel vulnerable and afraid about the prospect of being forced to attempt IVF; it might even be enough to stop me from trying. I had to say something, I had to tell him. It was now or never.

I steeled myself to utter the words, sat taller as I gathered the strength to say it, finally to say it. I looked up, my resolve strong. And that was when I saw it – the guru was glancing at his watch. I was about to trust him with the most shameful secret of my life, the one thing I struggled to discuss with any-one, and he was looking at his watch. Like a bored commuter or a company executive who has better places to be. I reacted much like a wild animal responding to human contact on the farm; I retreated like a rabbit down a hole. He had almost fooled me, but I wouldn't be fooled again.

"Is there anything else you'd like to add?" he asked.

"No. Nothing I can think of."

"Well," he announced. "I think you're in need of some nurturing yourself, some mothering energy. So I'm going to suggest you have treatment with Maggie. She's a very good practitioner and a lovely person. I think you'll get along very well together."

Oh. I thought I had waited all this time for an appointment because I was going to be treated by the guru himself.

'Ha,' a rogue thought broke in. 'You can't be interesting enough for the likes of him.'

I instantly tried to dismiss it, remain positive. I had been looking forward to this experience and, whatever the case,

Maggie sounded nice. And perhaps the guru was right. I was increasingly feeling the need for the kind of gentle nurturing he was describing. I wasn't sure how much longer I could battle along on my own; it was like simultaneously fighting on two fronts. I wasn't sure what would take a chunk out of me next – infertility or its friend and ally, the performance anxiety problem. And, of course, there was still that other unspoken lurking thing, which had been firing warning shots of its own for several years. If there was a time when I had ever felt more alone, then I couldn't remember it. I immediately made my first appointment with Maggie; if it was going to take £85 a pop to buy support when I needed it, then that's what I would do.

If I had actually kept a fertility accounts book, this was the time when the entries would really have started to pour across the pages. And the entry to beat all entries thus far? Two hundred pounds for a counselling session/preliminary appointment with the acupuncture guru. Yes, I had just shelled out near-on the equivalent of the minimum weekly wage to talk to someone about a psychological block which I had then failed to mention because I caught him looking at his watch in a disinterested manner. I knew in that moment that this was just a transaction, a timed exchange, but I still spoke positively about it afterwards. I might even have sounded a little excited, hopeful, when I met Chris in Regent's Park and we shared a barbecued sausage in a bun while I filled him in on my latest pilgrimage to Harley Street.

And it might have been expensive but what if, for the sake of that £200, I never got to have children? Anyway, MBNA had sent me a credit card with zero per cent interest until June 2007 – and they kept increasing the limit without me asking. I now had just over £15,000 available on my magic card. It was so helpful, the way the balance climbed but the monthly payments stayed low …

Seven years later, I take a much more cynical view of that £200 session, bankrolled by MBNA. Do you know what I think now? I think it would have been far more useful to my mental and emotional health if I had taken that £200 and spent it on shoes, or lipstick, or a night away in a plush hotel. I could have worn a fluffy dressing gown and had my face massaged by an in-house beautician. That's how you deal with a psychological block: you just be nice to yourself. Can I have £200 for that piece of advice, please?

FOURTEEN

THIS IS EMBARRASSING TO write. It is also unsettling and it makes me boil with anger and resentment. Not to mention that it makes me feel a little bit sick inside. Here I am typing at what appears to be the beginning of chapter fourteen and, still, a little bit of me is saying, 'Really? You're giving it a chapter of its own? Forget it! It doesn't deserve that much space in your life.' Unfortunately, my time in the Ten-Year Club does not make complete sense without it.

I am not embarrassed to write about this for the reasons you might expect. I am embarrassed because it just seems like one drama too many. I've already managed to lose three parents by the age of seven, one via desertion, one via adoption and one via a death that happened right in front of me. I've watched my one remaining parent struggle, financially and emotionally, to keep us afloat. My marriage has failed and my ex-husband has decided he preferred the chief bridesmaid anyway. I've been unable to have a family of my own and have spent years struggling with infertility and associated other delights. And that's just the potted highlights. I feel like the human equivalent of the fictional television village of *Emmerdale* – everyone knows it's had far too many murders, explosions, storms, accidents and affairs for such a tiny place. It's way out of whack with other, 'normal', towns.

Now here I am, about to throw another improbable storyline into the mix. I would have pretended this new thing had never happened – I would have left it like a discarded scene on the cutting room floor. But if you're going to write honestly about infertility, if you're going to truthfully convey the dirt it carelessly digs up, then there is no point unless you disclose everything. I don't want to be like those fertility 'experts' who give the impression that infertility is all clean and white, minimal and orderly like the identical buildings they operate out of. Sometimes they place a box of tissues on their desks, arranged at right angles and always white, but that's the only concession you will find to the fact that this hurts beyond all other hurts. This is worse than watching my father die, this is worse than losing my birth parents, this is worse than knowing that the love of my life has chosen my best friend to be the love of *his* life. Why? Because this is what no expert seems to understand: it is not enough for infertility just to be painful in its own right. Oh no. As the years pass, infertility will make sure that you encounter each and every one of those earlier pains all over again. It batters you over the head with what is happening in present time, it drags you back to the sorrows of the past and, just for good measure, it fills you with dread about what might happen in the future.

If it sounds like I'm furious with infertility, well, sometimes I am. But the thing I'm most furious about is that it has forced me into a corner on one last issue. It's been like those arguments, where you trade insults until someone says something so revolting that the other person cries, "I'm sorry, but you've really crossed the line now. That was a low blow!"

❧ ❧ ❧

I was eleven years old. Mum and I had driven for about two hours, to a sports event where I would be competing for the next few days. I was thrilled; I loved these trips away. At that age, I had never stayed in a hotel or a motel. We didn't have the money for those sorts of luxuries, but I didn't care because we did far more exciting things instead – sometimes we camped in a tent at the sports ground; sometimes we pushed down the back seats in the car and turned it into a bed for the two of us. I loved it when the rain would drum on the roof and I would read a book by torchlight. Or when Mum would say "eek!" as she scrambled out of the door and made for the toilet block, holding tightly to the towel that flapped above her head to keep off the rain. She would do a funny high-stepping dance through the puddles to make me giggle.

She was not like other people's mothers, who made a fuss when someone dropped food on the floor, or when a bit of mud found its way into the house. She laughed at these things; she liked a good adventure as much as I did. That year, though, we were not staying on our own in the tent or in the car; we were staying with some of our oldest family friends. They were the people who had gotten me and my brother Ray into this sport in the first place. I hadn't even turned five when I took part in my first competition; there's a picture somewhere of the four-year-old me displaying the prizes I won that day.

"This one came out of the ruddy womb playing her sport," the farmer next door used to say of me. At the age of eleven, nothing had changed. Just like in the early days, we would all be at the same event together – our old friends and their now teenaged daughter. There were three days of competition, but I would not be participating until the final two. We were only there for the first day because Mum was playing her familiar role as judge of one of the senior events. I would amuse myself at the stalls and sideshows that accompanied the competition and spend the rest of the time with our family friends.

The husband seemed a lot older than the wife to me. He'd been old ever since I knew him, and that was pretty much all my life. I'd never liked their house. It was stinky, partly because of all the overflowing silver ashtrays on sticks that dotted the lounge and partly because of the bug-eyed pug dogs that I was sure used to take a pee in the corner. Then they'd settle on the faded holey blankets that covered the couch and drip pug dog saliva onto the spot where someone might be about to sit. If it was down to me, I'd have preferred to sleep in the back of the car. But apparently our friends were looking forward to seeing us.

I could remember being in that lounge when I was five years old. We used to share a joke, the old man and I. "Here comes my girlfriend," he'd announce when I entered the room. "We're going to get married one day." He'd guffaw as I settled into his lap. "Aren't we?" Everyone would laugh. Wasn't it cute, how well we got on together?

That day, when I was eleven, Mum and I met him and his family at the sports ground; we'd left home at 6am to get there in time. Most of my other friends, who I knew from years of competing together, would not be arriving until the next day. So I sat quietly at Mum's feet for a time while she judged older competitors, then wandered off to find my own entertainment once the stalls and sideshows began to open. At some point, as so often on these excursions, it began to rain – not just any old rain, but the pounding sub-tropical variety that is said to come down in sheets or buckets, depending on which farmer you are speaking to. All I knew was that I was getting saturated. I made a run for the cars, parked in a giant horseshoe stacked several lines deep around the outdoor competition arena.

Right at the front, directly overlooking the arena, I spotted our friends' red car. It stood out not just because of the colour but because it was so old-fashioned, its sharp tail fins jutting out beyond the other more streamlined vehicles. I opened the passenger door and dived in, smiling. The old man was sitting at the wheel smoking a roll-up. If I thought his house was stinky, this was a whole new level of stench. His driver's side window was partly down and some of the smoke floated out into the rain.

"Well then," he said, and wound the handle that closed the window all the way to the top.

I wanted to see the competition, still going on out there in the squall, but he turned off the windscreen wipers and let the oversized raindrops pile up on the glass. We were enveloped in a smoky, rainy fog. He finished his cigarette, partly rolled down the window to flick the discarded butt out onto the soggy grass then closed it to the top once more. He slid across the vinyl bench seat towards me. "Come here."

Oh, I thought. He wants one of the hugs we used to have when I was little. Doesn't he realise I'm too old for that now?

His arm snaked around me and pulled me close. I could feel his white whiskers against my cheek. He needed a shave. Then suddenly his mouth was on mine, slobbery and stinky like his disgusting dogs. I felt sick, confused, scared, like my insides had started shaking. Surely this was not normal? No one had ever mentioned anything to me about this sort of thing. I knew I shouldn't accept lifts from strangers and that if anyone suspicious approached me when I was out riding my horse, I was to gallop away. But what did I do now, with this man I trusted? Who wasn't a stranger? Who I didn't want to get into trouble with? Or be rude to? Whose lips were all over my face?

'Oh my God,' I thought. 'What if other people in other cars can see? They'll think I'm loose, they'll think I'm dirty.'

He was emitting a low groan that sounded like contentment, his hands were moving under my clothes and I was pinned to the seat, trapped against him with nowhere to go. I thought I might vomit, just from the feel of his saliva on my mouth. The assault went on and on, I didn't know how to stop it. He made comments about my physical development that made me sick to my stomach. I fretted about the other people in the other cars. They mustn't see this; I knew that. So that meant for sure that it shouldn't be happening. It was wrong. He was wrong. It was all wrong! I couldn't breathe, he was too heavy, why was he touching me there?

Eventually, when I could take the violation no longer, I wriggled my face away, now wet with saliva. "I've got to go. Mum will be looking for me," I said in a trembling voice.

"You come back and see me," he rasped. "You come and see me tonight. At bedtime. Just you and me, no one else needs to know. Okay?"

"Okay. Can I get out now?"

"Remember not to tell anyone. It's our little secret."

And he winked at me, flicking the windscreen wipers on, clearing the front window as I finally escaped into the remnants of the rain. Mum. I had to find Mum.

I ran, on shaking legs that I couldn't seem to control, to the judges' area. She smiled at my arrival then fastened her gaze once again onto the contestants, and I sat at her feet, nestling in tight against her legs. I made myself small and still, a guilty bundle of badness. I was an awful person. I had done something really, really wrong.

When the competition ended, everyone else in the judges' area moved gradually away. Mum was packing up her bag, taking her time as she chatted to Carol, another of our friends who lived nearby. Carol said, "Would you watch my things, May? I need to spend a penny. My poor old bladder thought that last round would never end."

She trotted off, wincing.

"Well," said Mum, turning to me as she stretched her arms above her head. "Now that's out of the way, we can get going to Tina and Con's. Ready?"

A rogue tear broke loose before I could stop it.

"Loulou? What's happened? What's wrong?"

She pulled me into a hug and the tears emerged in gulps against her best judge's jacket.

"Has someone been picking on you? What is it?"

I nodded. "Someone picked on you?"

I nodded again, miserably.

140

"Come on now. You're going to have to tell me otherwise I can't do anything about it."

"It was Con," I managed to whisper into her chest.

"Oh him. He's a grumpy old sod at the best of times," she said. "What's he done now? Just ignore him, Lou. That's what you do with people like that."

"I caaann't," I cried.

"What?"

"I can't ignore him. He says I have to go and see him tonight," I confided in a rush.

I felt her soft, cuddly, motherly body become rigid.

"He says what?"

Fear and desperation surged, but still I couldn't find, didn't begin to know, the words to use when telling her what had happened. My voice dropped to a mumble as I said the least embarrassing thing I could think of. "He kissed me. In the car. I'm not supposed to tell anyone, but he said I have to go and see him at bedtime."

"He did, did he?" Her voice had turned to steel. "Well, I'll tell you something. You won't be doing that."

I looked up to see Carol wandering back in, looking markedly more comfortable now that she had made her convenience stop. "It's okay," Mum said. "I'll be looking after you, don't you worry. Just sit here for a minute and dry your eyes while I talk to Carol. Here. They gave me a can of Fanta – that will make you feel better."

I sipped the syrupy drink and watched Mum and Carol speaking in low, serious voices in the corner. I still felt guilty and sick that I had done this thing. I put the drink down after a few half-hearted gulps.

Eventually Mum came back, followed by Carol, who gave me a hug. "Come on Loulou, we can't have you upset. You're our little ray of sunshine."

I forced the corners of my mouth into a doleful smile.

Soon Mum and I were walking back to our car. "I'm afraid you're not the only one this has happened to," she said quietly.

I looked up, confused.

"Carol just told me. Something similar happened to Anna when she was staying at his place. She won't go anywhere near there now."

Mum had told her? How embarrassing! And he'd done it to Carol's daughter? But why hadn't Carol told someone, why hadn't she warned them? I didn't understand any of this. Perhaps, I thought, she didn't want to get Anna into trouble.

We drove through the countryside for about twenty minutes to get to the last place on earth I wanted to go. I felt so guilty, so gut-wrenchingly sorry, and deeply ashamed of this thing that had happened. It must be me, I realised, as we travelled in silence – I was a bad person. Look at all the people in my life who had already left me; they knew what they were doing, those parents of mine who never were. No wonder they didn't want me. During that tense drive, it never occurred to me that we could cancel our visit to Tina and Con. I knew we didn't have the tent or even our sleeping bags with us. Where else would we go? Paying for a motel was out of the question; we'd only afforded the petrol to get here in the first place because I had won some prize-money at a previous event.

Before we reached our squalid destination, Mum said I was to sleep with her that night, in her bed; I was not to share a room with Mish, Con and Tina's daughter, like I normally did. Mish had a bright orange giraffe poster on her bedroom wall and there were lines drawn on it, inch by inch, which we'd once used to mark how tall we'd gotten. It was the only thing in the entire house that I liked. It wasn't even a house, come to think of it, more one of those pre-fab classrooms that people just dumped anywhere when the proper school buildings had run out of space. I stayed close to Mum when we walked in the door.

Later, at dinner, I had to sit opposite Con. I refused to look at him and, when he spoke to me, I refused to speak back. I sat silently, staring at my plate of mince and boiled vegetables, swimming in a shallow pool of greasy water.

When Con asked me something in a jokey tone and I didn't reply, he gestured angrily across the table and jeered, "Look at her! Sitting there, sour as a lemon."

No one came to my defence.

When would dinner be over? How did I swallow my food when I felt this sick?

When the others had finished – finally – and the women were busying themselves with carrying dirty dishes to the kitchen, I made my escape. I slipped out through the back door and nearly tripped over Mish's pushbike, leaning drunkenly against the steps. Immediately, I was sitting on it and pedalling furiously out of the driveway and down the road. I didn't know where I was going; I just didn't want to be in that house. A few hundred metres down the road, the dusty metal surface was suddenly transformed into a tarmac bridge over a water-fall. I came to a halt there, stood at the bridge railings and watched the water tumbling and tearing at the rocks below. Normally it scared me, that wild place where it looked so easy to drown. But today I didn't care. I pushed off again on the bike and rode in arcing, aimless circles, round and round, in the middle of the bridge. I needed to keep moving; the anxiety that surged up my throat, through my stomach, down my legs could not be kept still.

I was tracing a wobbly circle in the centre of the road when a figure appeared just around the bend, beyond which sat the house of my nightmares. It was Mum! She must be coming to comfort me after what had happened at dinner. Then, as she got closer, I realised that her mouth was set in a tight, hard line. I knew that look, you didn't want to mess with it. She took hold of the bike, bringing me to an abrupt halt.

"You've got to pull yourself together," she ordered, guiding me off the bridge and onto the side of the road.

If I was going to tell her what had really happened, then that was the time to say it. But still I said nothing; I couldn't bear for her to know that I had done these things. So we walked back to the house, where I tried not to look like a person who had just been sexually assaulted, even though I didn't yet know that was the name for what had taken place.

Mish was upset when she heard I wouldn't be sharing her room that night. "But I was going to tell ghost stories," she complained. "We always do that."

Con sneered at me. "She's a little baby. Got to sleep with her mummy."

The next day when I was competing, his car was parked in exactly the same place. From behind the steering wheel, his knowing eyes bored into me every time I passed that spot in the arena. *I know what you've done.* I did not perform well enough to win any prizes.

Three years later, I was taken out of high school one morning to attend Con's funeral. He had set his bed on fire with a cigarette; that didn't actually kill him, but the shock hastened things along and he collapsed and died not long after. As we walked out of the crematorium after the funeral, Mish, now sixteen, was sobbing, grabbing on to people's shoulders for support and almost wailing their names as she did so. I looked around. No one else was crying.

❧ ❧ ❧

What fertility experts don't seem to consider is that perhaps, to some women, IVF does not feel like a straightforward medical procedure. Depending on what has happened in your past, the unpalatable truth is that it can feel like another violation.

That is why I did not rush into IVF the moment I realised we couldn't seem to have children naturally. It wasn't just the apparent cost and it wasn't just that our doctor said it would probably tear our relationship apart. It's because I wasn't sure whether I could allow myself to be that vulnerable again. I didn't want to lie still while someone else took control, perhaps pulling cells out of me, then later placing them back in. I couldn't be that compliant, that trapped; I have to keep moving to feel safe, even now. Here's something else my doctor didn't know: pre-infertility, I had not had a smear test since 1990. There was no logical reason not to return for a repeat test when it was due; I had never had an uncomfortable or painful experience during a smear, and I always made sure they were carried out by women only. But, despite all the evidence, all the publicity about the dangers of cervical cancer, I had never brought myself to do it again – something about it returned me to that day in the car, when all control was taken away from me. When I felt exposed, both because of what happened inside the car, and because of what people outside the car might have seen.

On the day I went to have my internal fertility scan at the hospital, my legs shook all the way there and all the way back again. There is only one thing in the world that could have caused me to have that scan, and that is my desire for a child of my own. I wouldn't take a five-minute smear that could potentially save my life, but I would undergo a lengthy internal scan if it might lead to me having a family. The question I have wrestled with is this: am I strong enough to cope with a procedure as invasive as IVF? Which is more powerful, the fear I have carried since I was eleven years old or the desire that has now fuelled me for a decade? In 2006, I didn't know the answer. Until I knew for sure, all I could do was try to heal my fertility problem naturally.

FIFTEEN

OUR NEIGHBOUR'S CAT MARCHED into our flat with his tail in the air, like a celebrity who expects nothing less than access all areas. I looked up to see Chris trailing in his wake, speaking into his mobile phone and giving a wry shrug that let me know Angus had outwitted him once again in the battle of the doorstep. "He just gets in," Chris would explain, "no matter what I do. I don't know how he manages it."

Once he had gained entry – either by stealth or by sheer force of will, depending on his mood – Angus then expected an official welcome, befitting a creature of his status. First of all, he would leap up, standing on his hind legs while he repeatedly head-butted your hand. Then he would flop onto his side in the uniquely louche manner of a Burmese cat and demand that his belly be tickled until he tired of it. After that, he would expect you to drop what you were doing, sit down and provide him with a warm lap, where he would carry out his fastidious ablutions before falling asleep in an arrangement of head, legs and paws that tended to be entirely comfortable for him and entirely uncomfortable for you. That was on a good day. On a bad day, Angus simply did his best to tear apart the flat and its contents.

"Hello Angus," I said from the kitchen. "I'm sorry, I can't adore you today, I'm cooking dinner."

He had obviously intuited this for himself; he followed Chris, still talking on his phone, into the lounge. When no welcome was forthcoming there either, he ankle-tapped him from behind, which at least caused him to turn and waggle a finger at his assailant. Chris set off in the other direction, towards the bedroom; Angus appeared at speed from behind the couch and threw both paws around his leg in a lopsided rugby tackle. Chris leapt across the floor and, struggling not to dissolve into laughter down the phone line, rolled his eyes at me. Angus disappeared to one of his hiding places while Chris removed his shoes and sat down at the table.

"Argh!"

I poked my head around the corner. It appeared Angus had just bitten Chris's toes, right through his socks.

"No, no, everything's fine, Mr Connor," he was saying, while wildly waving his left foot in the air. "Apologies for the interruption, it was just a little … er … accident."

He finished the call shortly after. "Trust Angus to attack me while I'm speaking to my dreaded accountant."

"Well, you let the little Tasmanian Devil in," I joked.

"But I was so careful this time. I thought he couldn't possibly have snuck in."

"Oh well," I said, returning to the kitchen. "You've let him in so you're in charge of him."

"I need a drink," he announced, heading for the fridge. He poured a glass of wine while I kept one eye on the lounge.

"Angus is chewing the speaker cables. Oh! Yuck."

"What?"

"I'm fairly sure he's just sprayed on Bruce Springsteen."

"He's what?"

"You know that anthology you've got in the special case? Yeah, well, he's just backed up to it and shaken his tail at it for all he's worth. I don't know if anything came out but—"

"Angus! Angus? Come here you little vandal." Chris abandoned his glass of wine and rushed into the lounge. "Where's he gone now? Oh hell. Did you see him?"

A black tail disappeared around the corner of the stairs that led to the spare bedroom in the loft. Chris followed in hot pursuit. "Angus. Don't even think about it. Anguuus."

There was a brief pause. "Lou! Lou, you'd better come up."

I sighed and turned down the oven. "What is it now?" I asked as I reached the top of the stairs.

Chris was leaning precariously out of the skylight that had been cut into the steep slope of the roof. "He went out the window! I couldn't stop him."

"What? Has he fallen? There's only a tiny bit of guttering under there."

"No, I looked. There's nothing on the ground – he must have whipped straight up over the roof."

We scurried to the other side of the room and peered as best we could through the skylight at the top of the stairs. A tell-tale black ear was visible just above the apex of the neighbouring roof.

"Phew," said Chris. "But what are we going to do now? Should I get a ladder? Should we call for help?"

"Well, he's not going to fall now he's got over to that side," I reassured him. "Knowing Angus, he'll come down when he's ready, probably right about the time my chicken comes out of the oven."

We spent ten minutes crooning and calling to no avail then decided on a change of tactic and retreated back downstairs to pretend to eat dinner. Sure enough, the roast was barely out of the oven when Angus's distinctive yowl floated down from above. Chris abandoned his still-empty plate and ran upstairs.

A few minutes later, he returned with a smug-looking Angus in his arms.

"He's so clever," he said. "I couldn't reach him, but he knew he had to jump down to me. He got the message just like that." He ruffled the fur on Angus's head, lowered him gently to the floor then offered him a piece of roast chicken. "What a clever boy."

"Hey," I laughed. "You've just rewarded his bad behaviour."

"Well, I thought he might be traumatised," said Chris. "Poor little thing."

"Traumatised? If anyone's traumatised it should be us."

We finally sat down to eat and Angus jumped into Chris's lap, uninvited. "You do realise," I continued, "that when you have children, this is exactly what they'll be like?"

"They will not," Chris said indignantly. "I shall go to great pains to make sure my children have excellent manners."

"Yeah," I said. "But there's one problem with that – they'll have your genes."

"Hey, what do you mean? I've got great genes."

"Well, who was it that buried an entire canteen of cutlery in their mother's garden? Who shot their grandmother with a rocket left over from fireworks night? Who—"

"Oh no," Chris interjected. "Mum talks far too much. I've got to stop her telling you these things."

"Who," I persisted, "got in a strop with their mother while staying at a posh hotel and asked the *manager* to deliver her a note of complaint?' Who does that when they're seven?"

"All kids do that type of stuff – you must have done it yourself."

"No, I did not. I was an absolute angel compared to you. I just threw the odd cowpat at people, but everyone did that where I came from."

"Yes." Chris snorted. "That sounds like life in the colonies."

I was making a concerted effort to keep things easy, to keep the laughter going. Bless Angus and his antics. This was such a relief, a momentary lightening of the strained and strangling atmosphere that seemed to have settled permanently around us.

In the initial ten-day period after my appointment with the acupuncture guru, Chris and I had had two failed attempts at sex around ovulation and one successful attempt just after ovulation, interspersed with four heated arguments about our lacklustre efforts at conception. I know this because I was becoming so worried about the growing tension between us that I started noting all of these events in my diary, almost as if I wanted to see if I was imagining it or not. The mental and physical exhaustion I was feeling after having different versions of the same row, throughout night after night without any real sleep, should have told me all I needed to know. But I didn't know what to do, how to fix it.

I was having weekly acupuncture sessions with Maggie, handing over £85 a time in the hope that it would improve my fertility and yet we were able to have sex only once or twice a month, not necessarily when I was ovulating. I tried not to make a fuss about ovulation, not to even say the word. I tried to take the pressure off by saying it would be fine to have sex every other day at my fertile time, when secretly I wanted to do it every single day of the month if that was what it took.

I had read about a woman who struggled to conceive her third child and that was exactly what she informed her husband they would do – every day for a month and, presto, suddenly they were pregnant. I could never tell Chris that. He would undergo any number of tortuous discomforts rather than forcing himself to make love to me every day for a month. It was as likely as a thirty-seven-year-old getting pregnant from one attempt at sex when she wasn't even ovulating. It was never going to happen.

At acupuncture, it didn't take Maggie long to pick up on the fact that something was very wrong. She was warm, intuitive, funny, kind; precisely the sort of woman I could imagine being friends with. That proved particularly fortunate because, with this new type of treatment, she remained in the room with me throughout.

Now that I come to explain the treatment, I realise I didn't pay much attention to it – it was my chats with Maggie, the emotional support she provided, that I really needed. She carefully explained it all to me – I knew about the way she inserted fine needles or sometimes burned cones of herbs to stimulate meridian points – but the information is long gone from my mind. When it comes to infertility, it seems I have held on to the emotions involved – or they have held on to me – while letting go of the detail. Yes, I have gradually lost sight of whatever it is that might actually get you pregnant.

One afternoon at acupuncture, I was so drained by the rows, the constant effort of trying to conceive while Chris seemingly did his best *not* to conceive, that I let down my guard; I told Maggie what was really happening.

"Is it true," I asked, "that you can tell if a woman is pregnant just by the change in her pulse?"

"Yes, that's right. It's a very noticeable shift, the pulses become very lively. That's why we can often tell that a woman is pregnant even before she knows it herself."

She smiled. "You never know, maybe next week I'll be able to show you exactly what I mean. Yes," she confirmed, glancing at my chart, "that would be about the right time for it to become apparent."

"I doubt it," I said glumly. "Not unless it's an immaculate conception."

"Oh dear. What's been happening?"

"Nothing." I laughed nervously. "That's the whole thing. Chris has …" I faltered. How should I phrase it? "Stage fright, I guess you'd say."

"Oh Louise," Maggie said gently. "Is it the stress in general do you think? Or is it the pressure of ovulation? Some men do struggle with that."

"I wish I knew. I don't think it's just about trying to conceive, though. He's been like this ever since we met."

Oh," she said again, patting my shoulder. "You know, life really is a lot less complicated when you get a bit older and the only things you're looking forward to at night are a mug of hot chocolate and a good book."

This was why I liked Maggie so much; she had seen the tears swimming in my eyes and instinctively knew that now was not the time to push me further. She understood that it was a big deal for me to have actually said it and that, next time, I would be ready to say a little more.

After the session, I walked to a nearby department store in search of a mirror; I wanted to ensure any evidence of prospective tears was wiped from my face before I started work. However, I took a wrong turning on the way to the restrooms and emerged from an escalator to find a sea of bedrooms for babies stretched out before me. I stopped dead, not wanting to move forward but too late to avoid it: the nursery furniture department. Beautifully-crafted wooden cots and matching miniature sets of drawers, tiny mattresses with multi-coloured bears on the covers, woven Moses baskets, fat moons and stars dangling from mobiles at the end of cribs, rugs with stencilled penguins waddling across them. Pregnant women, with their expectant bumps and their equally expectant partners, browsing.

I saw the first cot, the white wooden bars, the tiny blue pillow at one end and my throat and stomach seized. I stood at the end of the little bed, instinctively reaching out to touch it, and it felt just like grief, the yearning and longing for someone to be there when they are not. Except the person I was missing, until I almost couldn't breathe, was someone who I might never know. What if he, or she, never came? What if I never knew them, never saw their face? Never tucked them into a cot just like this? I wanted to curl up on the floor with the stencilled penguins and cry. When I jolted back to present time, I realised I already was crying. I dropped my hand from the cot and kept my head down towards the floor while, heavy with grief, I dragged myself to the bathroom. Finally, it was safe to lean against a cubicle wall, doubled over in pain as I sobbed and hiccupped into a wad of toilet paper.

Back at home, the fights continued. At least one or two a week, through May, June, July and on into August. I don't

152

know why we bothered; the script was almost always the same. It would have been far less taxing to have recorded the first row and played it back to each other a couple of times a week, in the hope that someone might – finally – get their point across.

During each of those summer months, I began to dread ovulation almost as much as Chris apparently did. It didn't matter that I hadn't said, 'Today is the day!' he seemed to sense it and there were far more false starts than triumphant finishes. I was beginning to become afraid to even try, but what other choice was there if we wanted to have children? It was not as if we had time to wait it out. In a couple of months, I would be thirty-eight years old.

I tried to hide my disappointment whenever sex came to an angst-ridden halt, with Chris shaking and sweating above me. He would start out hopefully, confident almost, but I could always sense when it was not going to happen. It didn't feel natural. It felt as if he was willing himself to believe 'it's going to be okay this time' – like one of those mantras you repeat over and over in the mirror in the hope they will affect reality. "I am a happy and healthy size ten. I am a happy and healthy size ten. I am a happy and healthy size ten." Yet a year later, a size fourteen is still staring back at you, happy, healthy and just a little bit wobbly. It was the same with sex, except you didn't need to wait a few months to see if the mantra had worked its magic. Unfortunately, there was no denying that, some days, the more Chris touched me, the more intimate he became with me, the faster his desire appeared to shrink. Still he would continue to bump against my groin, fighting with his body the battle that could only be won in his mind.

"I'm just a bit hot," he would say, his words urgent and agitated. "Let me cool down a bit and then I can try again." Or, "I'm probably just tired today." Or, "Maybe that sore throat took more out of me than I thought." Or, "Maybe I ate too much dinner tonight." Or, "I haven't done enough exercise lately, that's what it is." Or, "I've done too much exercise lately, that's what it is." Or, "I just need to get my strength back."

He would look to me, anxious for reassurance, and I would wait by his side, trying to gulp down my emotions, trying to appear calm so that he wouldn't get even more upset. I wish I could say my thoughts in those moments were the thoughts of a mature woman who understood human psychology and, indeed, biology. But I am ashamed to admit that my thoughts were neither sanguine nor secure. What I was actually thinking was: 'I must be really bloody ugly, I must really, seriously turn men off.' Also, something about the whole experience made me want to cover myself up, to get my clothes back on as quickly as possible. Somehow, I didn't want him to see me; I was repulsive, I belonged under cover.

However, much sharper even than the lingering sense of shame were the fear and anguish that clutched at my throat as I realised I might never become a mother, not if we continued like this. Afterwards, even if I just turned over and tried to go to sleep, it would lead to a row.

"You're upset with me," Chris accused after our latest abandoned attempt at conception, this time on a Tuesday night in late summer.

He leaned over me, crowding my space.

"Sweetheart, don't be upset. It's silly. This is silly."

"Silly?"

"No, no. It was just the wrong choice of word. I don't mean you're silly, I mean it's silly to let this become a big thing."

I lay curled in a tight ball on the edge of the bed, resolutely facing away from him. "Okay."

"Sweetheart, why are you being like this? We can try again tomorrow. I'm probably just a bit tired from work tonight. Please don't be like this."

I sighed sadly. "I just really want to go to sleep."

"But you're angry with me. Look how far you've gone across the bed to get away from me. You don't even want to touch me."

"I'm not angry, you don't understand—"

"You mustn't say that! You mustn't say these things."

"Well, it's just hard sometimes. It's—"

"Honestly! How can you say that? I'm so much better now. I've made such great progress. I'm doing so well. We have a great love life, you know we do."

He never asked how I was. Why hadn't I noticed? He just rushed to tell me how I should feel, as if stage-managing the optimum response.

"Oh God, this is so pointless."

"Listen to you," he barked. "You're really angry. Why are you being like this? It's just one time, you said yourself it can happen to anyone."

I felt my fingernails digging into the flesh on my upper arms as I curled tighter into myself.

"It's not just one time, Chris. Even you must know that."

I inched further away, my bent knees now suspended beyond the edge of the mattress.

"That's a really cruel thing to say," Chris protested. "You're going to knock me back now. You know how well I'm doing with this. Why do you want to turn it into an issue?" He was propped up against the headboard, hands and legs fidgeting so that the mattress shifted and shook beneath me.

"I can't believe you would say these things," he continued. "You said a blip like this could happen to anyone. You said that and now you're going back on it."

"Well, maybe *anyone* who cared about their partner would get off their arse and do something about it."

Chris flung aside the duvet and leapt out of bed in a frenzied whirl. "That's a horrible thing to say. You're just being spiteful now. How can you tell me last week that I've made such great strides with this and now you tell me I'm useless?"

"I never said you're useless! And last week I was trying to encourage you."

His voice began jagging through the dark, from one end of the room to the other. "Well, why can't you encourage me now? What about when we were in Melbourne? You said I was the best lover you'd ever had. I thought that meant something. Now you're not even giving me credit for trying to do it."

It stung, hearing, after already seeing the evidence for myself, that I had become a woman who men had to make a supreme effort to love.

"Oh, so you're *trying* to bring yourself to make love to me."

"I didn't mean *trying*, I didn't mean it like that. I have made love to you, many times. I know we've only managed it once this month."

"Once."

"Well, it only takes one time to get pregnant. It's not like we haven't done it at all, you know I'm always there ready to try. You're making me feel hopeless now."

I retreated back into silence then and, the more I kept quiet, the more Chris talked, as if racing to fill a void or bail out a sinking boat. His words hammered away at my head until the hurt, because that's what it always started out as, gave way to frustration.

"You're being really unfair," he complained. "I'm not the enemy – I want you to become a mother more than anyone."

"Ha!"

"I do want you to become a mother, I want that for you more than anything. I've been with you every step of the way."

"No you haven't!"

"How can you say that? That's a dreadful thing to say. Why are you being so horrible? I don't deserve this."

"Forget this. Forget the fact that we can't have sex when we should, it's—"

"We do have sex! How can you say we don't have sex? Why are you always so critical? You're really upsetting me now—"

"I'm making *you* upset?"

"Yes. You should be supporting me, helping me with this. Why must you always make things so difficult?"

I unfurled from my defensive position in an explosion of limbs and surged upright in bed. "You bloody wanker!"

"How dare you speak to me like that?" Chris shouted back. "I don't deserve this!"

I wondered if the neighbours could hear, I wondered if they thought, like I did, 'Oh great, here we go again.' I wondered if they had also grown sick of hearing Chris proclaim what a wonderful love life we had.

Silence, again.

"Louise, don't go quiet. Louise? — Oh right. If this is the way you want to be."

I slumped back down into the sheets, sprawled on my stomach, and began to cry quietly into my pillow.

"I can't believe this," he said. "I can't believe you're doing this again."

"It's not going to happen." It was a muffled plea, almost to myself. "How can it ever happen?"

Chris's voice shot across the room like a punch. "I don't need this in my life, Louise, I really don't."

"Huh! You think anyone needs this in their life?"

"Right, well if this is what you think of me, then I'll pack my things and leave in the morning. I'll be gone before you get up."

I heard him collide with a chair as he barged his way out of the room. "Argh! Fucking hell. Honestly."

The script then ran like this: Chris paced up and down the flat, sighing dramatically and muttering, "For God's sake" or,

"Really!" loud enough for me to hear. At around 4am, he would launch himself back into bed, tossing, turning, banging his pillows against the mattress, getting up again, pacing some more, flopping back down and graphically making the point that he was *upset*.

Generally, I cried forlornly into my pillow and fretted that I would never be attractive to anyone, that the lack of sleep would throw my cycle off, that we were wasting another precious ovulation, that I might be getting too old to ever ovulate again, that I would never have a baby, that I would never be a mother.

How did I explain to someone who was too afraid to hear it that conception requires sex just before, during or after ovulation? And even then, even if you managed that and you were a mere twenty-four years old, you still had only a 25 per cent chance of conception per cycle. I was nearly thirty-eight; apparently my chances were less than 15 per cent, and dropping by the month. What were the odds of conception, I wondered, when you're two years off forty and you've had sex once, six days after ovulation? The answer did not bear thinking about.

I would get up the next day, feeling more hungover than I ever did when I drank alcohol, and, as futile as it seemed, I would go to acupuncture. I had to do something – anything – to improve our chances.

In early September, after four consecutive months of wasted ovulations, of opportunities that we watched sail past, the same argument played out again. It was only two nights since the last time; I couldn't be bothered to even repeat the lines that were always mine, in response to the lines that were always his. It boiled down to this:

Me: "If we ever want to be parents, we need to resolve this problem before it's too late."

Chris: "There is no problem."

I threw my pillow and sleeping bag down on the couch and left Chris pacing the hallway. I did not want to be in the same room as him, something of an understatement given that, the way I felt that night, there was nowhere I could have gone on this earth that would have been far enough away from him. There had been a subtle but disturbing change – I was increasingly finding that this issue wasn't just preventing us from connecting with each other, let alone trying to have a family, it was playing tricks with my mind. All the angst about sex, the way it now seemed contentious and unnatural, was increasingly dragging me back to a place I thought I had left behind. Infertility had stirred it up and this was further fuelling it, bringing into sharper focus the face of a predatory old man who I had done my best to erase for good. The familiar feelings of shame and fearful anxiety were back. Still in the background, but back, tormenting and unsettling me. Why wouldn't Chris do something – anything – to stop it?

The next day, I awoke in the grip of a raging black mood. What was the point? All this effort I was making to have a family – for what? Why did I even bother? It was a waste of fucking time.

Chris had gone out, continuing his pacing on a larger scale along the Thames, no doubt. I scragged back my hair, pulled on a t-shirt and sweatpants, ripped my debit card from my wallet, threw my handbag to the floor. I slammed the front door as I left, kicked the pavement with every step as I walked. Ten minutes later I was back, in possession of six cans of cider and two packets of cigarettes. The crack of the tab on the first can was the most satisfying sound I had heard in quite some time. I took several long, meaningful swigs, the only alcohol that had passed my lips in four years. At least I actually liked cider. Cigarettes, not so much. Still, I opened a packet, flinging the plastic wrapping to the floor, and immediately lit up. I took a deep drag, enjoying the foul taste and the sharp sensation in my throat and lungs. I was glad that it hurt. Everything else hurt didn't it?

I finished the can of cider and took pleasure in squashing it under my foot, leaving the dregs to dribble out on the carpet. Who cares? Who cares about anything? Another cigarette, another pile of ash flicked into the remains of the plastic wrapping on the floor.

I was halfway through the second can when I heard the door open. Right, I thought. Maybe now he'll realise how devoid of hope I feel.

Chris walked into the lounge and looked at me as if I was a house-breaker who had just painted a mural on his wall using the medium of dog poo. Angry didn't cover it.

"What are you doing?"

"What does it look like?"

"For goodness' sake, you don't even smoke. And you don't drink anymore either."

"Well, I do now. Sure as hell can't see any reason not to."

He tutted loudly. "Look what you're doing to my couch. Really!"

"Your couch," I exclaimed. "Your couch?"

"Ach! You've splashed it with alcohol. Honestly —"

"Stuff your couch. What about what you're doing to me?"

I leapt up, spilling more cider as I went. "Your girlfriend is falling to bits in front of you and you're worried about your bloody couch. That is so typical!"

A minute earlier, I had barely mustered the motivation to lift a half-empty can to my lips; now I was overcome by a fury so forceful that I could not control the energy that pumped and surged in its wake.

I stormed to the kitchen. "It was one fucking *tiny* drop of cider. It was nothing. Nothing!"

I grabbed a wine bottle from the box of empties by the door, lifted it above my head and hurled it against the far wall. The glass was still shattering when I picked up the next and flung it even harder in the same direction.

"Stop!" Chris shouted from somewhere behind me. "You'll hurt yourself."

"Oh, *now* you're worried that I'll get hurt." A third bottle went flying. "Well, you should have thought of that a bit earlier."

Shards of glass piled up on the floor, some skidding towards me, others bouncing off the walls and cupboard doors. A glass missile hit a terracotta bowl, instantly cracking it from end to end.

"You're going to get glass in your eye!"

"I don't fucking care!" Crash. Another bottle landed in a crescendo under the kitchen window. "Go check on your couch. That's the only damn thing you're worried about."

Chris lunged towards me.

"Don't touch me! I don't want you anywhere near me." Smash. Smash. Smash. Smash.

After nine bottles, I ran out of ammunition. I kicked a pile of glass with my bare foot.

"Don't! Don't do that. What is wrong with you?"

"What the hell do you think might be wrong with me? You still don't get it. Of course you don't. Just go to work and get away from me."

Chris tutted angrily again, picked up his bag, walked out, slammed the door and ran down the stairs.

I heard him open the front door to the building. Then, to my almost instant shame and embarrassment, I heard a voice, from somewhere just below what I now realised was our open kitchen window.

"All right Chris?"

"Good thanks Norm."

"Off to work?"

"Yes, off to work I'm afraid. See you Norm."

Why had I forgotten that our landlord was painting the front of the house? That his ladder was leaning against our kitchen wall? The realisation jolted me out of whatever mania had taken hold.

Still shaking, I surveyed the carnage that spread from one end of the kitchen to the other. Who was this mad woman who threw wine bottles and swore at people? She was nothing like anyone I knew. Chastened, I began to sweep up the glass, belatedly quiet, in case Norm could hear. Maybe infertility was having more of an effect on me than I thought. Another understatement. Infertility was shredding me, from the inside out, leaving a pile of damaged parts of myself that I didn't recognise. I was just beginning to realise, to fully understand, that, whatever the outcome, a markedly different person was going to emerge at the end of this struggle to have a family. And I wasn't entirely sure it was going to be someone I could like. I wrapped up the broken glass and picked out of the carpet the tiny shards that had ricocheted into the hallway. It was okay; tomorrow I would go to acupuncture.

I turned up for my lunchtime treatment session with Maggie before starting work the next afternoon. She focused on my lower back, the warmth generated by the burning herbs seeping through me, drawing me off. Even my bones felt exhausted; I just wanted to sleep for a month.

We didn't speak much. Maggie knew, with no need of an explanation, how drained I was. Later she asked gently, "So, how are things this week, with Chris?"

"The same."

"Oh, I'm sorry to hear that," she said. "You've been very, very low lately, I know. I've been rather worried about you." She paused. "You know, if you ever want to have a cup of tea before work, anything, I'm always here."

I smiled my thanks. "It's happened for the last four months."

She instantly understood what I meant, even though it was some time since I'd felt able to mention it. "Would he speak to anyone about it, do you think?"

"I don't know. He went to the doctor once, when we first got together. But now he says everything's fine."

I sighed, confused. Maybe it *was* me, maybe I really was the one who made problems out of nothing.

Maggie was speaking again. "How long have you been together? I don't think I've ever asked you."

"Nearly five years."

"So this has been an issue that long?"

"Yep."

She gave a sympathetic murmur. "Just a thought really, but I was wondering whether speaking to one of my male colleagues might help. They're used to working with men on these types of issues, and acupuncture can sometimes be very useful."

I felt myself rally, buoyed by Maggie's concern. "That sounds a good idea. I might get up the courage to mention it. He's a bit funny about sperm tests, too, so anything, really, that could help …"

"I was going to check whether he'd had his test yet," Maggie said.

I shook my head.

"No. He finds it too embarrassing. You know, providing a sample to order. It stresses him out."

"Well, he should count himself lucky he's never had an internal scan," Maggie said with a laugh.

"Tell me about it. At least no one has to even see his bits."

After we'd finished giggling, Maggie spoke again.

"I think," she said quietly, "that it might be time he got himself together."

※ ※ ※

I opened the door to our flat and was greeted by the sound of water being vigorously splashed onto the sides of the bath. A whistled tune that sounded like it wanted to be a Beatles song carried up the hallway.

"Chris? Is that you?"

He emerged from the bathroom, wearing only a pair of swimming shorts, cleaning cloth in one hand and bottle of disinfectant in the other.

"What *are* you doing?"

"I'm cleaning the bathroom. I had so much energy left after I finished work that I thought I'd do it."

"But it's midnight. And you never clean the bathroom. Do you even know what to do?"

"Of course I know what to do. I'm not completely useless you know. Come and look."

It appeared a typhoon had struck our bathroom; there was water on every surface, including the floor, which was littered with every beauty product we owned, and a waterfall of bubbles was cascading from the empty medicine cabinet.

"It's amazing," said Chris. "I can't describe it. I feel like a completely new person, I really do."

Acupuncture, it seemed, had caused him to become hyperactive. That day, he had been for only his second appointment with Maggie's colleague Justin.

"He says I respond to it incredibly quickly, my system is really responsive. It's unbelievable that it can have such an impact," Chris enthused. "I can't tell you how different I feel, it's like a burst of energy, almost electrical."

"Well, I don't know what Justin's done to you, but if he can get you to clean the bathroom now and then, it's worth the money."

"He said my pulse picked up so quickly. Some people take much longer to respond, but my body has really taken to it."

"Did he burn the herby things?"

"It was like an electrical current, that's the only way I can describe it. I can't tell you how energised I feel. It's great that you can fix something just like that. Justin says …"

When I could get a word in, I asked how often he would be going for treatment.

"Justin says it won't take long. You know, since I've responded like this. So I'll probably just go once a month soon. Keep it topped up. It's great to know I've reacted to it so well."

I felt like acupuncture was only just managing to hold me together; on some days the sheer effort of ordinary life threatened to overwhelm me. How had Chris been transformed so instantly? He was a hot, bustling, talkative advert for yang energy. Meanwhile, me and my cold yin energy continued to shiver silently in the dark. He hadn't seemed to notice.

"I mean, it's fantastic. To know that I can have such a simple treatment and it can all be behind me, I can be completely changed. Transformed! I can't remember when I last had this much energy."

"Well, it's not like you ever sit still at the best of times," I said.

"Yes, I know. But this is different. Justin says …"

Luckily, the powers of acupuncture extended beyond domestic chores and all the way into the bedroom. Chris was suddenly Casanova himself, albeit restricted to one woman only. He instantly took it upon himself to become the Ovulation Monitor.

"What day is it? Are we up to day twelve yet? Shouldn't I be doing my duty today?"

"We did it yesterday. It's fine, really. Have a rest 'til tomorrow."

"No, I think we should do it today. Of course, if it's okay with you?"

And before I knew it, I was swept off my feet and Chris was strutting around afterwards like a barnyard rooster. Maybe this month, I thought. Maybe this month, I'll finally get pregnant. How could you have this much sex and not get pregnant?

For a month or two, Chris, now undergoing regular treatment with Justin, was almost evangelical about acupuncture, to the point of suggesting that perhaps he could retrain as an acupuncturist and use his new-found energy to help heal other people.

And then. With prolonged infertility, it seems there is always the 'and then'. It happened again. Chris, buoyed up by his recent transformation, had steered me to the bedroom, not because I was ovulating but because he wanted to. Somehow, for some reason, he faltered. Instantly, he became overheated, clammy, and the panicked look returned to his eyes. We ended up lying side by side, unsure of the right thing to say.

"It's like a demon," Chris said quietly. "That gets into my head."

Acupuncture, the magic bullet, had failed to fire and his confidence had leached away.

Later that day, I found him sitting on the floor in the spare room, his head in his hands. He looked over at me sadly as I sat down beside him. "I'm no use to you, am I? No use at all."

"That's not true. You know I don't think like that."

"I'm sorry," he said. "I really thought I'd cured it this time."

I sensed Chris had finally stopped battling; something had changed, something had punctured the ferocious denial that prevented him admitting the existence of the problem. Sitting on the floor in the spare room, we talked like two people who were not in the habit of flinging insults and accusations back and forth a couple of times a week.

"I thought acupuncture was the answer," he said. "I thought that voice was gone forever, you know that voice that gets in your head and says, 'You can't do this. You're going to fail.' I thought I'd shut him up once and for all."

"I'm sorry. I do understand, you know. I might not be a man with equipment that has to do its thing, but everyone's scared of something. I get it."

Chris shook his head, fingers pressed tightly against his temples. "But I'm not scared of being with you. How could I be? Please don't think that. I'm just scared of failing. And once the thought gets in there, I can't stop it, it takes me over."

I reached over and stroked his arm. "I know."

"If I could just stop the doubt getting in there."

I nodded. "It's horrible isn't it? I get that every time I hop on a tube train. I think, 'This time I'll stay on it when we get to the tunnels.' But I never do. Last station before it goes underground and I'm straight out the door. So much for being vaguely normal."

He managed a smile. "I'm glad you're not angry with me."

"I've never been angry about the fear thing," I said. "Look at everything I'm scared of – tubes, planes, elevators. I can hardly blame you for being afraid of something."

"But sometimes you get so upset."

I scrabbled around for a way to explain myself without making it worse. "It's only because I want us to find a way to deal with this, or at least try to. I know you can't help the issue … it's just your attitude to it."

Chris heard the catch in my voice and reached for my hand. "I know. I don't mean to get the way I do, it's just a defensive thing. I know it doesn't help."

I felt the familiar heat radiating from his fingers as they tightened around mine. "I don't mean to be the way I am either. I know I shouldn't take it personally."

"It's never been about you," he said. "Genuinely, I couldn't stand it if you thought that."

We hugged and smiled apologetically at each other before I kissed the side of his face and hauled myself up from the floor.

"Wait here a minute."

I scurried downstairs to the kitchen and returned with two mugs of tea and a plate of chocolate biscuits. I didn't want Chris to move from that spot on the spare room floor; it had taken nearly five years to have this discussion and I didn't want anything, even a minor change of scene, to suddenly bring it to a halt.

"Well," I began as I sat back down, "it's conception sex, isn't it? It always causes problems you know."

"Huh. Yes …"

"It's true though, isn't it? How is it supposed to be spontaneous? Let alone fun. I bet most people find it gets a bit old after the first year or two."

"So it's not just me then?" Chris sounded hopeful.

"No way. It's me as well sometimes, if you must know. Honestly, there are days I'd prefer a massive bag of crisps and a bottle of wine."

"Well thank you very much. You're too flattering."

We joked about it for a while then Chris suddenly became preoccupied once more. "You know," he said sadly. "I really don't understand it, why I would suddenly fail."

"Mmm." I tilted my mug to my lips, even though I knew it was now empty; I wanted to slow down my thoughts, ensure I said the right thing.

"I don't know that it helps," I said after a time, "to keep calling it a 'failure'. It's lovemaking, not a university exam."

He gave a wry smile.

"I know it's different for you," I ploughed on. "The thing I don't get is why, if you know this might be an issue, you wouldn't have a Plan B. Viagra, hypnosis, anything at all really so you're not going to stress right out if Plan A doesn't work. Plenty of men need a bit of help now and then – it doesn't have to be a big deal."

I gently squeezed his hand, once, twice, an old signal of ours. "It wouldn't take much, you know, to make it a lot easier for yourself."

Chris scooped up the last chocolate biscuit, broke it in two and offered me half. "You see," he said. "This is why I love you.

No one else could talk to me about it like this. You make it seem so doable, so logical. It's like you put it into perspective for me."

He thought for a moment. "You're right, of course. I should have a Plan B. I don't know why I haven't done that, but I will. I should have done it much earlier. I'm sorry."

"It's okay," I said. "I know planning's not your strong point. This is exactly why our kids are not going to boarding school when they're seven years old. They're going to stay at home and learn to think for themselves."

Chris chuckled. "Don't worry. No child of mine is leaving home at seven."

I waddled across the floor on my knees, pulled the duvet off the bed and tucked one half of it underneath us, leaving the other half draped over our legs. We talked on until we were shrouded in darkness, cocooned in the loft where the orange glow of the streetlights outside could not reach us. Now that we had found a way into this discussion, neither of us seemed able to leave it, almost as if we were afraid that it would be like exiting a maze and never finding your way back to the central point within. It didn't occur to me, in that intimate moment, that a shock could still be discovered, further along the maze.

"Maybe," I offered eventually, "you need to think about what was going on when it first happened. Was it just that you'd lost your confidence after your divorce, do you think?"

Chris considered the question for some time. "It was a bit earlier than that," he finally admitted.

"Oh. How do you mean?"

"Well, there was something. At the Stag's Head."

"That pub you showed me – in Oxford?"

He confirmed it with a murmur. "The women used to stand around the bar laughing about the men they'd slept with, making fun of anything they got wrong."

"I know, you told me. That was rank!"

"Well, I got involved with one of them."

I groaned, a little louder than I meant to. "Sort of," he added quickly. "Only sort of. She already had a boyfriend."

Chris had now become a shadowy figure in the darkness. I couldn't see his face. It was just our voices, murmuring back and forth. He finally confided that he and the woman from the pub had ended up together in a pool shed one summer night, but things had not progressed as expected; he had lost his nerve at the crucial moment.

"And were you worried she'd tell everyone at the pub, was that it?"

"That was part of it, but I thought since she had a boyfriend that was a reasonable excuse not to go through with it." He hesitated. "No, I don't think she did tell anyone. Actually, she wanted to see me again – she kept saying we had unfinished business."

"Huh. And did you finish the business?"

There was silence in the loft. I heard a tube train rattle by at the end of the garden as I waited for Chris to continue.

"No," he said at last. There was another long pause. "The truth is, I didn't try again for years." His voice dropped to a hoarse whisper. "I was afraid I'd fail again."

"Oh! You mean you gave up on it?"

"Yes."

"Completely avoided it?"

"Fraid so."

"How many years? You know, until …?"

"Too many. Far too many." He sighed deeply. "Think double figures."

"How awful," I blurted out. "No wonder it built up into such a big thing in your head."

An old familiar stab of unease made itself known in my chest and I instinctively reached for safer ground.

"That's exactly why you're supposed to get straight back on a horse if you fall off. Leave it for too long and you'll never get on again."

"Of course," Chris replied, his voice gaining strength. "That's what they say, isn't it?" He gave a rueful laugh. "Damn, I wish I'd got straight back on that wretched horse."

I forced myself to keep things light. "I don't suppose this is the right time to make a joke about riding?"

We laughed in tandem. "Thank you," he said quietly, "for being so supportive. It means a lot."

We sat there in silence once more, Chris's arm around me while I rested my head on his shoulder. Eventually, trying to sound casual, I asked the unsettling question that had begun marching in relentless circles around my mind.

"By the way," I said, "how old were you? You know, with that woman in the pool shed."

"Hmm," he mumbled. "We were both twenty-one, twenty-two, something around there."

Tension twisted and surged, tightening its grip. I had to know, but I didn't want to know. "So. Um … and … it's happened on and off ever since then?"

I sensed rather than saw that he was nodding his head in the darkness.

"But it stops here. I've got a lot to think about, a lot to do to resolve this, I know that."

I worked it out. This issue that had been plaguing both our relationship and our attempts to become parents had been in existence since I was seven years old. It had existed nearly my whole lifetime. I had believed it was a much more recent thing. Maybe, I had thought, I was responsible for it, maybe I was not mature enough in my response to it, maybe I had not been supportive enough, maybe I was not attractive enough, maybe the information I passed on about trying to conceive had put too much pressure on him, maybe …

I realised, for the first time, what I was dealing with. And I wasn't sure whether to hope that it could be resolved or to fear that, after thirty years, it never would be. I couldn't understand it. How could you let something that affected a relationship so deeply go on for so long? How could you, in all of the years between your twenties and forties, fail to come up with a Plan B, another option to take the pressure off?

If you had peered into the loft that day and observed us, nestled together under the duvet on the floor, you would have assumed a certain level of closeness and contentment between us. What no one would have seen, and what Chris didn't realise, was that I was now thrown into turmoil, caught between denying and acknowledging that old jolt of emotion, that instinct that whispered, 'This isn't right.'

There had been two lies, then, at the start of our relation-ship. One about Chris's age and the other about this issue. "Just since my divorce," he had said. "Just the last couple of years." And it had taken months of stonewalling to even have that discussion.

Perhaps I would have paid more attention to these realisations. Perhaps I wouldn't have been quite so keen to play them down. Who knows what I would have done if I wasn't thirty-eight years old and already worried that it was too late for me to have a family. But if I listened to that instinct, if I gave up on this relationship and the lies it had been built on, could I ever be a mother? It wasn't as if Chris would be a dreadful father; he'd be loving and kind with his children, I knew that much. And sex didn't matter, really, once you became parents, did it? Wouldn't I be too tired to care about it anyway?

It was like negotiations for a corporate takeover happening inside my head; what would I concede? What trade-offs could I accept? At the time, I was not even aware I was doing it.

The drive to conceive had begun to consume anything that made sense. Infertility 1, Rational Thought 0. Or maybe it was Performance Anxiety 1, Infertility 0. I was too caught up in it all to even know.

Sixteen

"Have you signed Adam's card?"

I looked up from my computer screen at work. "No, not yet. I don't think I've seen it."

Our office manager leaned over my desk. "Right," she whispered conspiratorially. "Well, Rusty's got it at the moment. You'd better get in straight after him. The presentation's in twenty minutes."

It was the seventh 'Congratulations on your new arrival' card that I had signed in the past three weeks. We were just one department of forty people within a much larger organisation and yet seven of my male colleagues – seven – had produced babies at around the same time. How did people do it? How did they have these perfectly choreographed lives where they left school, went to university, got a job, got married, bought a house, had a baby (and then another approximately two years later, followed by perhaps a third or fourth, depending on their preferences for family size)? It was the path all seven of these men had followed. Now they were in their early to mid-thirties, they had their mortgages ticking along and, bam, right on schedule, out popped a baby. I might have coped more philosophically with one or two at a time, but seven? Surely the fertility Gods were playing some sort of cruel game. "Don't drink that!" people used to joke as their workmates filled plastic cups at the office water cooler, "there must be something in it."

'No, there's bloody well not,' I would think to myself. 'I can assure you of that.'

I was grateful for one small mercy, though – since my colleagues were nearly all men it meant that, while they might be reproducing at Olympian rates, at least I couldn't see the evidence of it. At least I was not surrounded by pregnant stomachs, at least I didn't have to listen to conversations about stretch marks, morning sickness and what was the best buggy to buy. And men didn't tend to enquire about whether I thought it would be 'my turn' soon. Even so, it was getting increasingly draining to be constantly confronted with the evidence that, for most people, conception was just another simple tick on a list of life achievements. I couldn't seem to get any of it right. First of all, I'd gone and got divorced and now I couldn't have children. I was operating outside the guidelines.

I prepared to leave work that night weighed down by the gnawing fear that I would never receive one of those cards congratulating me on my fertility. It had been nearly four years, double the amount of time I had allowed for in my worst case scenario. Clearly, I knew nothing about this at all.

"What's up Louise? Can't be that bad, can it?"

On the other side of the room, the office manager was counting off on her fingers the names of all our new fathers. "First, it was Tim, then Jeff, then Richard, Will, Mike …"

I looked up, my despairing thoughts interrupted, and saw that it was my colleague Jonathan who had enquired about my wellbeing. "You look miserable," he stated bluntly but accurately.

"Oh," I said, my mind racing through the options as I sought an acceptable explanation. "It's nothing. Just my back. Too many sports injuries. You know, it seizes up now and then."

"You need my osteopath," he replied, swigging from one of the beer cans that were sometimes handed around late at night. "He's the best you can get, I've never seen anything like it."

"Really? How do you mean?"

He swivelled round in his chair. "The mother-in-law put us on to him. He's a bit of a baby whisperer."

"He's what?"

"It was when we'd first had Ruby, we knew she wasn't quite right. In herself, I mean, so Vicky's mum thought we should take her to see him. She kept going on about his amazing reputation for treating babies. What do you call it?"

He paused to search for the right term. "Cranial osteopathy, that's it. Really gentle. He also treats horses," Jonathan added. I brightened at the unexpected mention of the animals I had spent my childhood with. "He can deduce for himself what's wrong with you – you don't need to tell him. That's why he's so good with the horses and babies."

"Really? Did it work, whatever he did?"

"Yeah, definitely. Ruby was like a different baby afterwards. But the really interesting thing was Vicky. She'd been feeling off-colour since the birth, but, you know, we thought that was to be expected. He picked up on it, though, without anyone saying anything."

Jonathan described how the osteopath had suggested his wife also might be in need of treatment. "She lay down on the table, he felt her stomach and instantly told us that the placenta hadn't been fully delivered. To be honest, I thought 'Oh yeah' but he did some work on her – and the next day, sure enough, the rest of the placenta came out."

"Wow."

"I know. Vicky said the heat coming out of his hands was like nothing you've ever felt. Anyway, he's the man you need for your back. Only trouble is, he's in the midlands."

"Oh well, I wouldn't mind that. I've not been up there for years."

"You don't know what you're missing." He laughed. "Hang on, I'll Google him. Did I mention he's French?"

"He's sounding better and better," I joked.

"Not you as well. You should have seen Vicky's mum with him." He shook his head. "Not what you want to see from your mother-in-law. The poor guy's only in his thirties."

I travelled home with the French osteopath's details in my bag, Jonathan having scribbled them on the back of a memo about the state of the office kitchen. I might not have been miserable about my back, that was true. However, the reason it had sprung to mind so quickly when I needed an excuse for my pained expression was that it was almost constantly uncomfortable. Thanks to all the sport I had played, my spine, from base to skull, had been battered throughout my life in a range of imaginatively excruciating ways. I had sometimes wondered, when grasping for solutions to my childless state, whether it could possibly have any bearing on my fertility problems.

Now, at last, this seemed like a piece of synchronicity. Information that I needed, that might help me get back on track, had been randomly volunteered at a time when I least expected it. Could this be it? Maybe it could be. Hope sprung anew. *This* would be the key. This would be the vital piece of information that led to me getting pregnant!

At home, I told Chris the story of Jonathan's baby and the late delivery of part of the placenta.

"He's French," I added. "I can't pronounce his last name. How am I going to ring up and make an appointment when I don't know how to say his name?"

"Is there anything you don't worry about?" Chris laughed as he studied my piece of paper. "I see the boys are still refusing to clean up after themselves."

"Huh?"

"Your kitchen. Who's the culprit then?" He turned the memo over. "Oh!" he exclaimed, reading the details from Jonathan. "Samuel."

"Yes, that's right. At least I know how to pronounce his first name."

"Yes, but remember what Sebastian said?" Chris gazed at me intently. I drew a blank, a fact that was obviously reflected in my expression. "Sebastian? The psychic? In Brighton?"

"Yep," I said. "Course I remember him. It was only January, wasn't it? Yes, January."

"But you haven't remembered what he said." Chris paused as if waiting for me to catch up with his thoughts. "He said that you would have a little boy …"

"Hmph."

"… and that someone called Sam would help you. A male Sam remember?"

"Ah." The point he was making finally dawned on me. "I thought he meant Samantha, but he said no, it was a man."

"It's a sign," Chris said contentedly. "I know it. You've got to say, it's an amazing synchronicity."

"Huh, that's funny. I was just thinking about that word on the way home."

"There you are then," said Chris. "You've got to see him." He hugged me tightly. "I've got a good feeling about this."

⁂ ⁂ ⁂

I observed my torso in a mirror that hung on the wall a few feet away. My upper arms looked like someone had taken a vat of semolina and sculpted it into a matching pair of turkey drumsticks. This was how I still viewed my body: something to be critiqued and, in the case of my upper arms – always too large for the rest of me, even when I was slim – covered up and hidden away from polite society.

"Do you see?" Samuel asked, standing behind me and critiquing my mirror image in a far more helpful way. "Your right shoulder is several inches lower than your left. It is no wonder you are experiencing these problems."

Despite the many moments I had spent damning bits of my body while studying it in the mirror, I genuinely hadn't noticed. However, once he pointed it out, I realised my entire torso was lopsided.

I had taken Samuel through a lengthy list of all the injuries I could remember suffering. There was the cricket ball that had slammed into the base of my skull after being thrown with full force from only a few metres away. That had required several months in a neck-brace. Now it felt like a heavily-weighted brick was permanently sitting near the point of impact on the right side of my neck. There were myriad falls from horses, including being knocked unconscious three times in three months as a teenager. There was the time I narrowly escaped paralysis after being catapulted into the air when a horse had bolted with me, aged eleven. Later, I had also landed on a table-top fence that I was supposed to be jumping, shoulder and hip slamming helpfully against a ten-inch slab of wood. Then there was touch rugby, another concussion, another tumble flat on my back …

Samuel took all this in his stride; he was used to treating not only top racehorses and showjumpers but their riders too. He had no doubt heard worse.

Before I lay down on the treatment table, Samuel had me stand in front of the mirror while he instructed me to turn my head to the left, then the right, to lean forwards towards the floor and to slide my hands as far as possible down each side. On the right side, in particular, I barely moved.

When the treatment began, he started with my neck, cupping the base of my skull in his hands and gently rocking from side to side.

"I wouldn't say this is the worst neck I have ever seen," he announced. "But it comes very close."

The warmth generated by his hands was indeed astonishing; it was like having a pain-relieving heat pack placed at the site of an injury. If you could somehow package it up and market it as a product for crocks like myself, it would be an instant sell-out. I could already feel that the combination of the warmth and the slow, soothing, manipulation was encouraging my neck to unlock from the rigid position it had possibly maintained for as long as twenty years. After working on it in this way, Samuel then asked me to relax and deeply inhale. In one rapid movement, he deftly rotated my head to one side. I heard, and felt, a loud click. It was the sound that heralded the departure of the constant heaviness at the base of my neck; it had been there for so long I had half-forgotten it wasn't normal. Here was something that felt like progress.

Having spent two hours travelling to the appointment, I decided it was no time to be coy about my main reason for coming. It wasn't the pain caused by my catalogue of old injuries, it was the question of whether they were now affecting my chances of conception. I explained that we had been trying to start a family for nearly four years. I was getting used to telling people this now, saying it out loud and managing to look composed when, most of the time, the very words made me want to cry with either sorrow or frustration.

Today, however, it was worth the temporary struggle to keep my emotions under control. Samuel's response was enlightening and encouraging. "People often overlook these issues when they have fertility problems," he said. "But issues with the back and spine can affect your entire system. To begin with, just think how many nerves are running through the spinal cord."

Then he said something that really got my attention.

"I have known patients who believed they could not become pregnant. They might try for as long as eleven years to have a family then they might come for treatment for, perhaps, a frozen shoulder. Two months later, they will come back and say, 'Samuel, I'm pregnant! I can't believe it.' I always say, 'I *can* believe it, I have seen this happen before.'"

Samuel pinpointed at least two issues that could have a subtle, but powerful, bearing on my fertility. I was aware of one of them, but hadn't even noticed the other. "Your right hip is twisted and immobile," he explained. "This is affecting the position of your womb and also blood flow to the area. This part of your spine has fused but, at the top of your back, where you have another injury, your spine has become too mobile."

He applied light pressure to one of the vertebrae between my shoulder blades. "How long ago did this injury happen?"

I was perplexed. "I don't think I've ever hurt that part of my back."

He gave a knowing look. "There has been a definite trauma here," he said. "Do you find it difficult to take a deep breath? Does it feel as if you struggle to completely fill your lungs?"

"Yes," I replied, surprised that he would know this. "I often feel as if I can't quite get my breath all the way in. It's a weird sensation."

He nodded. "There is a blockage here that is affecting your breathing. You will notice the difference after treatment, your breathing will be much improved. It is important for fertility, and for your health in general of course, that oxygen is able to flow freely. We do not want you taking only shallow breaths."

Samuel was gently kneading and manipulating the point between my shoulder blades when I suddenly remembered something.

"Oh!" He stopped what he was doing and gazed at me. "I'd forgotten. I fell down some stairs in Oxford Street. When I landed, my upper back crashed against the edge of a step. It hurt like hell."

"I can tell this," he said with a smile. "You see, this is why I like working with horses. They do not say, 'No Samuel, I have not been hurt there.' I just treat them. It's simple. With humans, they will be adamant. 'No, you are wrong. I have never hurt my neck.' Then a month later, they will come back and say, 'Oh, I forgot about the whiplash in the car accident.'"

We both laughed.

Samuel moved on to my lower back, fused in its intractable and uncomfortable position. Again, he gently manipulated it before applying deep pressure to an area near my right hip. I could feel ripples of energy emanating down my legs and up to my shoulders as the tension slowly ebbed away. Later, he 'crunched' both ends of my back, moving around the treatment table and using his body weight to apply pressure as he worked to straighten the kinks in my crooked spine.

"Tomorrow you will feel as if you have been hit by a truck," he said, sounding more matter-of-fact about it than I felt. "But it is better for you that we do this all at once. I do not like you to have to keep coming back for treatment when I know I am able to relieve your symptoms in one session."

When I finally stood up again, we repeated the exercises in the mirror. Before treatment, I had barely been able to force my hands beyond my knees when I bent forward. Now my fingertips were almost touching the floor. I felt free to make fluid movements in any direction I wanted. This was what normality felt like. How could I have forgotten? I wondered if this might be precisely my thought if I was ever blessed with children. Would there come a day when life itself flowed freely again? When I wondered what all the fuss had ever been about?

"Look," said Samuel, studying his work in the mirror. "Your shoulders are even. See here. And your hips, they are back in balance."

"Wow," I said, moving my head from side to side in amazement. "I can actually see over my right shoulder."

He smiled. "You might not thank me for it tomorrow, but in a couple of days you should be aware of some major improvements."

He was right. It was suddenly as easy as it should be to breathe properly and gone as if they never existed were the dull, heavy backache and sharp, searing headaches that had bothered me for years. It was as if someone had turned back time; it felt like a body that was creaking towards forty had been replaced with the fluidly functioning body of my twenties. In short, joy to the world.

When I got home that night, aching all over and ready for a gentle lie-down, Chris studied me intently.

"You look taller," he exclaimed.

"I know. Isn't it amazing?"

The price of this life-changing transformation was £30. I thought ruefully of the Harley Street acupuncture guru who had charged £200 for a consultation that achieved precisely nothing in practical terms. I could have had six-and-a-half treatment sessions with Samuel for that amount. But that was the thing: I didn't need another six sessions. "I don't want my patients paying for extra sessions that they don't need," he said. "You will be fine. Just come back for a top-up if you ever experience any problems."

It says everything that I have consulted many experts during my time in the Ten-Year Club but, of them all, Samuel is the one who I still see. I suspect he has a gift for healing that extends beyond the abilities of a skilled osteopath. A year after that first appointment, I returned for treatment, having wrenched my back playing tennis. We were discussing fertility again, along with my ever-growing list of concerns about what could be wrong. Samuel placed his hands on my stomach.

"There is nothing to worry about here," he said. "You have one small fibroid, on the left, but it is out of the way, it is not in a position that would cause any concern."

I just smiled, unsure what to make of the information he'd imparted in such a natural, low-key way. No matter how hard I probed my stomach, there were no lumps or bumps to be felt externally. And Samuel had placed his hands there only lightly. However, not too far in the future, I would be astonished to receive a scan report that echoed him almost word for word. Having already benefited so greatly from his abilities, I shouldn't have been surprised.

Sometimes infertility does you a favour after all. Sometimes it leads you to people you'd never otherwise have found. Samuel's human patients range from new-born babies to pensioners in their nineties; his animal patients include many breeds of horses, dogs, cattle and even rabbits and a few sheep. He doesn't trumpet his skills in glossy magazines or national newspapers. He doesn't need to; thanks to word of mouth, that oldest form of advertising, he is booked out two months in advance. Finding him was even worth signing seven 'Congratulations on your new baby' cards. Which was just as well because a month later, there was an eighth.

"Graham," our office manager announced excitedly. "Twins! There's definitely something in the water round here."

SEVENTEEN

By OCTOBER 2006, THE fourth anniversary was looming. Four years since we had started 'trying without trying' for a family. We had knocked on many different doors, considered many different approaches to conception, but still we had not worked out how to become parents. It was time for a big decision. After three years and ten months, we had had enough. There was only one thing for it … we would move to Switzerland.

As I write this, I get visions of my mother slowly shaking her head and sighing, "Not an ounce of common sense between them." I imagine it would appear that way to many people. Indeed, if we had been in full possession of the facts, the move to Switzerland would have been written off as the poorly-timed, madcap idea that it probably was. Like sensible people who knew what they were doing, we would have stayed in London, waiting to begin the one free round of IVF for which I could still qualify until the age of thirty-nine. If we had been sensible people who knew what they were doing, we would have joined the NHS waiting list the previous year, after our visits to the doctors. Unfortunately, our GPs had neglected to pass on this crucial information – perhaps they were on a mini cost-cutting drive – and we made the fatal mistake of assuming they had told us everything we needed to know. "It will be expensive," they said, "and you are not guaranteed success at the end of it."

I had long ago worked it out: at a stretch, we might be able to use our credit cards to fund one round of fertility treatment. But there was no money – or rather, no credit available – for a second attempt. If our one attempt failed, then we had failed for good. Given my body's lifelong rejection of anything that resembled prescription medication, I couldn't believe that pumping it full of fertility drugs would be of any use to us now. And, of course, there was still the question as to whether I could actually go through with it, whether I could cope with being in such a vulnerable position after the assault I had experienced as a child.

It was no surprise that, through the gloom, Switzerland – the place we had each dreamed of living one day – soon emerged as the brightest option. And there was a certain degree of method lurking within our madness. There had been a lot of talk about our lifestyle since we had sought help for our fertility problem. Everyone, from our spectacularly unhelpful GPs onwards, agreed that there was too much stress in our lives, not enough sleep, not enough regular meals; even the days we worked were not set, but moved haphazardly from one week to the next, depending on the demands of a seven-day rota. In the fortnight before we left for Switzerland, I had eaten dinner at home only once. On the other thirteen nights, I either ate a sandwich at my desk about 9pm or filled up on toast after midnight. At 2am, my body would still be coursing with adrenaline. I didn't really blame it for not managing to fall pregnant. Lifestyle, I thought. That's the answer. It's obvious.

Here is another embarrassing admission to add to the pile: I genuinely believed that, once we moved to rural Switzerland, I would fall pregnant. There would be fresh air, healthy food, earlier nights and, well, who could fail to fall pregnant in such a place? There would be a certain symmetry to it, this return to the simple country lifestyle I had thrived on as a child. It seemed natural that this would be the setting for my own entry to family life.

Furthermore, there was another potent factor making its presence felt; we had spent too long focusing on what we *didn't* have. This constant pursuit of something that continually eluded us had placed us on the fastest route to unhappiness. We both knew it was time to flip it on its head. It was time to take advantage of the things we *could* do precisely because we didn't have children. So we had flown to Geneva, viewed only one house to rent in the surrounding countryside and signed up on the spot. The plan was that we would commute back to the UK for work – after all, the flight was only one hour thirty minutes; on bad days it could take that long just to get from one side of London to the other.

Back at home on the night we had signed up for our new life, Chris sat me down on the sofa, looked straight into my eyes and said: "Lou, are you absolutely sure you're okay about the flying?"

"Yes," I confirmed. "I'll do it."

"You're sure you can do it four times a month? That's all that's worrying me. I don't want you getting yourself into a state about it. It's not good for you."

"I'll do it," I repeated. "It'll be fine."

"Well, if you're absolutely sure. It's just that, on the plane today … I know I mentioned this on the train earlier and I don't want to go on about it, I honestly don't, but you couldn't speak. You didn't reply to anything I said all the way from Geneva to Gatwick."

"Oh, were you talking? I didn't notice." I laughed to let him know I was joking. "I know I was quiet. But at least I wasn't hyperventilating into a paper bag."

"Hmm. Well, I'll be straight with you – it's the one thing that worries me about this move. But if you say you can do it?"

"I can. I promise. I'll get more and more used to it and that will make it better."

"Okay," he said. "That's good enough for me. Let's move to Switzerland then."

With Chris suitably reassured – or at least pretending to be – we each went ahead and negotiated part-time contracts that would allow us to fly back to London for work on alternate weeks. I left my hostile workplace behind and we both transferred back to the office where we had worked Saturdays together when we first met. We would initially travel up on a Wednesday, work Thursday through Monday, and return on a Tuesday. In between, we would have seven glorious days of freedom on a vineyard in Switzerland. That was the thing I focused on when I block-booked budget flights for weeks in advance even though I was totally, utterly, completely and irrevocably afraid of flying. I can see my mother again: "You *do* like to do things the hard way," she says.

※ ※ ※

From the moment we started packing to the day we finally arrived at our new home, our departure for Switzerland was about as shambolic as our unsuccessful attempts to reproduce. The day before the furniture removers arrived to transport most of our possessions to a storage facility somewhere in the north of England, I had gone to work and left Chris in charge. Over the preceding days, he had been at work while I cleared and packed the bulk of the flat.

"You need to empty the spare room," I instructed. "I'm going to put the stuff we're taking to Switzerland in there. Then there's all that shelving in our bedroom to sort out. Pack those two rooms and we're almost done."

"Okay," he said, "the bedrooms. Got it. That sounds easy enough, I'll get through that in no time."

"Don't forget all the junk under the bed!" I called as I walked out of the door.

Eleven hours later, I returned from work, exhausted by the type of day that had reminded me exactly why I was so eager to escape to Switzerland in the first place. I found Chris in the lounge, surrounded by teetering piles of CDs. A quick reconnaissance revealed that both bedrooms looked precisely the way they had when I left at lunchtime. "What *have* you been doing?" I snapped, dispensing with any sort of greeting.

Chris looked up from his spot on the floor. "I've been alphabetizing the CDs. Hell of a job. Taken nearly all day, but I'm getting there."

"But the movers are coming in nine hours. At 8am. You have remembered?"

"Don't be like that sweetheart. I'm going as fast as I can."

"Let me get this straight," I fumed. "You have devoted an entire day to making sure that Bob Dylan is packed before Paul Weller, but you haven't touched either of the bedrooms – at all."

"I did! I took down the portable TV from the wardrobe."

I threw my work bag to the floor and stomped straight back out the door. It felt like my head would explode if I didn't get some fresh air right that minute. Eventually, head still intact, I returned to the flat, where I spent four hours overseeing the packing of our remaining possessions.

I think about that night sometimes when I'm smarting after another argument about fertility, usually brought about because I feel let down by Chris, unsupported when it comes to any tangible help. I realise, it's not only fertility, it's anything practical; he just doesn't get it. He does everything back-to-front, why should this be any different? And then I think: shouldn't he try? If he really wanted a family, wouldn't he try?

❧ ❧ ❧

Two days after our furniture disappeared to a storage facility we had never even seen, we set off for Switzerland twenty-four hours later than expected. This was because we had only just bought a cheap second-hand car, specifically for this move, and we had been more than a little optimistic about how many possessions we could cram into it. With the date for our departure slipping back by the minute, our landlord, Norm, was clearly starting to wonder if he would ever get rid of us. He hovered apprehensively as we stood in the driveway, the car full to the brim, yet still surrounded by piles of clothes, pillows, duvets, pot plants, coat hangers and a vacuum cleaner that we had been unable to squeeze in.

"It's no good," declared Chris. "We'll have to dump it."

"No! We'll do it," I said firmly. "We've just got to think about this."

"Hmmph," Norm interjected, before turning on his heel and slamming the front door behind him.

In the end, I drove to a car accessories store and had an ugly but expensive roof box fitted. That took care of the clothes and bedding. To fit everything else in, I sat in the passenger seat while Chris stacked our possessions all over and around me. The back of my seat was tilted forwards and my knees were hard against the dashboard; my feet were resting on the vacuum cleaner and a collection of sword-like leaves belonging to my favourite yucca plant reached through from the back seat to intermittently stab me in the head. As the driver, Chris had slightly more room, but there was another yucca plant behind his seat, shaving his ears all the way to Geneva.

It was the first long journey we had made in the car and it was so overstuffed that we were unable to see through any of the back three windows. We set off at 5am and, for the first couple of hours at a steady 40mph, laughed our way along the road. Then, since we had to proceed so slowly, we missed the ferry at Dover. Having transferred to the next one, we finally emerged at Calais at around 11am. There's still time to do it today, we reassured each other; eight hours to go, maybe nine – we'll be there in time for dinner.

However, it seems that in life as in fertility, we have a profound problem with getting from Point A to Point B. Why is it always us lost in the no-man's-land in the middle? On this occasion, it might have been that we were bullied off the autoroute by aggressive convoys of trucks who did not appreciate our presence in the slow lane; it might have been our lack of navigation skills when we took to the B roads; it might have been that we got fed up with each other after about twelve hours and started bickering. Whatever it was, we finally gave up driving at about half past midnight and fell asleep in the car outside a service station in southeast France, still about eighty miles short of the Swiss border.

It was the next afternoon before we slowly and painfully arrived at our new home. My lower legs, from knee to ankle, were swollen to several times their usual size; even on long-haul flights from Australia or New Zealand, this had never happened before. But, in our own ridiculous way, we had arrived. Our new life, the life that would surely give us the family we so desperately wanted, had begun.

We were now living on a vineyard to the north of Lake Geneva, between Lausanne and Payerne. Our English land-lords Mary and Ian lived in a converted barn across the lawn and, for less than half the price of our flat in London, we had the original farmhouse, complete with four bedrooms, three bathrooms, two living rooms, an expansive kitchen, a games room and a swimming pool. I had immediately noticed that there was a cot in the upstairs lounge. Was it too much to hope that one day it might be our child who slept in it, who peered through the bars at us, who gurgled with delight when we picked them up from within? It was going to happen, I knew it.

When this house was just a three-room building, the owner of the surrounding vineyard and his five siblings had grown up here, happily bundled in together. It had always been made for a family, it was a family home for family people. And somehow, despite there being scores of properties available for rent in Switzerland, we had found this one, the one made for us, at our first attempt. After such a long hiatus, perhaps things were starting to go our way.

Our lifestyle improved immediately. With time on my hands, I began to remember how to cook from scratch and we ate nearly all of our meals outdoors, where we had the choice of three different dining sets, offering three different views of our glorious surroundings. We swam, read books by the pool, played badminton and volleyball on the lawn and took long walks through the grapevines, accompanied by Dudley and Duke, the pair of black Labradors who belonged to Mary and Ian but became our frequent companions.

Having grown up on a farm in the southern hemisphere, I had spent six years in London pining for animals. In Switzerland, as I contemplated my future family, or lack of it, I felt comforted by experiencing something closer to my own upbringing. This was where we were meant to be, I knew it.

❧ ❧ ❧

"Oh my God! We're never going to get down from here."

My knuckles clenched tighter around Chris's wrist. My head swivelled from left to right and back again, like a frenzied meerkat sensing a predator on the horizon. "I can't see anything. I can't see. Is everything okay?"

I could tell Chris was also tense, but he did his best to mask it. "It's fine sweetheart. We're okay, I'm sure this happens all the time. Look at the crew, they don't seem concerned."

I could see only one of the flight crew and she was reclining in a seat across the aisle. "She's ten," I snapped. "What would she know? And she's reading *Heat* magazine. That's hardly professional is it?"

All around the aircraft cabin, I could feel other passengers starting to fidget, starting to wonder, like I was, if we were ever going to land. It was the third time we had commuted to London from Switzerland. On the previous flights, I was jittery, as usual, but had done my best to cope with it by burying my head in Chris's chest, closing my eyes and making reassuring mental lists of *Worse Places to Be*. Each time we landed at our destination, I released my grip on whatever body part of Chris's I had been clinging to and congratulated myself on becoming just a bit more normal, a bit more like other people who took business flights every day and thought nothing of it. I was going to become strong-minded like them, that's what I was going to do.

On this third flight to Gatwick from Geneva, I had turned and smiled at Chris when the pilot's voice filled the cabin as he introduced himself and his crew. He was from the southern hemisphere. He had the same accent as me and, for some reason, this voice from home helped calm me down. It needed to – I was more jumpy than ever because the flight had been delayed by an hour and a quarter, giving me plenty of time to survey the crowded waiting room, wishing I did not have to share such a small space, and consequently such a small plane, with so many people.

I should have known that a delay at one end would lead to a delay at the other. Just another detail to add to the ever-growing list of 'things I should have known'. Still, none the wiser, we eventually embarked and I told myself I just had to hold my nerve for one hour and thirty minutes. I counted it off in five-minute segments, like a time trial, obsessively checking my watch while other people ate peanuts and read newspapers.

When we reached the point at which I could make out the lights of England's south coast, albeit eerily subdued by the heavy cloud cover closing in around us, I thought, 'Don't worry, we're almost there. Nearly there now.' I checked the time again; we were due to land at Gatwick in around fifteen or twenty minutes. I could keep the looming panic at bay for that much longer, but only just. Half an hour later, we had descended right into the cloud cover and, for the past twenty-five minutes, had been bouncing around in the swirling darkness, so thick that I could barely make out the flashing light on the end of the wing. I didn't know where we were, there was no chance of catching a glimpse of any landmarks or, God forbid, any other planes. It was like being shaken up and down inside a giant chocolate milkshake. I tightened my grip on Chris, noticed that drops of fluid had sprung up across the palms of my hands; so it was true then, your palms really did sweat when you were nervous. No, not nervous. Terrified.

Another twenty-five minutes, bumping in what felt like aimless circles through the impenetrable murk, and you could sense changing feelings in the cabin; rising impatience among the calmer fliers, rising nerves among those who just wanted to have two feet on the ground. Was there a problem with the plane? Why didn't we seem to have a landing slot? Why were we still up here? Why didn't someone tell us something?

Suddenly, we dropped out of the roiling cloud and into an overcast evening. We had descended further than I realised; there was the airport terminal, there were the lights on top of the building, almost level with us. Thank goodness. This never-ending ride on the ghost train of the skies was finally over. I slumped forward in relief and waited for the reassuring thud of landing gear on tarmac.

It never came. In one horrifying instant, I was thrown back into my seat, the engines were roaring and we were climbing at what felt like an almost vertical angle. *No, no, no! This isn't right.* One minute we were landing, the next we were taking off again. In an adrenaline-fuelled rush we shot back up through the menacing clouds; it felt like clinging to a rocket speeding skywards on Bonfire night. The front of the cabin loomed above us as we powered upwards, the plane as close to bolt upright as I had ever seen a commercial passenger aircraft.

I could see passengers up front turning to look at each other, wide-eyed with either fear or surprise. The young French woman on the other side of Chris began to cry.

"Don't worry," he said to both of us. "I'm sure it's okay. It will just be precautionary."

His leg was jiggling; I knew he didn't mean it.

Despite juddering through the churning ocean of dense cloud, we made the most rapid ascent I had ever experienced. Chris bundled my head into his chest and wrapped his arms around me; I was now rigid with fear. "It's okay," he repeated. "We'll be landing soon. Just hold on a bit longer. It's all okay."

Sure enough, our urgent upward trajectory started to even out. Shortly afterwards, the intercom crackled. There it was – finally – the voice from home. "Sorry that we were not able to land as scheduled. I was not quite happy with the positioning that air traffic control had given us. We are currently being allocated another landing slot and I'll have you back on the ground within five minutes."

Positioning? Air traffic control? Was it a near-miss? I can't see anything! What's happening?

"Nothing major," Chris whispered, leg still jiggling. "Just routine, I'm sure."

I held my breath and hid my eyes in the collar of his jacket until, eleven excruciating minutes later, we repeated our bumpy descent through the darkness. By now I was petrified. I can't take any more. Please land safely. Please land. Airport lights again, getting closer, closer, lower, lower. Bang. Wheels on runway. Taxiing past the terminal. Don't relax yet. We haven't stopped yet. Is it over? Please let it be over.

Chris, visibly relieved, kissed me on top of the head as, against all my wildly imagined expectations, we pulled up to our landing gate. "For goodness' sake," he groaned. "I know your country's full of mad drivers, but I didn't expect to find one in charge of a plane."

The stricken silence that had settled around us was quickly filled with bursts of nervous laughter and the buzz of animated chat. We heard a familiar accent boom through the cabin as another of my compatriots opened an overhead locker behind us. "Geez mate, that was full-on! I was fair shitting myself. Bet he was a bloody boy racer back home. Bloody shithouse budget airlines."

I had nothing to add; I still couldn't speak.

By the time we eventually ordered burgers for dinner in London later that night, I was better able to express my feelings. "Look," I said, displaying my trembling hands as evidence. "Look at that."

"I know, I know," Chris soothed. "But it's over now, you mustn't worry about it. Look, we're both fine aren't we? We got there in the end. I know it wasn't much fun, I'm not surprised you found it a bit unsettling."

"Well," I continued. "I am *never* getting on another plane again. I can tell you now I won't be able to. And what if I was actually pregnant and this happened? What about that?"

"Come on," Chris said patiently. "Let's not think about that now. You just need a good night's sleep then you'll feel better about things tomorrow."

"No I won't! I am not getting on another plane in my entire life. It's a nightmare." Chris opened his mouth to speak. "Anyway," I continued, "you didn't like it either, I know you didn't and what if we get another lunatic boy racer like that driving us around in the sky? No. I don't know how I'm getting back to Switzerland but I'm not flying."

Chris ignored my protestations and prepared to take a bite of his burger. "He might have saved us from a very dangerous situation for all we know. Of course, I wasn't completely relaxed either, but—"

"See," I cut in. "You said it could have been dangerous."

"I didn't mean that, I just meant—"

"Well, it doesn't matter what you meant because I'm not doing it." I pushed away my untouched plate of food. "I can't."

Chris put down his burger and reached for my hand. "Look at me," he said. I glanced up, snuffling into my serviette, and found him gazing intently into my eyes.

"This is important," he said gravely. "I hate to see you so panicked and afraid. If you don't want to fly, then we won't fly. Okay? You don't have to do it, we'll find another way. Just, please, don't worry anymore. We're having a relaxed new life, remember?"

I forlornly returned his gaze. "Sorry," I whispered. "I know I'm a loon."

"You're not a loon. You're a country girl; of course you like to feel the earth beneath your feet. It's quite natural. Now, come on. Let's think about something else. I bet I know what you need – how does a chocolate brownie sound?"

This is another conversation that I remember sometimes when we've been arguing about fertility and I wonder why we ever decided to be together. When I can't think straight and doubts attack from every angle, I look back to that time and a voice says, '*This* is why you wanted to have children with him. *This* is why you knew he'd be such a good father.'

Chris never once said *I told you so*. I spent the weekend typing assorted departure dates and times into various websites, trying to find a way we could afford to take the train home to Geneva. Finally the realisation dawned that it was cheaper to book return tickets rather than a single journey. So that was it. We were now committed to travelling up and back by train. And there would be no refunds on the flights I had booked in advance but would not be taking.

After five days in our former 'Saturday' workplace, which we again shared since the move to Switzerland, we started our journey home on a Eurostar train that left for Paris shortly after 5am. I was not looking forward to the Channel Tunnel, which I had traversed on several other occasions, but it was not the time to let that show. I forced a bright smile and secretly counted time, minute by minute, during our twenty minutes beneath the sea bed.

"Okay?" Chris asked halfway through.

"Great," I replied. "*So* much better than flying."

We emerged into a clear morning at Calais and I started to think excited thoughts about how I could now enjoy our stay in Switzerland without the lingering dread about travelling back and forth.

"If I book quite far in advance, it won't be that much more expensive than the flights," I said. "I should have thought of this in the first place."

I looked over at Chris. He had fallen asleep.

I gently shook his shoulder as we approached Gare du Nord and, bleary-eyed, he followed me over the concourse and down to the RER line, which would take us across Paris to another station and another train, this time bound for Geneva. From there, it was a three-and-a-half hour trip through France and onwards across the border; unfortunately, our car was still parked at the airport so that added another short train ride to the journey. However, by 2.30pm Dudley and Duke were welcoming us home, the country dogs delightedly frisking us with their noses as they inhaled the tantalising mixture of scents we had carried back from the big city.

Chris, who had just worked seven shifts in five days, resumed his sleep in the lounge.

"Sorry," I said when he finally awoke around 8pm. "About all this extra travelling we've got to do now. Are you peeved off about it?"

"Sweetheart," he mumbled, still half asleep. "Of course I'm not annoyed." He leaned forward to kiss me on the nose.

"You can't help the way you're made. No need to say any more about it. Anyway, I quite like the train; it's a good way to see the countryside."

Please let me have children with this lovely understanding man, I thought as I walked through to the kitchen to cook dinner. *Please let us have a family together.*

Eighteen

It was noon in mid-January 2007. I lay in bed staring at the ceiling, wondering what it would feel like to want to get up. I needed to move yet it seemed I was stuck, not just in that moment, but in life. This is the fifth year, I thought. The fifth year and still no progress.

Rural Switzerland might have been awaiting me outside but, on some days, that was no longer enough to rouse me from bed. I just lay there and counted tiles on the bedroom ceiling, back and forth, first in one direction then the other. *Two, four, six, eight, ten, twelve. Two, four, six, eight, ten, twelve.* From our local village, the midday church bell sounded across the fields as it had done for centuries, calling in for lunch the workers dotted among the grapevines. I could see across to the stone church spire if I sat up, but I remained motionless. It was like being in a trance, just staring and counting while everything else remained frozen. I had spent so long wondering which way to move that it now seemed I had forgotten how to move at all. *Two, four, six, eight, ten, twelve.* Then Chris's voice carried through from the lounge: "Hey," he called, "Dudley's here." I slid, rather than sprang, out of bed, but I was moving, at last I was moving.

If it wasn't for Dudley and Duke, this might have been the time that infertility finally consumed me, leaving no trace of who I had been before. But 'the boys' would come nudging and snuffling, wanting snacks or a walk through the vines or just a scratch on the chest, and, somehow, I couldn't say no. Dudley would waddle in like a little black bear, full of joy for no reason at all, and Duke would plant a paw in my lap, gazing at me with chocolate-fondue eyes. Sometimes, when no one was listening, I would chat to them endlessly. "Do you have any idea how irritating men are?" I would say, or "What do you think I should do, boys?" They might not have answered, exactly, but they were still vastly more helpful than many of the humans I encountered during my time in the Ten-Year Club.

That January, if I was really going to take them into my confidence, I might have told them that what was truly weighing me down was the absence of hope. Once again, Chris and I had not managed to have unprotected sex at any stage, let alone around ovulation, so unless a mighty big miracle was about to occur, there was no chance that I could have conceived. Even on a good month, the odds of success might now be reduced to one in a million, for all I knew, but that was still better than no chance at all. Someone had to win the lottery, didn't they? However, January 2007 was one of the months when I didn't even have a ticket. We might have been in Europe, with Paris, the capital of romance, just up the train tracks, but we were once again practicing natural family planning. Chris had inexplicably gone from having sex twice a day in a hotel room in December to being too afraid to have it at all in January. I couldn't understand it. He couldn't understand it. But what he did say was that it wasn't a big deal and he was sure it would be fine the next month. I'm thirty-eight, I thought. How many months do you think I've got? However, I didn't say it out loud, not even to Dudley and Duke. Some things you're conditioned to keep secret, even from a pair of Labradors.

On the last weekend in January, we were invited to a birthday party at Mary and Ian's, our landlords across the lawn. Somehow, I had been socialising less and less since this struggle with infertility. I was increasingly finding it easier all-round to isolate myself from other people. To start with, there were basic irritations like all the questions that arose at parties about why I didn't drink and the pained looks that followed. It was almost as if people were deeply insulted that I was not 'properly' joining in.

I had learned to prepare a list of stock answers in advance. "Oh, I overdid it a bit last month – thought it was time for a detox", or "I'm on antibiotics unfortunately", or "I'm on a diet, no alcohol allowed". Perhaps one day, the question would be asked one too many times. "What? Not drinking? One won't do any harm! Seriously? You're not drinking?" Perhaps, finally, I would do what I really wanted to, which was pour my glass of sparkling mineral water right over my inquisitor's head while loudly announcing, "Actually, I'm infertile and have been for more than four years. Thanks so bloody much for reminding me of that while I'm out here trying to have some fun. And, by the way, do you have any idea what alcohol can do to a reproductive system? No? Well, let me tell you …"

And the 'why don't you drink' question was not the only tripwire at social functions. Right after the 'not drinking' observation would come the grenade that was so casually lobbed into every conversation: "So, do you and Chris have kids?" There's an added poignancy to that question when you're in your late thirties, a sort of uncomfortable beat that follows your answer as the interrogator tries to work out whether you just didn't want children or whether you're infertile. No one ever says, "Oh well, plenty of time" like they might if you were twenty-eight; they just look a bit baffled, as if they don't understand you and your life choices. I had grown tired of pasting on a smile and trying to think up a reply that put everyone at their ease – and if there's one thing that really makes you want a drink it's supremely fertile people enquiring after your own non-contribution to the fertility stakes.

So, you might have thought I was not much looking forward to the party at Mary and Ian's. Actually, I was looking forward to it very much indeed. When I think about that now, that very fact should have taken up a lot more of my attention. My eagerness to attend the party had a lot to tell me about my relationship with Chris but, yet again, the things it wanted to tell me did not necessarily chime with the things I wanted to hear. Because what I was really thinking when we got that invitation was, 'Phew! This might be it. This might be where I meet the one who actually *wants* to be with me.' The extent of my delusion could be summed up by the fact that it was a seventieth birthday party and would largely be attended by seventy-year-old people.

We were seated at the end of a table with what Mary described as "all the other young-uns". It felt unusual to be in an environment where I was still thought of as young and strong instead of ageing and frail, so miserably decrepit that I was no longer able to produce a single egg worth fertilising. I perked up a bit and looked around. Chris was seated opposite me beside Jenna, Mary's niece, blonde, beautiful without trying, and in her late twenties. Next to me was Jenna's boyfriend, Greg; early thirties I would have guessed. On the other side of Chris was Rena, Mary and Ian's prospective daughter-in-law. A year or two older than me, she was the only one who knew we had really come to Switzerland to have a family. When we first met, she had spoken openly of her own fertility struggles and we had bonded over tales of the excruciating things fertile people say and do when they hear you can't have children. Maybe that's why, on that day, I told the truth when everyone started passing around the wine.

"We're still trying to conceive," I whispered across the table to Rena and Jenna. "Maybe one day I'll be able to have a drink again."

An English neighbour from a nearby vineyard lurched past clutching two bottles of red from the village wine co-operative. He stopped to place one at our end of the table, then picked it back up and started pouring.

"Not for me, thanks," I said with a smile.

"Oh, I see. A white wine connoisseur in our midst. I'll be at your service shortly, madame." He gave a little bow.

"No, no, it's okay. I'll just stick with the mineral water, thanks."

"What?" he cried. "Mineral water?"

"Yep. You know, cheap date and all that."

"Well!" He sighed theatrically. "What's the point of living on a vineyard if you don't drink wine? You do realise we are here," and he swept one hand grandly around the room, "in one of the greatest wine producing regions of the world?"

"Yes, she does," Rena interjected. "Now buzz off and serve someone else."

We all laughed, including our would-be sommelier, who staggered off to find other guests to ply with alcohol. The party gained momentum while Dudley and Duke dozed side by side on their bed in the corner of the dining room. Every time I came to Mary and Ian's, I always thought the same thing: this is exactly what I want. Family gathered around a table, talking and laughing while a couple of Labradors wandered in and out or snored on the floor. That was it, my idea of bliss. It seemed such a simple wish and yet it remained so far out of reach. I wondered if I might not have been better off pinning my hopes on a chateau in St Tropez, or a hovercraft perhaps, because for some reason those over-the-top fancies were starting to seem more realistic than my one basic wish. I didn't feel like I was asking for much in my desire to have a family – I just wanted to share in something that everyone else seemed to achieve without a thought – and yet at the same time I knew I was asking for everything.

'Stop it!' I ordered myself at the party. 'This is supposed to be fun.'

I turned to Greg and made a possibly over-enthusiastic enquiry about his line of work which, as it happened, turned out to be really quite interesting. Across the table, Chris was leaning slightly away from Rena and slightly towards Jenna. He'd already had a couple of glasses of wine and was chuckling furtively while he and Jenna slipped pieces of smoked ham to Dudley, who had been alerted by the arrival of the first course and was discreetly soliciting donations from beneath the table. As the meal progressed, Chris's back swivelled inches by flirtatious inches, further and further from Rena's direction. I had seen this before. Once at a party, he had completely blocked me with his back while he set about casting his spell on a fifty-something woman and it had ended with her making a novel proposition: would Chris like to see her bathing naked in vanilla ice cream? He was horrified.

"Hell's bells," he gasped after making a hasty retreat. "She just came out with it. Why would she say something like that? I can't understand it."

"I can," I replied. "You gave her the massive come-on with your body language. And I saw you giving her crinkly eyes – what do you expect?"

'Crinkly eyes' was a seductive look that Chris deployed with anyone female, and also with himself. It involved a sort of puckering of the eyebrows, a twinkling of the eyes and a 'crinkling' of the skin beneath. Chris never looked in the mirror without adopting this expression; he regularly checked himself out in this manner in tube train windows, in the glow of computer screens and even while standing in front of me, angling to get the best view of himself in the lenses of my sunglasses.

At Mary and Ian's party, the crinkly eyes, fuelled now by a bottle of wine, were working overtime. Chris was 'stealing' an extra piece of cheesecake, sliding lower in his seat to conspire with the dogs and laughing endlessly with Jenna. I continued my conversation with Greg, my spirits dampened by the hurtful thought I couldn't keep at bay: *That's why he doesn't want to*

*have sex with me; I'm not young enough or blonde enough or thin
enough. I bet he'd have sex with her any old time.*

I noticed other couples in the room and the way they
interacted while still including others. Ben, Rena's fiancé, was
on hosting duties with his parents but, every so often, he would
appear at Chris's right, patting Rena's shoulder to check that
she was okay or kissing her on the cheek on the way past.
Sitting there, taking all this in, I realised something very
inconvenient: I wanted a Ben of my own. I needed a man I
could rely on when push came to shove. Because, truth be
told, infertility had not only left me isolated socially, it had
left me isolated in my own relationship. It was as if I was the
one carrying this barren burden while Chris spectated from
the sidelines. All I knew was that it was starting to feel a very
lonely place to be.

This party was doing nothing to help. Across the table, Chris
and Jenna had heads huddled together while peering under
a chair and guffawing with laughter. They were interrupted
by the arrival of simmering pots of coffee and by other guests
wafting past with the steam rising from their cups as they
took the chance to mingle with those at different tables. I was
chatting with a dapper white-haired man in a bowtie who had
materialised at my right. I smiled and asked what I thought
were pertinent questions, but my instincts were still focused
on the other side of the table.

I had no desire to cling to Chris, but how long had it
been now since he had even acknowledged that I was there?
Suddenly, I heard his voice, rising clearly above the thrum of
conversation.

"She doesn't miss a thing," he told Jenna. "I mean, I can't
flirt with you because she'd know. She watches my body
language and she knows. Nothing gets past her. Nothing!"

Instantly, I had to get out. "Do you know where the bathroom is?" I needlessly asked the man in the bowtie.

As I knew he would, he pointed to a door at the far corner of the room and I excused myself; I wouldn't be coming back. Just before reaching the hall that led to the bathroom, I detoured left and slid out of the front door and onto the driveway, barely visible now in the night.

Our farmhouse was cold, dark, empty. I threw off my shoes and curled up under a rug on the couch. It was about half an hour before I heard footsteps on the gravel, followed by the clicking and creaking of the front door. Chris shuffled over the threshold and fumbled along the wall before turning on the light.

"Sweetheart? Sweetheart, where are you?"

I remained silent. "There you are," he said. "What are you doing here? Are you okay? Don't you feel well?"

Chris leaned down towards me, reaching out to touch my shoulder, and I instinctively pulled away. "Oh, it's me! You're upset with me. Was it because of the wine – with the fertility? I didn't mean to drink that much, it just got away from me a bit. You know how hard it is sometimes. But surely one blowout won't have too much of an effect?"

Silence. "Oh, why won't you talk to me? Please tell me what it is, I hate to see you upset like this."

"Then don't do upsetting things!"

"What? *What?* I don't know what you mean." He squatted down in front of me, trying, and failing, to make earnest eye contact.

"You haven't got the first clue, have you?"

"Oh, don't be like this, please don't be like this," he urged. "I said I'm sorry about the wine. I know it's hard for you not being able to drink and maybe I could have supported you better by drinking less myself and—"

"It's not the wine. I don't care about the wine."

Chris stood up and pat, pat, patted the sides of his hair in the mirror above the mantel as he continued to speak.

"Tell me what it is, then – please. You know I'd never do anything to hurt you, of course I wouldn't."

"Ha!"

"Oh, why must you be like this? Why can't we just have a nice evening out?"

I threw my legs to the floor and drew myself upright on the couch. "Because I *heard* you. I heard what you said."

The claims and counter-claims flew around the room then; he denied saying what I had plainly heard him say – *I can't flirt with you* – and when I called him a liar, he denied that too.

Eventually, I leapt up from the couch, unable to contain myself any longer. "It still hasn't occurred to you, has it? You still don't get it."

"What? What don't I get? What is so terrible that it's led to this … this accusation?"

"Oh God," I moaned, sitting back down and letting my head sink into my hands. "Chris, we haven't made love for five weeks. How do—"

"That's it! I don't need this. You're throwing this back at me again," Chris shouted from the other end of the lounge. "You're just throwing it back at me. I've had enough of this Louise. Enough."

Again, he had steamrollered through my explanation before I could even get the words out. He was pacing, waving his arms, speaking in a frantic deluge, as unstoppable as a river rapid.

"Go on then!" I finally broke in. "Lose your temper. Have a hissy fit. You always do this. You ask for the truth then when I tell you it, you don't want to hear it."

My voice broke with emotion. I would never get through to this man; he would never understand.

"Lou! Really. I don't do it on purpose, you know that. We have a great sex life, you know we do, but you can't keep bringing it up like this. It makes me feel so useless. This is a really difficult thing for a man, you've said so yourself. I'm trying my hardest, I really am. I don't know what more I can give you."

I stared sadly at the painting on the far wall; sheep grazing serenely on rolling hills that were patterned by stone walls. Although it was a Yorkshire scene, it always reminded me of home. I should have stuck with a southern hemisphere man, I thought. I should have stuck with what I knew.

Chris was still speaking, the river rapid tearing through our lounge with no care for what was in its way. I gave it my attention once more and noticed there had been a change of tack in my mind's absence.

"I wasn't flirting with Jeannie …"

"Jenna," I snapped. "Her name is Jenna."

"Well, see," Chris said, attempting a smile. "I don't even know her name. How could I be that interested in her? You know I'd never do anything to hurt you on purpose. You know I always do my best for you – for us."

While Chris was doing the equivalent of dancing around the boxing ring, showing off his footwork and punching the air for effect, I saw my opportunity to deliver the knock-out blow.

"Okay," I said. "If you're so intent on doing what's best for us, then how come you haven't bothered to take another sperm test?"

"Oh, this is so unfair!" Chris gave a backhand swipe through the air, as if swatting the question away. "This really isn't on, Louise. I'm going to take another test, I've told you that. I'm going to do it, you know I am. Really."

"Yes, but you said that in 2005. Now it's 2007 and—"

"How dare you?"

"What? How dare I tell the truth?"

I was seething now, challenging him defiantly about the thing that, deep down, rankled and prickled and hurt most of all.

"You know how hard it is for me," Chris exclaimed. "I'm doing everything I can, I can't do any more. I've told you I'm happy to do another sperm test, you know I'm happy to do it."

"But you can't be happy to do it otherwise you would have *done* it."

"Honestly! You know how hard it is. I thought you understood that. This is beyond ridiculous."

I rose from the couch, pulled my shoes back on and walked to the door. "No!" I yelled over my shoulder. "The only thing that's beyond ridiculous is you. You need to take a good, hard look at yourself."

Whenever I bit back like this, I saw a moment's insecurity flicker across his eyes. "Lou, there's no need to speak to me like this. There's no need to go. It's not easy for me, that's all I'm trying to say. Really, I'm—"

I slammed the door and ran back out into the night.

It's not as hard for you, I thought to myself, as it's going to be when I meet a man I can actually rely on. It was a thought that had begun to breach the surface with uncomfortable frequency, just lately.

2& 2& 2&

As I counted the months until my thirty-ninth birthday, I realised it was time to stop fantasising about other men and to start being proactive. Chris and I talked, once again, about sperm tests and why he was so reluctant to take another one. It was stressful producing a sample to order – what if he missed the deadline? What if he couldn't do it and that would mean his performance anxiety had reached a whole new level? What if, given the circumstances, he didn't produce much at all? It was awkward carrying his sample across London – and what if the whole sorry thing was to no avail because there was a traffic jam or a broken-down train and he didn't get there on time? On the other hand, it was unthinkable to conjure up a sample in a clinic while people wandered by on the other side of the door. It was embarrassing handing it over, having your most intimate bodily fluids scrutinized by a stranger, invariably a woman. The whole thing was one big anxiety-producing, terrible task that he had kept putting off and off and off.

"I'll hand it over for you," I said. "All you've got to do is collect a sample in a hotel room with only you and me there. What makes you think you can't do that? You've done it before after all."

"I know," he said. "You're right, of course. I'll do it – I'm happy to do it. I give you my word."

Somewhere deep down, I must have already realised that he wasn't really going to do it at all but, churning around in the maelstrom that infertility had become, I kept thinking and hoping that soon we would have conclusive test results, soon we might know exactly where to focus our efforts. We'd start to move forward any day now, when he took the test, and we could cross that basic thing off the list once and for all.

I knew Chris well enough to know that his entire sense of masculinity was tied up in the words our GP had originally said to him: "You have enough sperm to fertilise the whole of the UK." He was clinging to that, as if it made him somehow more of a man, and batting aside my enquiries as to whether his UK-wide army of sperm was actually moving anywhere or whether the troops were entirely stationary. As far as I could tell, he really thought it didn't matter. That had to be the explanation, didn't it, for why he was dragging this out for such a painfully long time?

At some point in 2007, I started to become a Really Angry Person. At the time, I blamed infertility, my heartless challenger for nearly five years. However, now I know differently – now I know that I was tied up in hopping mad knots because I had inadvertently handed over to Chris far too much control over my future. Although we both professed to want a family, it was by no means a team deal. I ran around looking for information and health-food supplements and alternative therapies while he did the opposite of helping me. He was the one who determined whether we had sex or not – and if it was 'not', then there were no other options since he had not even begun to look for a solution. Now, despite all the efforts I had made to help him arrange it, he had taken nearly eighteen months to *not* undergo a sperm test. I had never, in all my younger years of fending off men, imagined that the day would come when I was so desperate beyond description to *just bloody interact with some sperm.*

I had always been adamant that it had to be with someone I loved but, almost without realising it, I now began extending the parameters of my fertility research into less familiar territory: I began seeking information on sperm donors. This wasn't being driven by my mind; it was as if every cell in my body was actually screaming, 'Emergency. Emergency. Wake up. Act now!'

Even ovulation seemed to be happening more obviously; it was as if my reproductive organs were doing their utmost to get my attention while there was still time for it to matter. Sometimes this seemingly primal drive made it hard to think straight. It was as if my body's overwhelming urge to reproduce over-rode all rational thought or query. Like whether I ever *could* reproduce.

All I knew was that I wanted to be pregnant beyond all wanting. I found myself fixating on sperm, the often missing ingredient, in a way that would have horrified my younger self. I began straying into dangerous territory when I lay in bed at night, inconsolable again because we had just missed another ovulation, another chance to have a family. Dark and selfish ideas found their way in, fraudulently offering themselves as seemingly sensible solutions to all this angst: I would have a one-night stand with a stranger (although I wasn't entirely sure I even had what it took to attract a man, these days), I would go ahead and sleep with one of the men at work who sometimes got a bit drunk and started sniffing around for sex, I would buy sperm from anyone who offered it online (was that even possible?). In the cold light of day, I wasn't going to do any of those things – of course I wasn't – but I admit there was a part of me that thought, 'I wish you were a bit bolder, I wish you had the guts to do this.' Ultimately, though, all arguments, whether for or against this madness, were always outstripped by one thing: the memory of my five-year-old self being told where I came from. They spoke about my teenage mother, but not my father. There was a gap where he should have been and throughout my life it had grown larger. I couldn't make this same choice for my own child; a father whose identity could never be mentioned.

In early February 2007, I put aside all these tortuous thoughts, ignoring the tangled avenues they led me down, and came up with another of my 'make do and mend' solutions. This idea, I thought, would neatly and painlessly bring to an end our lengthy stand-off over sperm tests. I had discovered that, a year earlier, a fertility testing kit for home use had been launched at a high street chemist. Its arrival meant that Chris could test the potency of his sperm in the privacy of his own bathroom – embarrassment factor nil.

"Look," I announced, waving a newspaper article in front of him. "You might not have to cart a pot of sperm all over London after all."

He brightened immediately. "Is it accurate then, do you think, doing it at home? Would it be the same as, you know …"

"It says 95 per cent here. Maybe we could just use it as a sort of pointer."

"It's not some suspect thing off the internet, is it?"

"No. It's at Boots. I'm going to do one, too. Well, not a sperm test, obviously. One that checks my eggs."

"Boots? The chemist?"

I nodded.

"Great," he said, relief written in every line of his face. "Let's get it."

The next time we travelled to London for work, I took a bus to Oxford Street and sidled up to the personal care items in a glossy and cavernous branch of Boots. There it was: £79.99, a sperm test for him, an ovarian reserve test for me. Given that this repeat semen analysis had taken so long to arrange, Chris was not the only one overdue for a test. My initial results now dated back to 2005; every article I had read since then seemed to shout 'failing ovarian reserve, failing ovarian reserve', like a flashing red light warning of danger ahead. I worried endlessly that, over the past eighteen months, my ovaries had decided enough was enough; they'd done their job perfectly well for thirty-eight years, it was now time to go into retirement. Every time I ovulated, I felt a swell of gratitude, followed quickly by a frisson of fear: what if this was the last time? What if there were no eggs left now? What if there were some eggs left but they were all hardened and damaged with age, not worth penetrating even if you could?

I pondered these immediately unanswerable questions as I waited for day three of my cycle to tick around – that was when I could take the test, thereby discovering a little more about whether my fertility had measurably declined since 2005.

Day three of my next cycle turned out to coincide with a budget hotel stay in central London. Before going to bed on day two, I laid the test kit out on the only table in the room, next to the plastic kettle and sachets of long-life milk.

"What *is* that little contraption?" asked Chris. "It looks like a melted-down Dalek."

He broke into a monotone impersonation: "Exterminate … ex-terminate!"

"It's not funny." I laughed. "It doesn't look anything like a Dalek – for one thing it's plastic." I eyed the kit, which actually looked exactly like a pregnancy test, sitting there next to the shabby array of tea-making equipment. "Maybe a melted-down Dalek's arm," I said dubiously before breaking into a fit of giggles. "Oh no! What if it tells me all my eggs have been exterminated?"

"Ha," said Chris. "Someone should make these things with sound effects to deliver the results. Why has no one thought of that?"

"You-are-an-old-bat. You-have-been-exterminated." I chimed in with an impression of my own.

"You-have-no-sperm. Give-up-now," Chris batted back. "You-must-surrender."

We rolled around on the bed, laughing and coming up with sillier and sillier judgments for the benign-looking ovarian reserve kit to deliver.

Only another nine hours or so and I really would know what it had to say. When the time finally came, I awoke to find Chris already sipping tea in bed.

"Good luck," he said as I scooped up the test from the table, read the instructions for the umpteenth time, and took it into the bathroom to pee on yet another stick.

I emerged to find a fresh cup of tea waiting for me.

"What now?" asked Chris.

"Cross your fingers for half an hour," I replied, double-checking the exact time on my mobile phone.

"Don't look so worried sweetheart, it'll be fine. You're far too young and beautiful to be exterminated."

"Well," I said. "You haven't seen my ovaries. Anything could be happening in there."

"It'll be fine," he repeated. "I feel it in my bones."

I watched the last five minutes tick around, behaviour that I usually reserved for time spent on aeroplanes. "Okay," I pronounced at last. "Time's up. Urgh, why did I say that? What if time really is up?"

I returned to the bathroom to learn my fate, picking up the instructions again to ensure I didn't misread the verdict. It seemed, these past few years, that I was forever handing over my hopes to little plastic sticks doused in my urine. Immediately, I looked for a line in the control window to show that the test had worked. Yep, it had worked all right. Now for the big one, the line I was really interested in, the one that was supposed to appear in a second window. One line – or one plus another lighter than it – indicated normal ovarian reserve. However, the appearance of a second, darker line would herald the news I dreaded – it would let me know my reserve was no longer at the normally expected level. I peered down at the test kit, carefully placed on the bathroom sink. I checked it, then checked it again, and once more for good measure. Yes, I was definitely seeing things clearly. It definitely looked just like the illustration on the instruction sheet.

I returned to the bedroom.

"Guess what? One line!"

"Oh," said Chris, obviously trying to take his cue from my expression. "Is that good news then?"

"Yes." I beamed. "Yes, it is."

"See," he said with a grin, "what did I tell you?" He got up from the bed and encircled me in a tight hug. "I knew it. I knew we still had time."

I flopped back down onto the bed with relief. Maybe we could still solve our fertility problem after all. Even, I thought, if it takes IVF. Technically, I still didn't know if I could really go through with it but part of me was already cautiously inching along that path. Suppose we could manage to pay for it? Suppose it was a viable choice? Could I choose it or would my core fear of being so vulnerable and exposed prove too much to overcome? I didn't know, but I was starting to fully understand that there is no drive stronger in this world, when it arrives, than the natural drive to have a child. It remained the only force I could think of that had a chance of competing with the dark voices from my past.

Chris interrupted my thoughts. "I'll do my sperm test when we get back to Switzerland. You'll have to talk me through it, though. You know what I'm like with instructions."

"It's fine," I said. "I'll run it like a military operation."

"Hmm," he replied. "That's precisely what bothers me."

We both laughed. Discussing each other's bodily fluids like this was hardly romantic and it was not exactly fun to have to do it, but sometimes you could feel a sort of drawing closer, a peeling away of layers that led to an exclusive bond between the two of you. I knew, right then, that we were both feeling it, that we loved each other more because we could still laugh, sometimes, at this intensely painful challenge we found ourselves facing.

Of course, in a day or so, I would be worrying again: what if these home tests didn't really work? What if *everyone* got one line? What if next month, or the one after, was the time when my fertility levels would take the dramatic cliff-top plunge that everyone seemed to describe once a woman reached my age? What if they already had and I just didn't know it? What if, what if, what if?

I was encouraged, though, to know that perhaps – finally – we were about to cut through the confusion surrounding what was wrong with us. The picture would be much clearer when Chris took his own test. Knowing the outcome – one way or the other – would make me feel that we had actually made progress, that the choices ahead of us were more obvious. It might be a lone life raft in an open ocean, but it would offer the sliver of security that I so badly needed. After an indifferent start to all of this, I thought Chris was beginning to understand.

On the train back to Switzerland, he wanted to know how the home test kit worked. "I don't completely see how it could match what they do in a laboratory," he said. "It can't be that simple, can it?"

"It's a really clever little thing," I answered. "Well, that's if it works like they say it does. You know it's supposed to be 95 per cent accurate?"

We shared one of those looks reserved for couples who are scanning each other's thoughts on their own private wavelength. "Don't say it!" I joked.

"You were thinking it, too."

"Yeah, I know. Hard to help it after all this time, isn't it? You just automatically think, we're bound to be …"

"… in the five per cent who get a duff result," Chris finished off, laughing.

"Exactly. Why is it, do you think, that fertility stuff never goes our way?"

He rolled his eyes. "I wish I knew, I really do. But, come on, let's not give up. Let's assume it's going to work for us. For one thing, it wouldn't take much for it to be better than the appalling lack of information—"

I sniggered. "What?" he asked. "What?"

"Sorry. It's just that when you say," and I adopted the poshest accent I could muster, "*appalling*, then I know a rant's coming on. You go all Lord Snoot of Snootsville."

"Well, it was appalling. Our GP never should have … *who* did you just say I sound like? Come here you! This is how we deal with southern hemisphere upstarts."

He made a lunge for me across the seat, emerging empty-handed after I leapt out into the aisle. Such were the joys of travelling in an empty carriage on a 5.30am train.

"I'm going to sit down that end," I pointed to the far doors, "if you don't behave yourself."

"If *I* don't behave myself? Well, that is rich."

And so it went on, through the outstretched fields of northern France.

Eventually, after brokering peace for long enough to share a warm croissant, we returned to the original subject.

"I read an article," I explained, "that said medical researchers have designed this test so that sperm have to swim through a sort of obstacle course. It's the same type of barrier they'd encounter if they were trying to get through a woman's cervix."

Chris pulled a face. "All I know is that I'm glad I can do it in my own bathroom."

"Better tell your boys to start lifting a few weights and doing a few stretches," I said with a chuckle. "They've got a tricky swim ahead of them."

"Nothing we can't handle," Chris replied. "You will talk me through it, though, won't you? You know what I'm like with instructions …"

If, during that cosy, companionable moment on the train, you had told me what happened next, I wouldn't have believed you. But, really, what did I expect? After all, I knew Chris better than anyone.

NINETEEN

OF ALL THE TIME that I've passed in the Ten-Year Club, the moments I'm most proud of are the ones that I've actually enjoyed – when, despite the pressure and the doubts and the uncertainty, I've gone ahead and had fun anyway. It sounds such a simple thing, but it's one that no longer comes quite so naturally when infertility has you by the throat and you start to feel that all the truly good parts of life have been put on hold. Should I fly long-haul to visit my family? No! What if I conceived that month? What if the flight interfered with my cycle? Shall we go out to dinner? Or away for one of those romantic weekends we used to have now and then? No and No. We might need the money for fertility treatment. Shall I visit my old friend in Dorset? No. Not that weekend – you're ovulating. You can't miss ovulation.

And so it goes on. Somehow, almost by stealth, it feels that life has become one long list of things you cannot do. When fertility says no – no you can't have a baby – it almost convinces you that everything else in your life has also become a big fat 'no'. Suddenly, there seem to be limitations everywhere, all lined up behind the one major limitation like taxis on a rank. When I look back over the past ten years, I rue the fact that infertility came calling, but more than that I rue the fact that good things in life were still happening and sometimes I didn't see them. If it wasn't for the slightly left-field decision to move to Switzerland, I wonder whether I would have experienced any joy at all during vast swathes of this ongoing struggle to have a family. Perhaps it was the one thing I did right in all of this, turning the question on its head: what *can* I do since I don't have children?

Deciding that I would achieve one long-held goal while pursuing another might just have been the thing that brought enough joy into my confusing new world to motivate me onwards. I might not have had children in 2007, but I still knew that I was in a very fortunate position. As I eyed the fifth anniversary of our infertility, I had at least found an avenue of escape, a way to ease the pressure that relentlessly built with each passing month. I still worked punishing hours when I was back in London and adrenaline flooded in with the stress of the job, but we had created an air pocket, a safe place we could go to get some breathing space. For part of each week, the external pressures that could finally have suffocated me existed elsewhere. And, more than that, I had progressed onwards, savoured a new experience, at a time when life felt stagnant.

So, in the summer of 2007, Chris and I did something that had gradually begun to feel very unfamiliar – we had fun together. It was like getting a memo that reminded us: despite all the arguments and recriminations and insults, you can still make each other laugh until it hurts.

In Switzerland, we stayed home most of the time because that was the cheapest thing to do. We played volleyball, tennis and badminton on the grass. We ate dinner sprawled on the lawn and lunch under a tree. We walked the countryside in the daytime, admiring the vines and the yellow stone houses, and in the nighttime, admiring the stars. I found a glow worm in the garden and named him Sirius.

In bed at night, my mind still churned with anxieties about fertility, forever trying to unknot our problems, but during the day I remembered how to live.

If I look back in my diary, I can see that I noted the dates of my cycle, the days we had sex and the days when we tried to, but did not succeed. I'm surprised now to see that those days have 'failed at ovulation' – Chris's term for it – scrawled across the top of the page. I'd forgotten about that. My memory is of joy bubbling back through our relationship, like a spring through barren ground. One day in July, we drove to the hypermarket and, for reasons that we were unable to translate with our trainee French, returned home with the free gift of a bright pink Winnie the Pooh ball.

Chris, forever trying to look suave, even in shorts and a t-shirt, looked comical just holding it. "What are we going to do with this thing?" he asked, chomping on a piece of ham as we unloaded the groceries.

"Well, you seem very taken with it," I answered. "Look at you bouncing it on the bench."

"Habit," he said. "You get a ball in your hand, you've got to bounce it ... Hang on, you won't tell anyone at the office about this will you? I know what you're like."

"Ooh good. Something else to bribe you with. It might make a good volleyball. Or we could always play 'donkey' with it," I added in jest.

"What?"

"Donkey. You know ..."

He looked blank. "Every time you drop the ball, you get given a letter of the word. 'D' for the first drop, 'O' for the second – first one to collect them all is a donkey."

He raised an eyebrow. "I think you just make up half these games so you can laugh at me. Like that 'Final Card' thing."

"*Last* Card."

"Yes, that one. I'm sure you just make up the rules as you go along. I can never remember any of them."

"I *do not* make them up," I protested from within the pantry. "It's not my fault you didn't play any kids' games at your posh school."

"Of course I did," Chris said indignantly. "You know how much I loved sport."

"Yeah, but you got the cane if you missed a shot at cricket. Didn't you ever do anything just for the fun of it?"

"That was never really in the schedule," he said.

"Urgh! I hope you don't think our children are going to be brought up like that."

We took the pink ball, Winnie the Pooh on one side of it and Piglet on the other, and started casually throwing it around on the lawn. I fired it high above Chris's head and watched as he made a hopeless leap for it.

"That's D." I laughed. "You dropped it."

"Hey! I didn't drop it – you didn't throw it properly. That was not a proper throw."

"Sorry, it's the rules. What can I do about it?"

"Right!" Chris retorted. "Take that then, rule girl," and the ball flew past several feet to my right. "I believe that makes you an 'O'."

"How can I be an 'O'?" I cried. "I haven't even been a 'D' yet – and you've got the nerve to call me a cheat!"

Inevitably, 'Donkey' soon became a little too tame and we moved on to highly evolved versions of the game called 'Wanker', 'Tosser' and 'Dickhead'.

Ian stopped on the driveway as he drove past, winding down his window to call a greeting across the lawn. "Have the pair of you been on the sauce?" he enquired with his usual dry humour. "I haven't heard two people guffawing with such gusto since Madame Toussaint fell off Donald's kitchen table with her bloomers on her head." He waved merrily and drove off, leaving us wondering who Donald was and what exactly had occurred in his kitchen.

Having moved from 'Donkey' to expletives to the names of people we loathed, we were both covered in sweat and grass stains.

"Okay then," I said eventually. "Let's end this once and for all. Nicholas Chalk, winner takes all."

Nicholas Chalk was a man begging to be parodied; it was unfortunate that we each relied on him for our employment because he was the most obsequious, petty, Machiavellian, ridiculous person we knew. He fawned, almost to the point of bowing and scraping, over people who mattered and took unseemly pleasure in playing mind-games with the rest of us. One moment you were in favour and had regular work, next minute, due to some imaginary slight or other, you were out of favour and didn't. He got his kicks from watching how you coped with it.

Chris immediately started up with his Nicholas Chalk impressions. First the walk, part swagger, part flounce, then the comments: "How dare you disrespect my spreadsheet? Mere plebs must not touch my spreadsheet!"

Just as Chris expected would happen, I fell into fits of giggles and was immediately incapable of catching any throw that came my way.

Soon enough, Chris had collected only the 'N' and the 'I' but I had accrued every letter bar the 'K'. Damn! I was about to become Nicholas Chalk. Masquerading around the lawn, Chris wound up his comic impersonation to the point where my sides ached and I could take no more. He launched an underarm throw, knowing that nothing further was required since I couldn't stand up straight for laughing. However, just as the Winnie the Pooh ball left his hand, Dudley appeared in a black flash from behind the pool shed and, with unexpected athleticism, snatched it out of the air. The look on Chris's face sent me to the ground in a shaking heap of snorts and chortles. I had to wipe the tears from my eyes as he pursued Dudley round the lawn, like Mr Bean herding geese.

"Go Dudley. Go!" I cheered.

Chris sprinted past, back in character now as Nicholas Chalk.

"Stop it," I pleaded. "I'm going to wet myself."

Unfortunately, I realised I really meant it. I made a desperate run for the bathroom, but had to abandon it halfway and squatted down behind our car, much to Chris's amusement.

"That settles it," he gloated. "I've won."

"No you haven't," I claimed with as much dignity as I could muster. "Dudley saved me. Yay for him."

Later, as we lay like starfish side by side on the grass, Chris reached out and stroked my hand.

"I could never be like this with anyone else," he said contentedly.

"Me neither."

"I really do love you," he whispered.

The tree frogs started singing in Ian's pond and we dozed off, as companionable as two people could be.

I know that both of us have always remembered that day, but I don't know whether it was because of the fun we had together or because it turned out to be the last burst of sunshine before summer ended.

Maybe, I think now, Chris and I would have been better off having just a holiday romance. I could have gone back to my normal life afterwards and daydreamed about the sweet, funny, kind man who never raised his voice and who would have undoubtedly become a great lover in time. And what story would he have built up around me? Maybe it's both of us, I think, maybe pressure warps us both. I can feel myself blaming him for mutating into a darker form under the strain of a challenge like infertility and then I remember something Jai said to me, just as we were breaking up. I had thought it might help salvage the relationship if we focused on positive things about each other, so I asked him: "What's the best thing about me that you'll treasure from our ten years together?"

Do you know what he said? – "You were fun on holiday."

Maybe Chris isn't the only one; maybe I'm not much fun to be around in real life either.

Perhaps the reason the next stage of our ongoing skirmish with infertility hurt so deeply is that it came within weeks of that day with the Winnie the Pooh ball, when we reminded each other of the people we could be. It was too easy, I guess. Anyone can be nice to you on a sunny day. The question is, what do they do when the weather turns nasty? Do they offer you shelter or do they snatch it for themselves? Unfortunately, I was about to find out.

TWENTY

CHRIS DID NOT USE the home-based testing kit I had bought for him in early February. He was happy to do the sperm test, he said, relieved in fact that he could do it in his own bathroom. He would do it next week, when we got back from London. He would do it next week, when he wasn't so tired from travelling. He would do it next week after I'd talked him through it first. He would do it next week, definitely. He'd do it tomorrow and that was a promise.

"I *am* going to do it," he would declare, affronted, if I ever said something like, 'Oh, don't forget, you've got your test to do.'

"Yes," he would snap, bristling at my interference. "I haven't forgotten. I'm going to do it tomorrow."

After six months' worth of next weeks and tomorrows, I finally lost patience.

"Do you even *want* to have children?" I demanded, smarting with frustration and disappointment.

"Of course I do, sweetheart," he declared. "I want nothing more than to have children, you know I do."

"Well, you've got a bloody funny way of showing it."

He launched in then, immediately. "Really, Louise, I can't take this! I feel like I can't do anything right. Why must you always be so critical of me? I've told you I'm more than happy to take the test. I was going to do it tomorrow and now you've made an issue out of it and made me feel like I've let you down. I had it all planned, I was going to do it tomorrow morning."

Crack, crack, crack, his words reverberated around the room like shotgun-fire, no room for a breath between each new blast. "You know I wouldn't let you down on something as important as this. How can you say I don't want children after everything I've done to help us have a family? Why must you think so little of me? Why?" And he paced and sighed and tutted.

I was daunted by this tactic when I first met him. I'd barely argued with anyone in my life; I was a novice when it came to this type of conflict. I even still wondered, immediately, if perhaps it wasn't me who had got things wrong. Chris never wondered that, not immediately. I began to realise, too slowly as usual, that he had one default setting: he was beyond reproach.

Well, not this time he wasn't, I was certain at least that I knew that much for sure. In a flash, indignation took over, spilling wildly across our faded room at a B&B in west London.

"Don't even try to turn this back on me! It's not going to work so don't damn well go there."

"Lou!" he interjected, looking momentarily stricken by the force with which I spoke. "Don't get yourself so upset. There's no need for us to be like this."

"Exactly," I snapped.

"It's hard for me," Chris broke in again, desperate to talk his way out of trouble. "You have to understand that—"

"Understand? What the hell have I been doing if it's not understanding you?"

He tried to over-talk me again, to plough across my concerns with a verbal bombardment of pleas and excuses and justifications. I had been trying to become a mother for nearly five years, I would soon turn thirty-nine; I was no longer in the mood to be over-talked.

"Shut up and listen," I shouted, rounding on him with a surge of anger that had been building for longer than I even knew.

"I've waited and waited and *waited* for you to take another test. I've sympathised that it might be embarrassing for you. Then I've gone out and found you a way around that – and you won't even take it! I took mine six months ago – six months –

and I had to wait to do it on a certain day. How come I can do that, but you can't be bothered to shove a bit of sperm into a cup in the privacy of your own bathroom?" I raged on, gaining molten-hot momentum.

"I'm sick of hearing how hard it is for you! Have you any idea how hard it is being the only one who's actually trying to do anything about this? While you fanny around and make promises you don't keep? That you never ..."

I suddenly spoiled my new-found ability to deliver a verbal bombardment of my own by disintegrating into tears. "I just want us to have a family," I hiccupped. "And soon it might be too late and you're ... you're wasting all this time."

"Lou, I'm not wasting time. I'm not! I don't mean to waste your time. Don't cry – please don't cry." He made a move to comfort me.

"No," I said. "Don't come near me. I don't even want to see you. All you do is let me down, over and over."

"I don't let you down! I would never let you down. Please, I ... Oh, this is so silly."

"Shut up and get lost then if it's so silly," I said from the bed, where I had curled up in a dejected ball.

Chris left for the office and, after I followed an hour later, I ignored him all day. I knew how it worked; these frozen impasses had been going on since the start of our relationship. I wondered if any of our colleagues had picked up on it. Just as well there weren't many other women there, I thought. They would surely have noticed. They might even have guessed that I didn't want to be in a relationship remotely like this one. It was either express my honest opinion and brace for the backlash or keep quiet and watch as any problems got worse. I couldn't seem to find the middle ground and fertility, with all its biologically-induced deadlines, was starting to push me, more and more often, into speaking up. I'll give infertility credit for this: it's beyond efficient at exposing any fragilities in your relationship. It likes to find the cracks, then crowbar its way in there and turn them into crevices. Deep, dark, isolated caverns that you could fall into and really hurt yourself.

❧ ❧ ❧

The argument about the test that hadn't been taken led – finally – to the test being taken. We were in London again. Chris was sorry. I was quite right to question why it had taken him so long to get this done. He had genuinely intended to take the test, but time had gotten away from him. He would do it now and everything would be okay. If I could just read the instructions and explain to him what he needed to do …

If my twenty-four-year-old self, on my first trip to the UK, had been offered a glimpse into the future there fourteen years hence, I would have been horrified; surely someone was playing a bad-taste joke on me. You did not go to a hotel room to sit on the bed while your boyfriend went into the bathroom and then emerged a bit red in the face, holding a dollop of sperm in a plastic container – that was just weird. You went to a hotel to lie around in a cosy couple, sharing nachos and chocolates, drinking red wine and making easy, romantic love after – or maybe during – a late-night movie.

Sometimes you even got carried away with the passion and caused a crack in a marble coffee table, which was exactly what had happened to Jai and me once. No! That plastic container would not be my future. Staring at someone's sperm? And you weren't even involved in producing it? Are you kidding me? When I was twenty-four, I didn't give a second thought to the latex-veiled contents of the used condoms that piled up in the bathroom bin. It wasn't mine to worry about. All things considered, it's probably best that I didn't know what I'd be getting up to in a London hotel room at the age of thirty-eight and three-quarters.

It was another plastic contraption, part collection pot, part testing unit, and another wait for the verdict. The little circular device in front of us was putting Chris's sperm through a type of obstacle course. If all was going to plan, it would now be forging its way through a barrier that mimicked the female cervix; the test would then measure the concentration of active sperm that was able to swim beyond that point. If the level was high enough, the test would be positive. Chris paced the floor while his bodily fluids faced their challenge.

"Remind me again, Lou. Which red lines do we want?"

"Two," I replied, instructions still in hand. "Doesn't matter how faint they are, just as long as there are two."

"Would that mean there were enough swimmers to reach an egg?"

"Yes, I think so. Not just reach it, but fertilise it." I grinned reassuringly. "There might even be enough there to fertilise the whole of the UK."

Chris stopped pacing and plonked down on a chair, one knee instantly jiggling. "What if he was wrong? What if I don't get two red lines?"

"It'll be fine. Don't worry about it. I mean, look what a great swimmer *you* are. You'd swim all day long if you could."

He smiled wryly. "I know. It would be ironic, wouldn't it, if my sperm just sank to the bottom."

We looked across at each other and simultaneously burst out laughing.

"I didn't mean *your* bottom!" Chris snorted.

"Well, that would explain the problem." I chuckled. "They could get lost in there for years."

"Oh no. What if they've got my sense of direction? That would be a disaster."

"Don't worry," I said again. "It's probably my body causing the trouble. I'm probably just karate-kicking your sperm right back out again."

"Yes," he laughed. "That sounds about right."

Ten minutes later, time was up. "You look first," Chris prompted from the far side of the room.

I took a deep breath and peered down into the results window. At first glance, it seemed as if there were no red lines at all. I squatted down for a closer look. This was very confusing: definitely no red lines.

"What?" asked Chris. "What is it? It's bad news, isn't it?"

"Weeelll ..."

"Just tell me. It's okay, really. I knew something would be wrong anyway. I knew it."

"Um." I scanned the instructions once more. "I don't get this. Have a look at it. Can you see any red lines?"

Chris took his reading glasses from the bedside table and tentatively approached the test unit. He bent over to study the results window. "No," he said. "There's definitely nothing there."

"That's what I thought."

I handed him the instruction sheet. "See. It says one red line for bad news, two for good. Trust us to get no line at all, that's just typical."

Chris inspected the device once more. "Definitely no line. Nothing." He paused. "Did you push the right button?"

"Yes," I said, grabbing the instructions to double-check nevertheless. "Stupid thing hasn't worked. All that sitting around for nothing."

"Hell," said Chris. "My sperm must be an extraordinary kind of awful if it can't even get the test to register its presence."

We laughed about it then and, shortly afterwards, walked arm in arm to the tube station. The argument, inevitable though it was, would wait until later.

⁂

I had been brooding on the situation. I was tetchy, irritated, annoyed. How were we ever going to have a family if Chris didn't buck up his ideas? I might as well not even bother. What was the point?

We were sitting outside in soothing sun that I had barely noticed. It was a public holiday in Switzerland a few days after the failed sperm test attempt. In the distance, a family of five straggled along the road in an unruly line of cycles, one parent at the front and one at the back, shepherding their young like swans across a lake.

"Hmph," said Chris. "All these people with all these kids. It's so easy for them. One, two, three. Just like that."

I didn't reply, although I was watching the family, too, thinking, 'Yes and I bet there's an exact two-year age gap between each of them. Simple!'

"I sometimes think things are meant to be a struggle for us," he continued. "Look how nothing's gone our way. We've had a duff doctor, duff test results and then a do-it-yourself thing that didn't work either."

"Well, we'll never know, will we?" I said coolly.

Chris glanced across at me. "What do you mean?"

"Maybe," I said, "it would have worked perfectly well if you'd used it six months ago when we first bought it."

"Oh. I see," he retorted. "I wondered when this was coming. I knew you'd blame me for it. A test malfunctions and it's my fault. I shouldn't have to put up with this, I really shouldn't."

It was like peeling a dressing off a wound. I was tetchy and irritated only because I didn't know how to express the pain that lay beneath. It had become so raw that I didn't know how to look at it, let alone soothe it. The anger arrived first, like some sort of protective reflex.

"You carted that thing back and forth for six months," I snapped. "On and off trains, jammed in luggage racks. You didn't even take it out of your bag. How *hot* do you think it gets in there in summer? Of course it didn't work. What did you expect? No wonder it bloody broke!"

I was weeping now, unexpectedly, because I had been sure I was more furious than sad.

"Why couldn't you just help me?" I managed between surging tears. "I just wanted to be a mum and now I'm nearly thirty-nine and it's not going to happen. And you ... you just think it's bad luck. It's not bad luck – it's not."

"Sweetheart!" Chris broke in. "We've tried everything we could. It just hasn't fallen our way."

"You haven't even tried," I whimpered. "You haven't even tried."

I was inconsolable, so much so that I barely heard Chris's urgent cascade of words, tumbling forth to tell me how much he had tried, how much he had done to ensure we had children.

"I stopped drinking beer," he said. "Look how much beer everyone at work drinks, and they've all become fathers. Sometimes it doesn't matter what you do."

It felt as if the core part of me, deep inside, was breaking in two. I was never going to be a mother, not if we carried on like this. It was completely and utterly hopeless.

"Lou," Chris pleaded. "Don't give up, you mustn't give up. It's hard for me too, you know, but we can't give up on this. There must be something we can do."

"It's all been about *you*," I stammered. "When is someone going to come along and help *me*? I've had to help you with your ... your issues about sex and I don't know if that's stopping us getting pregnant or not. Half the time we can't even try. It's so confusing because of that. Then I've had to help you about sperm tests that you don't take and now ... no one's supporting me," I finished. "No one."

"Urff!" Chris sighed sharply. "I'm sitting here doing my best to encourage you and that's what you say to me. I can't believe you can say these things when all I'm doing is trying to console you. It really is unnecessary."

234

He leapt up and stalked off, leaving me there on the ground in a pathetic puddle of tears.

After nearly five years, I was finally drained of all spirit. There was nothing left to fight either Chris or infertility itself. When I got up off the grass to go back inside, it was as if my body was hauling itself along; I was no longer in there. I saw without seeing and heard without hearing. None of it mattered anyway. None of it was worth the effort.

I remained in that state for the rest of that day and all of the next. While I was inert, Chris was a ball of perpetual motion. He disappeared down the driveway or through the vines on one long walk after another, frantically pacing alone as he always did when agitated.

Near the end of the second day as dusk came down, leaving the house in shadows, I heard the front door open. He was back. I sat on the couch in the half-light, staring straight ahead at nothing, willing him to disappear again.

Chris walked into the room, not stopping to turn on the light. With a bit of luck he would go upstairs and I could continue to pretend he didn't exist.

When he squatted down in front of me, it felt like the invasion of a protected zone. He placed a hand on my knee and looked searchingly up at my face, willing me to meet his gaze. I resolutely refused to acknowledge his presence. It wasn't hard; I wasn't there either.

"Sweetheart," he said quietly. "I don't want to be like this. Please talk to me. I've spent all day thinking about things."

He reached up to touch my cheek and I automatically ducked away. "Oh, Lou. Please. I'm not trying to fight with you, I just want to talk."

I focused on the silence that followed his words; there was a thrum to it, like being in a trance.

"Please forgive me," he said then, still squatted in front of me. "Please give me another chance. I know I've messed everything up, but please let me put it right. Everything you said is true, all of it. I just want to put it right. You deserve better than this, you really do. You deserve so much."

He began to cry.

"I'm sorry, I'm so sorry. I'll do anything to put it right. Anything. Please, please, just let me back in."

Eventually, tentatively, I re-emerged, like a hedgehog unfurling in slow motion. "I'm going to help you with this," he said. "I promise you that."

I had nothing to say, not right then, but we slept that night wrapped close together. We could discuss how to start again tomorrow.

Over breakfast the next day, with Dudley snuffling hopefully for crumbs, Chris reached out to take my hand. "This is important. I really want you to know that I mean this."

Dudley flopped down heavily onto his side, emitting a lengthy groan as he did so. I smiled. "I think Dudley's heard one of your talks before."

Chris smiled back. "I don't blame him. I expect you probably feel like groaning too, don't you?"

"I don't know. It depends what you're going to say – and whether you mean it."

"You're right to wonder," he said. "I've been no help to you at all, I know that."

"Well, not—"

"No," Chris continued. "You've given me nearly five years' worth of chances and I'm very grateful to you. I know I don't always show it properly, but I am. But it's hopeless, it really is. It's time now that we did something for you."

"It's not completely hopeless," I reassured him. "It's just hard, you know …"

"When you've got to focus on me all the time," he finished. "My issues and my disastrous lack of organisation. I've held you back, I didn't mean to, and I hope you know that."

I nodded. "I want you to be free to move forward now in your own way," he said.

For a moment, I thought he was breaking up with me. This was starting to sound like a more eloquent version of the 'it's not you, it's me' speech.

"How do you mean?" I asked doubtfully.

"I was thinking I could pay for you to go and see Belinda Cooper. It's the least I can do. You can ask about having tests or doing IVF, you can ask about using a sperm donor if you want. You can find out what options you've got and then it's up to you. I'll support you whatever you want to do."

I laughed. "Wow. I didn't think you knew who Belinda Cooper was."

Belinda Cooper was the eponymous head of one of the best-known fertility clinics in London. I had read one of her books; it lay in the ever-growing stack of fertility tomes that teetered upwards on my side of the bed.

"I do listen sometimes, you know." Chris raised an eyebrow as he grinned across the table. "You showed me that newspaper article on her, then you ordered her book that time and I know you were very taken with it."

"But a sperm donor? Are you sure? To be honest, I don't know if that would be right for me, let alone you."

"Well, that's the sort of thing you could ask about," he said. "I know you can't always rely on me and that's just not good enough anymore, I do see that. I mean, we could still carry on trying – if you wanted? It's just, we need to do everything we can to make sure you become a mother. You'd be a brilliant mum and I want that for you more than anything."

I got up, stepped carefully over Dudley's dozing form and gave Chris a hug. "Of course I want us to keep on trying. But if I could get to see Belinda Cooper – that would be amazing."

"Right," Chris confirmed. "Leave it to me, I'll get straight on the phone and book an appointment. I'm going to take charge of this – it's time I upped my game and got things done."

"Will you come with me?" I asked. "Whenever it is?"

"It's completely up to you," Chris said. "I really want this to be your thing. Of course I'd love to come, but only if it's what you want."

Hope sprung anew. For the first time in nearly five years of trying to conceive, I would be going to a fertility clinic. *This* would be the key. This would be the vital move that led to me getting pregnant!

TWENTY-ONE

ON THE MORNING OF our appointment at the fertility clinic, I was every kind of frustrated that it was possible for a person to be. My almost thirty-nine-year-old body was ovulating with a vengeance. This had started happening often throughout the past year – maybe it was a bonus of the Swiss lifestyle; more likely it was my ovaries making one final, desperate stand while they still had some precious eggs left in stock. I had never thought the day would come when I would be mentally conversing with parts of my reproductive system. However, more and more now, that's what I found myself doing. *Thank you,* I would think, *thank you,* whenever I felt my hormones and my ovaries seamlessly working together to produce multiple signs of ovulation. Then, other times, I would sense them, chugging along still, and I would think, *I'm sorry, I'm so sorry I've let you down.* Because my body seemed to be doing its best; it was my mind that got in the way and messed everything up. There were still biological resources available to me and yet, overtaken by so many conflicting and confusing emotions, I was unable to think straight about how to use them.

The problem with ovulation is that it fills you with overwhelming urges, it causes you to 'want' a man in every way possible. I wish I'd known this in my twenties – I would have thrown away my contraceptive pills, introduced my body to itself, and quite possibly saved my marriage. How could a couple grow apart when, for a few days a month at least, every cell in your system is demanding that you be together? It would certainly have been a good start, I think now. The way I felt when I was ovulating, it would have been very surprising indeed if Jai had been left with the energy to even glance in

Dana's direction. The primal power of natural urges: another nugget to add to my list of 'things I wish I had known'.

That morning of our appointment, it seemed especially ridiculous to be going to a fertility clinic and asking about how to get pregnant. I was ovulating to the point where I could barely stop myself from reaching out and grabbing any half-decent man who walked past and yet Chris and I were not capitalising on this seemingly miraculous surge. We were not having sex. That was okay, however, because I had come up with yet another plan as to how we might work around this. Time spent trawling the internet in Switzerland had revealed donor conception sites, where there lay a solution so simple that it made me want to slap my forehead for not thinking of it myself.

If Chris was struggling under the weight of his performance anxiety, he could take sex right out of the equation; all he had to do was go into the bathroom and provide a 'sample', which I would then send on its way to my cervix, using, of all things, a baby medicine syringe from Boots. There were now several of these little plastic vessels in the bathroom cabinet at home and several more in my washbag for when we were travelling. Simple. I would no longer have to worry about so casually wasting the gift of ovulation when it was presented to us and he would no longer have to worry about his fear of 'failing'. That alone would remove an enormous portion of the pressure that was bearing down as time threatened to leave us behind once and for all.

It had been a straightforward trip up to London the day before our appointment. However, straightforward still meant an hour's drive into Geneva, a three-and-a-half-hour journey north on the train, a dash across Paris on the RER, a two-hour Eurostar ride through the Channel Tunnel and a forty-minute bus trip to west London. And that didn't count time spent waiting around for connections. Then, around 7.30pm, we finally dumped our bags in another room in another B&B and wondered what we were going to eat for dinner. I was still ever conscious that this drawn-out day was all my fault. If I had only been able to travel by plane, like every other 'normal' long-distance commuter, then that was an extra three or four hours shaved off the day's proceedings right there. So I had sympathy for the fact that Chris was tired that night when we arrived at the B&B; it was more than eight hours since we had locked up the farmhouse and driven off through the vines that morning.

In the circumstances, the last thing I wanted to say was, "Um, I seem to be ovulating" or, "Er, I'm a bit ovulatory", but what choice did I have? I didn't know how often these opportunities would present themselves from now on. And I couldn't just 'spontaneously' throw myself at Chris; I knew he wouldn't be interested. All day and all evening, I mulled over how to bring up the subject of ovulation. I wished then, more than ever, that he had been involved in this endless cycle tracking, that he had taken note himself of when we should be trying, for the umpteenth time, to conceive. If only he would be the one to say something. Didn't he know that I remained horrified on every level at the thought of pressurising someone into bed with me? Another wish: that I could reach out for him and we would make love, naturally and carelessly, just because we wanted to be with each other, not because we had an agenda or a schedule to stick to. But there were too many layers of potential rejection wrapped up in that idea. I knew, deep down, that I could no longer take the risk. No, if I wanted to seize this chance to finally become a mother, then I had to say something.

I built up to it all evening, planning how I could casually bring it up. "Ooh, look. I'm ovulating. Fancy that," or, "Gosh, what a surprise. I didn't realise it was that time of the month already."

I just wanted to find the magic words that would transport away the momentary flicker of alarm that crossed Chris's face whenever he realised that I was asking him to procreate with me. I remembered, while wrestling back and forth with the issue, that there was always the DIY insemination kit. It was supposed to be for back-up, to take the pressure off when things went wrong. But I suddenly realised what I could say, so that I would feel less guilty for raising the subject and he would feel less press-ganged into service.

"Um," I started nervously. "You don't think you're up to producing a sample, do you?"

"A what?" Chris replied. "Oh. Are you ovulating?"

"Yes. Switzerland seems to be quite good for ovulation," I offered, trying to keep things relaxed.

"Are you sure?"

"As sure as I can be. It's a bit of a turbo-charged one, for some reason."

There it was, unmistakably: the flash of fear that escaped to the surface before Chris could command his facial features back into order.

"You don't want to be doing it with a sample, do you? Let's have a go at making love," he said. "There must be a better chance that way."

"Well, if you're sure you're up to it? I know it's been a long day …"

"Let's try," he said. "I'm happy to try."

I knew within thirty seconds that we would not be making love that night. I recognised the signs and I sensed that Chris did too. Again, I didn't want to be the one who brought it up, the one who said, "Look, I don't think this is going to work." It seemed kinder to at least leave that call to him. However, he shook and flailed and sweated and eventually I couldn't bear for it to go on any longer.

"It's okay," I said. "Why don't we just use a sample?"

"I can do this," Chris urgently insisted. "It's not that I don't want to do it. It's just so hot in here. The air conditioning's useless! Look at the sweat, it's pouring off me. I'll be okay, I just need to have a rest and cool down. Then we can try again, I'll be fine."

"No," I said, more firmly than I intended. "A sample will do. It's a big day tomorrow, let's just get some sleep, huh?"

"Are you sure?" Chris asked, instantly jumping up and making straight for our suitcases, lying open on the floor. "Have you got a syringe with you? Is it in here?"

"In my toilet bag. In the bathroom. Just bring it with you when you come back out."

"What can I use for—?"

I handed him a plastic cup from the bedside table and he disappeared behind the closed bathroom door.

I waited anxiously. Please let this ovulation not be wasted. Not this one, not this month; I might have been nearly thirty-nine but it was the most intense set of symptoms I had ever experienced. After ten minutes or so, the bathroom door shot open. Thank goodness. There was still hope after all.

However, Chris emerged empty-handed. "I just need a drink," he said. "It's too hot in there. Look at me, I'm bright red. Bright red! I don't know how they expect people to exist in this heat."

A stab of panic made itself known in my chest. This was a whole new development. Was it just because he was fatigued after all the travelling or was it because he was afraid? I wasn't sure how to work it out; I wasn't sure that he knew the answer himself.

"Look," I said. "Anyone can see it's not going to happen. Don't bother anymore. We can try again in the morning."

I slid into bed and turned out my bedside light.

"Oh," Chris said. "You're upset with me. Don't be upset, please. You've said it yourself, these things happen sometimes.

I'll be much better in the morning, I know it, I just need to cool down and get some sleep. Honestly, sweetheart—"

"I know," I replied, cutting him off before he could turn it into yet another lengthy, angst-fuelled discussion. "It's fine."

I turned my back on him and felt tears welling beneath my closed eyelids. Why? Why couldn't it just be simple? Every time something went our way – like this fiercely powerful ovulation – something else emerged to stop us in our tracks.

I couldn't bear all the 'what ifs?' or the desperate thoughts and emotions that relentlessly crashed against each other as I lay there, unable to put to use the desires that were overtaking me. It was the ultimate irony: Chris was the one with the ongoing issue, but I was the one who felt supremely impotent. I was sexually and reproductively frustrated all at the same time and the truth of it was that I would have given anything at that moment to have been lying in bed with another man. I was beginning to stop even caring who it was.

Chris was gently snoring now, oblivious to the distressing mental and emotional battles being played out on the other side of the bed. I threw back the duvet and padded across the floor to the bathroom; I shouldn't have drunk so much water while I was nervously preparing my 'casual' comment about ovulation. When I stood up again after taking the pressure off my bladder, I felt something brush my leg. I looked down; there was a clear string of ovulation fluid, like stretched egg white, reaching halfway down my thigh. I sighed heavily and threw back my head in despair. I was an idiot to have ever let it come to this.

The next morning, Chris immediately declared that he would like to 'try' to make love again. Despite nine hours' sleep, he was shakier than ever. It was okay; we would use our new back-up method. However, Plan B also failed and there was no Plan C.

"It's probably just anticipation about everything," Chris said. "It's difficult, you know, when you've got things on your mind. We can try again tonight, or tomorrow."

"Don't worry," I replied dismissively. "The best time's gone."

I turned my thoughts, and my hopes, to our appointment at the fertility clinic early that afternoon. What a relief. Finally, we could stop battling along in such a hapless way. Finally, I could talk through all of the options with someone who was an expert in this field. Surely with their help we could make some progress? We had to. It was obvious that we couldn't go on like this any longer.

As usual, there were introductory forms to fill in; we did this seated alongside each other in a Circle Line tube carriage, waiting with pens aloft for a station stop or a smooth portion of track. As well as the now routine information about our ages, health, lifestyle and conception history, the questionnaire also covered deeper issues like whether you had ever suffered from depression. Instinctively, I pulled back at that point, still unsure whether I should, or even could, trust a stranger with these intimate details. But how often would I get the chance to receive help from one of the most feted fertility clinics in the UK? I purposefully resumed writing, admitting to possible bouts of depression, not that I ever would have called it that, and moving on to questions about whether I had ever been verbally, physically or sexually abused. I ticked yes to everything; Chris ticked no. He skipped lightly through the form and was finished well before me.

"They don't really need mine anyway," he said. "It's your appointment. I'll just stay in the background." He looked over at me, still working my way through the list of increasingly personal questions. "Okay Lou? You know what you're going to ask about?"

"I think so. Mainly stuff about what other tests I should take – and I *really* want to know whether we could have

245

fertility treatment without the drugs. Oh yeah, and how much the whole thing costs." I paused. "It is still okay to ask about sperm donors? I mean, just to know how it works, that's all. Doesn't mean we're going to do it."

"It's fine," Chris replied, squeezing my hand. "Just make sure you ask whatever you need to know. That's what this is for."

"It's just because. Well. I don't know how long I could lie there like that, if we tried full-on IVF. With all those people around." I trailed off. "After what happened…"

"You just need to talk to someone about it," he said. "Then you can see how you feel. It's about time we got you some help with this."

"Thanks," I said with a smile. "I still can't believe we're going here." I reeled off the names of celebrities who had received treatment at the clinic. "They've all got children, haven't they? Mind you, you never hear about the people who don't go on to have children, do you?"

⅔ ⅔ ⅔

The waiting room was white. They always were. Artfully arranged on the far wall was an array of framed covers from glossy magazines, each one featuring either the clinic or its well-known director. Behind the reception desk were beautifully stacked bottles of the clinic's own-brand fertility supplements. Everything flawless, perfectly placed. We sat quietly; it was as if the pair of us had realised at once that we were now entering a far more advanced stage of infertility. Maybe, somewhere within this clinic, lay the answer to our childlessness. It was both daunting and exciting to be here.

The woman who emerged to greet us was dressed in white linen trousers, a white linen shirt and white Birkenstocks. It was left to a voluminous crown of unruly brown curls atop her head to rebel against the clean, colourless lines below.

246

We followed the white woman upstairs and into a room that might once have been a bedroom in this central London townhouse. Nowadays, the space was clearly designed for 'talking things through'. Chris and I sat side by side on a firm, low-backed couch that did not encourage lounging; I noted the obligatory box of white tissues on the coffee table before us, always set at a diagonal, in the same way that clocks in movies were always set at ten to two. The woman who sat down opposite us was not the eminent director of the clinic; the waiting list for an appointment with her had been too long to contemplate. This was Janet Brown, a senior colleague with years of experience in the fertility field. For our initial consultation with her, we had one hour. One hour and one hundred and sixty-five pounds, which is what it would cost. If this progressed as I expected, my notional fertility accounts book was about to be doing business at an unprecedented rate.

I reached forward to pass across to Janet Brown the forms we had filled in, aware that I was chattering anxiously as I explained that we had only just collected them from our postbox in London since we now spent most of the time in Switzerland. She set the documents aside on the low table and the familiar routine began. We had been trying to conceive for nearly five years, I told her, outlining almost by rote the tests we had taken in 2005 and the additional ovarian reserve test I had taken at home earlier that year. So far, I had had two different types of acupuncture, which had improved my cycle but never resulted in an actual pregnancy – as far as we could tell. Oh, and there was also the question of the inconclusive initial sperm test and, as to the length of time it had taken us to conceive, there had been, um, 'other issues' …

Chris broke in before I could think how to phrase it. "I'm afraid I've rather muddied the waters a little," he said quickly. "I've had problems with, ah, performing when I feel under pressure so we haven't always been able to try, er …"

"At ovulation," I finished for him.

Janet Brown immediately seized upon this and began questioning Chris about it. I felt him shift nervously, imperceptibly, next to me on the couch and instinctively jumped back in to the conversation to try to help him explain.

I told her the problem had existed at the beginning of our relationship in 2002, that Chris had been to see his GP to rule out physical causes and that it had been deemed a psychological issue. I had bought books for him to read, I said, and we had worked on it together by doing 'exercises' where – oh help, how did I say this? – he just lay inside me so that it would start to feel natural and safe. Embarrassed to be relaying such intimate details, I found myself mentioning something I had read about the concept of *vagina dentata*, the idea of a 'toothed' vagina, and the fear this could instil in some men. Ordinarily, I never used terms remotely like that; why, oh why, did I start babbling in this way whenever I was flustered?

I saw Janet Brown summing me up; 'I see', she seemed to be concluding, 'another amateur psychologist who has Googled a few terms and thinks she knows the answer to everything.' She informed me crisply that it was good that I wanted to help Chris, but that I shouldn't have done it; these things were best left to the experts. Well, I thought, good luck getting him to speak to one. I stopped talking then; this was starting to feel a bit uncomfortable.

She turned her attention back to Chris. It was quite common for men to be affected by the pressure of performing on demand when couples were trying to conceive, she said. However, once anxiety took over, it was physically impossible to have sex because the body's fight or flight response kicked in, diverting blood supply to essential organs. An erection obviously required increased blood flow to the area, but ...

We knew this because Chris's doctor had explained it to him in 2002. I waited for him to say, 'Yes, I understand the mechanics of it, I've been through it all before.' However, he remained silent and Janet Brown was already moving on.

"So you've been together for about five-and-a-half years and you've been trying to conceive for much of that time. That is quite pressurised."

Chris instantly agreed – it would be very difficult, he said, for anyone to 'perform' when their partner was so obsessed about having a baby.

What? Obsessed? It was like being ambushed before I could even begin. I tried to explain that we had been 'trying without trying' for as long as two years and that there hadn't been much fuss about ovulation at that stage. And, bloody hell, why was Chris letting her think this problem began and ended with our relationship – why didn't he admit that it had been going on for more than thirty years?

The discussion about the wretched issue continued and, as it gained momentum, I sensed the tension ratchet up, both within us and between us. This was partly because Janet Brown had an unnerving way of 'umpiring' our conversation as if she were a match official at the Wimbledon Tennis Championship. She would snap her head to the left if I spoke, gazing at me too intently for comfort, then snap it back to the right when Chris replied, placing him under the same intense scrutiny. As the pressure increased, we responded in vastly different ways. I opted for raw honesty, thinking there was no point paying £165 for this session, and this expert advice, if we were not going to convey the truth of the situation. Chris fell automatically into the opposite stance; he presented his social face, as if at a cocktail party. He even managed to deploy his crinkly eyes while answering questions about whether he awoke in the mornings with an erection.

I began to worry about how much of the hour had passed; fear and frustration, already simmering after the previous night, were beginning to overflow. When could we stop talking about this and just get on with things? Hadn't we already wasted more than five years on the subject, to no avail?

Chris was now speaking about his childhood and how he was sent away to boarding school at the age of seven.

"I think it made him a bit institutionalised," I interjected. "It wasn't normal. They didn't even meet any girls 'til they were about seventeen. I don't get it, growing up like that."

"Was your childhood quite different, then?" Janet Brown enquired.

"Totally," I said. "I was free to roam across the paddocks wherever I liked … to be independent, think for myself. I was so much more free."

"Louise thought I was gay," Chris suddenly added. "Where she comes from—"

"I did not!" I retorted indignantly.

"Yes you did. You accused me of being gay!"

"I did not," I snapped again, too upset to add that being gay was not something you 'accused' someone of, or to explain that I'd brought it up as sensitively as I could, offering support if he needed it. Now it just sounded wrong. And this ridiculous conversation was costing £165 and I was never going to find out what the hell I needed to do just to become a mother. Why did *everything* have to come back to him?

I cast a furious glance at Chris and saw that the crinkly eyes had become earnest, hurt. "Louise also said that men in the southern hemisphere don't have these problems."

"What?" Taken unawares, it was all I could say.

Chris and Janet Brown were now pondering whether his time at boarding school might have affected his confidence and whether that, in turn, had fed into his issues with sexual relationships.

"Well," he said, rearranging his eyebrows into a Hugh-Grant-does-intellectual pose. "Someone did laugh at me in class once."

"Ach," I groaned, rolling my eyes to the ceiling. What I was really thinking was, 'How pathetic. I'm the one who's actually *been* sexually abused and I don't carry on like this.'

Janet Brown fixed me with a cold, enquiring stare.

"Well," I said. "I just don't think you'd be unable to have sex because someone laughed at you in class once. It wouldn't affect me like that."

"Yes," she retorted. "But you're Ms Together."

What had she just called me?

With a sickening jolt, I realised she was judging us. She was judging us and she had taken sides. I thought 'counsellors' were supposed to remain neutral. What exactly was going on? I should have trusted my instincts and stayed well away from all of this 'baring-your-soul-on-a-couch' stuff.

Ms Together. It stung like vinegar in a wound.

And why wasn't Chris sticking up for me? Why wasn't he saying that I'd tried to help him over and over again, and that I hadn't had such an easy time of it in childhood either? Why wasn't he confirming that we weren't here to talk about this, that we'd agreed to put the issue aside before we wasted all our time and energy on it and it was too late to become parents?

Unbelievably, the session was degenerating into yet another of our rows about the same tired old problem, with Chris playing down the effect it had on us and cleverly, invisibly, passing along the toxic parcel until I found it sitting in my lap. Janet Brown and I were now not even pretending to get along and Chris was still acting as if he were exchanging social niceties with her. He and Janet Brown were like two people analysing modern art, peering earnestly at two dots on a blank canvas and extrapolating deeper meanings from it. Meanwhile, I was the philistine in the room, bellowing, "For God's sake! It's just two dots. Can we move on now please?"

At one stage, I said something like, "But you don't see how angry he gets if I try to bring this up."

However, that man hadn't turned up to this consultation; he had been replaced by a smooth operator who knew that talking about boarding school was the perfect ruse to avoid the real issue. In thirty minutes flat, Chris had taken two dots on a canvas, transformed them into something they weren't, and then sat back and watched while I was repeatedly admonished for clumsily, angrily, trying to point out the discrepancy.

Janet Brown had now decided that he was under too much pressure. "What I want you to do," she said, still twitching back and forth as if watching the tennis, "is to stop having sex. You need to take sex right off the agenda."

I thought I would burst into tears on the spot. I just wanted to be a mother; I didn't have any more time for *not* having sex. Didn't anyone understand? There was no more time for this.

Having been told that we shouldn't even try to be together, Chris and I instantly abandoned hostilities and shared a brief, sorrowful look. It was one of those times when we each knew precisely what the other was thinking. I knew he was remembering, just as I was, one of our touchstone moments, like the time we had made love on the floor while *You Do Something To Me* played on the stereo. It was blissful, complete, a level of intimacy we each felt we couldn't have experienced with anyone else. Now we were being told we shouldn't even try to reattain that closeness, to return to the people we used to be.

My conflicted feelings must have shown on my face.

"What's wrong now?" Janet Brown asked wearily.

"I just think it's sad that it's come to this," I replied.

Chris theatrically threw back his head, gasping and flinching as if I had punched him.

"Now you're just firing more arrows," Janet Brown accused, unable to disguise the antipathy in her voice.

No, no, no! He knows what I mean, I know he does.

I waited for Chris to say, 'It's okay, I know what she's trying to say. I feel it, too' but he remained silent. With one final shock, I realised what was happening: his priority was to remain out of the firing line; he would not step in to defend me in case that made him a target too.

The hour was nearly up. All I had gleaned so far was the name of a gynaecologist I could be referred to; I had no information about the tests we might take or how we might move forward using assisted conception. There were about ten minutes left and I didn't know when we would be able to afford an appointment like this again. I was afraid now of saying anything at all, but a looming sense of panic grew with every ticking second. I had to ask, I had to find out something.

"Actually," I began tentatively. "I was going to ask about sperm donors and how that might work."

Janet Brown glared at me. "What do you want a sperm donor for?" she snapped, "when you've got a perfectly willing donor sitting right here?"

"Ha," I muttered, furious that I was being stymied at every turn. "I wouldn't exactly say 'willing'."

That elicited another long, cold stare from Janet Brown, while I turned my own gaze to Chris, questioning why he hadn't intervened. Why didn't he tell her? Why didn't he say that we'd discussed this kindly and calmly and that we had agreed to enquire about it? Again, he was silent, enjoying the safety on his side of that infernally uncomfortable couch.

Janet Brown was winding things up now. We would need further consultations as a couple, but it would be more instructive if Chris also had some private sessions where they could work together on unravelling his issue. I could barely focus on the words but it seemed she was suggesting some sort of art therapy.

"I'd be very interested, in particular, to see your drawings," she told Chris, eyeing him intently.

I didn't need to look at him to know that this would not be happening; I could tell just by the oblique view I had of his right side that he was plainly horrified at the idea. In the meantime, Janet Brown continued, we were not to have sex, but we were to try to relax and enjoy each other's company.

Emotion surged up my throat, constricting, overwhelming; every part of me wanted to run from that room and leave them both there to continue admiring their pointless pair of black dots, all smiles and crinkly eyes. It took every ounce of self-control to force myself to stay for the final round of pleasantries.

As we stood up to leave, I briskly led the way towards the door. Somehow, I realised, Janet Brown was handing Chris a form for another sperm test, the one thing that this consultation had so far achieved in fertility terms.

She looked at me, like a head teacher dealing with a pupil excluded from class, and spoke with a faux-aggravated laugh. "And *you*. You need to stop obsessing, stop reading books and relax."

I made for the stairs and didn't look back. It was the final insult. I didn't read because I was obsessed; I read because it had always been one of the greatest pleasures of my life. And how else was I supposed to glean information about fertility if I couldn't afford to pay for it at a clinic like this? 'I'm not one of your fucking celebrities,' I thought, 'with thousands of pounds to throw at the problem.'

That was the last cognisant thought I had before the tumult of emotion broke loose, carrying me along in its path, not knowing where I was going or what I was doing. Tears already streaming, I ran down the stairs, straight past reception and out onto the street. It was left to Chris to stand in the waiting room, next to the glossy magazine covers that proclaimed the clinic to the world, and hand over £165. I hit the pavement and kept running, straight across the road, down the footpath on the other side and around the corner towards the shops and cafés on the high street. Escape, escape, I had to escape.

I know I ran through banked-up traffic and along crowded sidewalks, but I didn't see any of it. It was as if I had been overtaken by blind panic, the irresistible drive to get away from a looming threat while I still could. When, running without looking back, I saw an ancient stone church rising from the pavement, it seemed like the right place to go. I ran up to the heavy wooden door and flung myself inside. Chris would not find me here. I sat in a pew at the back, dropping my head almost into my own lap as I wept uncontrollably.

After nearly five years of infertility, it had finally happened: I had reached the point at which I couldn't take any more. I broke down, bent in two in the back of a church in central London. Other people were praying there, nearer the front. For the first time in my life, I admitted that I needed someone else's help. 'Please come and talk to me', I thought, 'please, please help me.' No one came; I sat alone in the pew for an hour, unable to stem the flow of tears. I would never be a mother. Wasn't it obvious? Hadn't I been kicked back nearly every time I had tried? It wasn't meant to happen, all along it had never been meant to happen. There was no quid pro quo for the fact I'd been adopted; there was no reprieve, no miracle treatment, I really would be childless. For my entire life, I would never have a family of my own to love. The thought took my breath away.

My body was inert, but my mind was still running. It whirred on, then, to thoughts about *how* I had been kicked back, *why* I had been kicked back and, nearly every time, the answer lay with Chris. The man who had been handed every privilege in life did not have it within him to let someone else stand before him in line. Even at a fertility clinic, even when it had been pre-agreed that it was me who needed to talk things through. That's when I felt it, the slow shift within that happens when anger begins to fill the void left by sorrow. I was surprised to find that I was going to get up off that pew and I was going to go to work in an hour, as planned. It was time to stop crying once and for all. Suddenly and surely, I knew exactly what I had to do.

⚜ ⚜ ⚜

Before walking into the office as if it was just another Saturday, I paid 20p to use the public toilets on Victoria Station and spent five minutes wiping away all traces of tears and reapplying my make-up.

As I was striding purposefully towards my desk, I bumped into Gavin, a colleague who was good friends with Chris.

"Hi Louise," he said with a smile. "Dragged yourself back from Switzerland, I see. But, hey, where's Chris?"

"I don't know," I replied firmly. "That's no longer my problem."

"Oh," he managed, momentarily lost for words. "I'm really sorry to hear that."

I turned on my heel and walked away. "I'm not," I said under my breath.

I logged on and began working immediately, immersing myself in the words before me on the screen.

After about ten minutes, I was interrupted by Chris, who arrived at my desk looking dishevelled and upset, still wearing his coat and with his satchel slung across his body.

"Where have you been?" he asked urgently. "I didn't know where you went. I had to stop to pay the bill and then you were nowhere to be seen. I've been worried about you."

"Get lost," I said, without looking up. "I'm working."

"Sweetheart," he protested. "It wasn't my fault. I didn't mean it to—"

"I'm *not* doing this at work," I hissed. "Just sit down, log on and get on with it."

He shot me a look that was part hurt and part disdain then stalked off to a desk on the other side of the office, thankfully ignoring his usual work station opposite mine. "What's this?" A colleague guffawed as he walked by. "Haven't fallen out, have you? I thought Switzerland was supposed to be neutral."

"No," I lied. "Screen's broken. We'll have to get by on our own for a while."

Chris might have created waves in my private life, but he was sure as hell not going to affect my career. I fully intended to bluff this out and ensure I at least appeared professional.

Later in the afternoon, I walked down the empty corridor to the women's toilets. When I came back out again, Chris was waiting for me.

"Why did you tell Gavin we'd broken up?" he demanded.

"Because we have," I said. "You seriously think I'd stay with you after that?"

"But Louise, this is ridiculous! How can you say that when we've been trying to have a family together? What about trying to have a family?"

"I don't need you. I'd be better off on my own." I defiantly stared him down. "I'm going to find a sperm donor."

"How fucking *dare* you?" he shouted.

"You absolute *cunt!*" I spat back through gritted teeth. I had never in my life been outraged enough to call anyone that word; it was another dubious first during this tug-of-war with infertility.

An hour later, Chris was at my desk again. I ignored him, resolutely staring straight ahead at words I was not reading.

"Louise," he whispered. "This is important. Please, just listen to me. I've telephoned to complain. I've spoken to Janet Brown and I've told her that she's had a devastating effect. I've let her know I'm not happy about the way she conducted herself. It was appalling."

I continued to gaze at the screen, refusing to acknowledge his presence. "I just wanted you to know," he added undeterred, "that I'm doing something about this. I've told her I *will* be following it up. A consultation at a fertility clinic should *not* cost you a relationship."

He waited in vain for a response, then gave an agitated sigh and thumped at high speed back across the office. I enjoyed a private smile at the thought of Janet Brown enduring one of his dressing-downs, of realising that he wasn't all crinkly eyes and mellifluous voice.

Later, I used my dinner break to spend £27 booking a last-minute room at a student hostel behind the Royal Albert Hall. I arrived around midnight, not knowing where Chris was and not caring.

As I lay in the single bed, almost within touching distance of the study desk on the opposite side of the room, I felt as relieved as if I had just been released from a chamber deep under the ocean. Finally, I could breathe freely once more. I walked to the window and looked out at the street-lit view of the Albert Hall. This was why I had come to London in the first place, this frisson I experienced whenever I saw at first-hand these treasures that I never could have imagined, growing up in a paddock in the middle of nowhere. A flicker of recognition slithered through my body; I remember now. This is what it had felt like when I lived in London on my own. I was free to breathe my own air and dream my own dreams. I skipped over the bit about having to pay my rent with a credit card advance and continued with my reverie. There was no one to hold me back, no one to trip me up when I tried to move forward. Yes, that's how it would be from now on. Just me, moving forward at last.

Twenty-two

I DIDN'T EXPECT A fertility clinic to make the pain of failed conception evaporate in a puff of smoke. I didn't expect it to hand me a gurgling baby bundle precisely nine months after my consultation. I didn't expect it, necessarily, to uncover exactly what was wrong with me. However, I did expect that someone who worked at a fertility clinic would understand what it feels like to be infertile.

It seemed I had failed to understand that fertility is just another business, with overheads and a balance sheet, no different from an engineering factory or a building contractor. Some builders might empathise about the discomfort caused by a leaking roof, some might not. It was the same with fertility treatment. Like all businesses, what it was really built on was the transaction that followed the consultation. You handed over your cash and you might, or might not, go on to have a family. If you did have a child, the clinic would certainly be pleased; after all your baby news would improve its overall success rate, the yardstick that could entice new clients. But would the clinic be pleased because, in creating new life, it had also handed your own life back to you? Who could tell? Much like choosing a builder, it depended where you went and who you saw.

After our consultation with Janet Brown, I was at first distraught and then disbelieving. Surely that couldn't have happened? Not at one of the 'best' clinics there was? When the initial flood of emotion had subsided, I went over and over it in my mind and still could not make sense of it. All I kept hearing was *Ms Together, Ms Together,* like a playground taunt chanting inside my head. Sometimes the chant morphed into *what do you want a sperm donor for?* Yeah, *Ms Together,* what do you want with a sperm donor?

I couldn't deny that Janet Brown must have felt as if she'd been hit by an express train that Saturday afternoon. Chris and I had built our relationship on animated conversation, and between us, we could bat words back and forth at an alarming pace. Even one of our most positive discussions could whip up, down and along at a confusing rate. I knew that as well as anyone; it was tiring sometimes, the way we talked.

I also imagined that, when Janet Brown went to work that Saturday, she didn't exactly expect to be confronted with a five-year-old argument about performance anxiety. And, in all fairness, no one told her that it was the last thing we wanted to discuss. I did try to say so, but the effort was clumsy, pressurised, flustered; I was easily dismissed.

She also didn't stop to read the introductory questionnaires we had filled in, so she didn't realise I'd already travelled a bumpy road and that the fall-out from those past challenges might influence the way I faced the current challenge. I wondered, when things got heated why hadn't she just called time-out, on the pretext of reading those forms? I couldn't conjure the answer to that, but I did know that she was given one piece of crucial information at the outset: we had been trying to conceive for nearly five years.

I could concede that, in my frustration and despair, I might well have come across as unpleasant, but staff at these clinics work with infertile couples every day. Can they not see that infertility is dark and messy and gritty? It's hardly clean white walls and framed magazine covers – why did they all choose white when infertility was the very opposite of white? Why did they arrange a box of tissues on a table as if that displayed some sort of understanding? For some of us, particularly those grappling with prolonged infertility, they'd be better off placing a punchbag in the corner. I see their glossy adverts and their luxury supplements and I want to shout through a megaphone: you don't know what pain looks like! I might not have sniffled into that blessed box of tissues, but it didn't mean I wasn't hurting. I want to tell them – we don't always cower and sob in the face of infertility, sometimes we fight back. Should I really have to explain to an expert in the field that infertility doesn't present itself in a neatly-wrapped package? Surely, if you knew someone had been trying to have a family for five years, then you might expect they could be riven with anger, frustration, maybe even a hint of resentment? Or were all the other couples who came here white and neat and perfect, too?

That Saturday afternoon at the Belinda Cooper Clinic, I had never felt so misunderstood. I didn't expect that an hour-long discussion would entirely go my way, but I *did* expect not to be kicked when I was already on the floor. Chris and I were the ones who paid £165 for that consultation but, afterwards, we were also the ones left to point out the obvious: if someone has been trying to conceive for five years, it is no help at all to call them *Ms Together,* or to admonish them for trying to glean information about their infertile state. Janet Brown might not have seen us coming, she might not have anticipated what would unfold, but surely, certainly, the number one rule would be to suspend judgment. How could she possibly know who was telling the truth? How could she possibly know what had really gone before? And wasn't the truth subjective anyway?

Maybe fertility clinics are so used to creating life, to playing God in a way, that some of the people within really start to believe they are all-seeing omnipotent beings. All I knew was that, with the wrong woman on the wrong day, a consultation like the one we endured could have had catastrophic results. As it was, a relationship was broken up, I was left distraught and Chris was left agitated and upset. We were not exactly about to 'relax and enjoy each other's company'.

It is now more than six years since that consultation with Janet Brown and it still has the power to invoke a range of deep-seated emotions. About once a fortnight for several years preceding our appointment, I used to take a shortcut down the street on which the clinic sits. I have never taken that shortcut since. Even now, I cannot bear to be in the vicinity of the building where one of my most difficult days was played out.

Janet Brown's approach caused a great deal of damage that afternoon, but what no one may have realised is that the worst damage was yet to come. And it is this: in the six years since that appointment, there have been dark, lonely days when I should have sought professional help – really needed to seek it – as I began to succumb, once and for all, to infertility. However, because of that searing experience, I have been afraid to reach out and ask, to tell someone that I'm not sure if I can cope. What would I do if they judged me so openly, if they saw me there in turmoil and sarcastically dubbed me *Ms Together*?

❧ ❧ ❧

It turned out that, after our consultation, Chris had spent his Saturday afternoon at work pacing up and down at the far end of the office while outlining his complaint on the telephone to not only Janet Brown but to Belinda Cooper herself.

"You have just destroyed a relationship," he told them. "Your badly handled session was the straw that broke the camel's back."

He demanded that his concerns be investigated and that someone get back to him with some sort of conclusion. Chris, who stuffed unopened bills into his dressing-gown pocket and mislaid umbrellas all over London, was nevertheless not a man to be trifled with when he had a complaint to make.

We did not see or even speak to each other for several more days. Thankfully, we were working different shift patterns for the rest of our stay in London and, Chris, despite realising I hadn't gone back to our B&B on Saturday night, had continued to sleep on Gavin's couch. He left voice messages on my mobile phone, but I didn't bother to play them. I was done with this relationship and I wasn't ready to hear what he had to say; Janet Brown might have taken pot-shots at me but, as far as I was concerned, he was the one who had repeatedly handed her the ammunition. They could cover their tracks as much as they liked after the event, but it was too late – none of us would get to take back what had happened.

Chris finally cornered me in the office on Tuesday night.

"Look," he began, "we really need to talk. There are things you need to know. Janet Brown has phoned me back this week – she admits she got it wrong." He eyed me nervously as if assessing my response, but I remained expressionless.

"At least tell me if you're coming back to Switzerland with me tomorrow," he said. "We can't just leave it like this."

I didn't know what I was going to do; that was the problem. All my belongings were in Switzerland – maybe it made sense to use my train ticket to go and collect them? I was starting to run short on the anger that had been fuelling me, and where would I go tomorrow if I didn't go to Switzerland? I realised how isolated I had become from anyone who could offer support. The more infertility dragged on, the more I seemed to be uncomfortable spending time with other people. The things they said about it! The questions they asked. I could just about manage being infertile, but I couldn't deal with some of the extraneous baggage that came with it. I liked hiding amongst the rows of grapevines in a place where no one could find me. I didn't realise then that a comfort zone is not necessarily comforting in the longer term.

❦ ❦ ❦

We got back together again. I don't know how, but we did. Even at the time, part of me knew it wasn't something I would have done in my twenties, when I was surrounded by family and friends and not the slightest bit interested in having children. However, I was committed to this path now – five years committed – and I didn't know how to get off it, not without jeopardising the slim hopes I still nurtured of raising a family. Maybe fertility is like an addiction; in the pursuit of your idea of nirvana, it ends up seizing control of you. It causes you to pursue it at all costs, even well past the time when it has ceased to be healthy. However, when you're going through it, when you're right there *in* it, you sometimes think as logically as a person suffering withdrawal pains. There you are, writhing around in agony, overwhelmed by the desire for the very thing that is causing you such torment. How is it possible right then to know what's good for anyone and what's not?

So, I found myself sitting at the kitchen table in Switzerland with Chris, going over what had happened in London.

"I genuinely didn't mean to hijack your session," he said. "That was the last thing I wanted to do."

"But you made the whole thing about you," I protested. "You took it over completely."

"That really wasn't my intention at all, please believe me." Chris's knees jigged in tandem under the table. "I just wanted to mention the performance anxiety, or whatever you like to call it, because I wanted to show you I was taking responsibility for it. Then she kept asking me all those questions and I really did *not* want to talk about it, you must know that."

I resolutely studied the swirls on the coffee mug that sat empty before me. "Well, you said a heck of a lot for someone who didn't want to talk about it."

"But Lou!" He tried, and failed, to hold my gaze. "I was worried you'd think I was trying to avoid it again if I said I didn't want to go down that road. I didn't feel like I had the choice and you saw what it was like – she kept on and on about it."

"Okay then," I said, trying a new tack. "Why didn't you stick up for me? Why did you just sit back and let her make those comments? It wasn't right and you know it."

Chris shook his head with a sharp, exaggerated flick. "I'm furious with her for saying those things, Lou. That was not the way I would expect a woman in her position to conduct herself."

"Yeah, well it's easy to say that now. You were the one who just twisted everything around to suit yourself."

"It wasn't like that at all, I wish you'd believe me!"

And so it went on, like the imaginary tennis match Janet Brown had appeared to be umpiring.

"You must still want us to be together," Chris attempted. "Because you looked so sad when she said we couldn't make love anymore. I knew what you were thinking, I knew you were remembering *You Do Something To Me,* on the floor. I was thinking that, too – we're more similar than you know."

I eyed him angrily across the table. "But you acted as if I'd kicked you in the guts. Even though you *knew* what I meant."

Chris pushed back his chair and stood up in a rush. "I don't know why I did it! It was just too pressurised. She shouldn't have even let it get to that stage."

"I knew you were thinking exactly the same as me," I replied sadly. "That's why it hurt so much. You made it look like I was just being out of order, but you could have told her … and you didn't."

"I'm sorry, " he said, eyes brimming with tears. "I'm so, so sorry."

After hours of batting the issue back and forth, it was clear that this was one tennis match neither of us could win. However, we had at least reopened the lines of communication. Later in the day, Chris told me about the phone calls he had made to the clinic and the response he had received. "Janet Brown phoned me back and apologised," he explained. "She said she'd been back over it, read through our forms, and realised she had got it wrong. She went straight to Belinda Cooper, put her hands up and told her that."

The upshot was that I had been offered a free session with Belinda Cooper herself. We could wipe the slate clean and start again from the beginning.

"Ha!" I cut in. "I wouldn't even *set foot* in that building, let alone speak to any of them. Not in a million years."

"Yes," said Chris, smiling wryly. "I rather expected that would be your response. I did think it might have contained a few expletives though."

Finally, we both laughed.

"Well, what did you tell them then? You know, without including the swear words?"

"I just said, 'I don't think Louise is quite ready to be thinking about another consultation just yet.' Or something like that."

For the first time in days, I smiled at him. "Thanks," I said. "For ringing them up. At least you gave it a go in the end."

"I just did what I thought was right," Chris replied, unable to disguise the relief flooding across his face.

He knew me well enough to know that normal service was about to be resumed. Sure enough, it was not long before we stopped trading allegations and began swapping apologies – in a manner of speaking.

"I'm not sorry about Janet Brown," I began with mock defiance. "Because you acted like a complete knob."

"Excuse me?" Chris interjected. "Are we not supposed to be making up?"

"Stop butting in and I'll get there. I was going to say I'm *really* sorry for calling you the c-word. That totally crossed the line. I feel pretty bad about it anyway."

"Not half as bad as Nicholas Chalk felt about it," Chris said with a grin.

"What? Nicholas Chalk? What do you mean?"

"You didn't see him, did you? I thought you were too angry to have taken it in."

I still didn't understand what he meant. "Nicholas Chalk came around the corner just as you called me an absolute *c-word*. Right at that moment," Chris finally revealed, looking a little too pleased with himself.

"No! He didn't?"

"Yes, he certainly did. I thought those high-waisted pants of his were going to fall right off, he looked so taken aback."

"Great," I groaned. "Now our boss thinks I'm a mad woman."

"And I'm supposed to be the bolshie one." Chris laughed. "They might not think you're quite so mild-mannered anymore."

"Oh great," I said again. "How embarrassing. How … *unprofessional*. I'm not going back to London next time – you can go on your own."

A few days later, we were lying together on the floor in a patch of sunlight and listening to music.

The next thing we knew, we were doing exactly what Janet Brown had banned us from doing. Bryan Ferry was purring 'Make you feel my love' and it just felt right. Natural. Like it used to be, back in the day when it was a different floor and a different soundtrack.

As we finished, Chris leaned back, still breathing heavily, and exclaimed to the ceiling, "Fuck you, Janet Brown!"

We broke into laughter, as if releasing the last vestiges of tension, then, still resting on top of me, he nuzzled his face into my neck.

Neither of us was thinking about whether we had just conceived a child.

"I've missed you," he whispered huskily into my ear.

TWENTY-THREE

IT WAS MY THIRTY-NINTH birthday. I wasn't thinking about opening gifts or sharing a celebratory drink. What I was thinking was: if I don't conceive within three months, I'll be forty years old before I become a mother. Forty. How had this happened? When we began trying to have a family, I had just turned thirty-four; I would never have left it until my forties to become a parent. Never. No, I was going to tread the sensible middle ground; I would have my family in my thirties. Throughout my twenties, I had feared it would be too early, that there might be resentments, both for me and for any child who arrived to find that their mother wasn't quite ready for them. However, I always knew that I would have my children before the age of forty – well before then. Wasn't forty practically middle-aged?

My own mother was forty years old when she adopted me and I was often aware of the generation gap yawning between us. It doesn't matter now that I am an adult, proud of her strength, resilience and independence. But when I was a teenager, it mattered. Ironically, as I edged closer to my forties, I wondered if it was fair to knowingly provide my children with an 'older' mother, to understand already that the generation gap might be too big for them too.

I had long been calculating how old my children 'should' be. If I had conceived immediately, in 2003, I would now have a four-year-old. I had thought about that with every year that passed, adjusting the age upward as one barren twelve months followed another. As I turned thirty-nine, another calculation emerged. How old would *I* be when my children started nursery, graduated from high school, got married? If they had children of their own, could I be an active, helpful grandmother? I did not want them having to spoon-feed their decrepit old mum at the same time as they were weaning a toddler. This was an example of the way that, even after nearly five years of infertility, I still believed I could control life if I thought ahead, if I planned for it. The flaws in my thinking are underlined by the fact that my mother, who is now in her eighties, still lives alone, plays competitive sport twice a week and drives herself to an exhaustive range of social events. Every so often, she sends a text message to say she has been pulled over and issued with a speeding ticket. If she does sit still, it's to drink a bottle of beer after table tennis. So much for being an 'older' mother. She has also outlived by many years some of my friends' much younger mothers, underlining the fact that there can be no knowing.

And yet here I was, still persisting with my speculation about a future that might never unfold. A helpful grandmother? So far, I hadn't even managed to entice sperm to meet egg, let alone fertilise it and begin the creation of a dynasty. Why did I always think I knew what was going to happen just because I had a plan and it appeared to make sense?

On my thirty-ninth birthday, I sensed panic looming just over the horizon, already altering the atmosphere and making it that little bit harder to breathe. Forty. Forty. Forty. There it was, I could almost see it. Any more than three months and my entire thirties would have passed without me entering motherhood. There were bound to be stats about it some-where, a percentage graph showing my diminishing chances of reproducing now that I was about to swap one decade for another. I didn't want to read those stats and definitely not on my birthday; it would be a bit like opening a card that read simply: 'You're doomed!'

I spent my birthday reminding myself that I was only one day into being thirty-nine – forty was an entire twelve months away. It made no difference; it kept poking its nose into my thirty-ninth birthday celebrations anyway.

Chris didn't notice; he had a bit of a swagger about him that day. We started out early, at 7am, to return the company car he had been using while working on a prestigious month-long contract in Switzerland. I had been travelling back and forth to London on my own; each time I returned, Chris was out at work, but I always found our fridge stocked with a specially-chosen selection of my favourite foods and a loving note left on the table. After our temporary break-up not long before, he had been making an effort.

On the night of my thirty-ninth birthday, we drove to a nearby village for dinner and fell immediately into our usual routine. As we neared the main road, Chris said, as he always did, "Just remind me, Lou – which way do I turn?" And, like a traffic marshal, I held my hand out to the right, our way of ensuring he did not negotiate the Swiss roundabout in the wrong direction.

This was one of his vague eccentricities, like the lost possessions and the unopened bills – he had no sense of direction, particularly in Switzerland where he was further confused by being on the 'wrong' side of the road. He also couldn't see that well at night, or necessarily recognise our regular driving routes. However, he insisted on driving that night, since it was my birthday.

We were nearly there, at the restaurant, and it happened in an instant.

As we accelerated towards a 'stop' sign on a B-route, a set of headlights loomed closer and closer along the curve of the road we were about to join. Still we didn't slow down; it appeared we were about to drive straight through the intersection and into a head-on collision.

So much for worrying about forty; I wasn't even going to see it. My reflexes kicked in. "Stop! Stop," I urged, without thinking.

"All right!" Chris raised his voice as, just in time, we jolted to a halt. "Why do you always have to be so critical of me? It's not necessary."

He snapped his head towards me, fixing me with a cold accusing stare. "For God's sake Louise!"

"Wow," I said quietly.

I had driven this road with Jai once, his arm hanging from the window of our camper van as we sang Bob Marley songs together. Suddenly the homesickness that had been building all day washed over me and I wished I could somehow slide from this vehicle to that, back to the safety of 1994. In present time, Chris was still speaking, fast and agitated, about how it wasn't his fault that we had nearly crashed.

"But no one blamed you for anything," I said.

Nevertheless, he was soon shouting at me on the honey-cobbled streets of one of the most admired villages in Switzerland. Before I had even cancelled dinner and driven home myself, tearful and angry as the row reverberated around the car, I knew with sickening certainty that, this time, it really was over. It couldn't have been any clearer if a handwritten message had dropped from the sky.

Luckily, people don't tend to ask how you spent the night of your thirty-ninth birthday; it's one of those 'nothing' numbers, no milestone, no big deal. That's just as well because the way I passed the rest of the evening represented a very warped coming of age – I experienced a panic attack. This had never happened before, even under all the previous years' pressure of trying to conceive.

However, the handwritten message from the sky had an addendum: I appeared to be ovulating. Once again, it was impossible to do anything about it.

No. No. No! This wasn't how it was supposed to be. This wasn't how life turned out for me. My breathing began to come in gasps and my heart was pumping as if I had just run all the way home. No! This couldn't be happening. I was never going to become a mother. No. No. No. *No*. How had this happened? How? How had I gone from living a normal life in my twenties to this? What had I done?

When I turned twenty-nine, I sang drunken karaoke and danced home down the street with my strong, funny, laid-back fiancé and a warm gaggle of friends who felt like family. That girl did not turn thirty-nine like this. That girl had options. My breathing grew faster and more laboured until I could feel my heart beating in my throat. Not only had I got things monumentally wrong, but there was barely time to do anything about it.

All I heard over and over, thrumming through my body, was 'No, no, no!' But it was too late, I couldn't stop it, the worst had already happened. How could I ever bring a child into this seething, churning relationship? I was an idiot. The stage had been set for me when I was twenty-nine; now, year by year, it had emptied out. I was just like one of those lottery winners who scoops the jackpot and blows it all within months. Would infertility always have ensured that I lost everything or had I done that myself? I heaved and gasped and rocked. I never thought it would come to this; somehow, pathetically, I had always believed that I would be a mother. In the end, I would be a mother. Now it was slipping away and I didn't know what to do to get it back.

Chris charged in and out of the room, not knowing what to do or say to fix his broken-down girlfriend.

He began with, "This is silly. It doesn't need to be like this," and moved on to, "Come on sweetheart, it's okay. I'll look after you."

"Look after me?" I gasped. "After that? Who does that? And this year of all years." I curled into a foetal ball, sobbing uncontrollably. "Don't you think I'm already hurting enough?"

"Please!" Chris rushed over and wrapped his arms around me. "I just want to make it right. Let me make it right."

I reared up in bed, shrugging him off. "I should never have ended up with you! Oh my God. What have I done?"

"It's not over," Chris promised. "It's not over. You could still have children. You don't know for sure that you won't."

"Your ego wrecks everything," I began to accuse before the same refrain took over: "What have I done? What have I done?"

And onwards throughout the night formed a darker thought: 'What have I become?'

The next day, I was at home, motionless, drained and heavy, and Chris was out walking again, as he always did when we argued. I ignored his call when it trilled through on my mobile phone, left it for ten minutes before I dragged myself over to listen to the message that had persistently bleeped for attention every ninety seconds.

At first, I was baffled. What was this? Then I heard a familiar voice in the background, above a humming noise that sounded like machinery in motion. I realised that what I could hear was a car, apparently being driven by Robert, our friend from the next village; he had obviously offered Chris a lift and now Chris had sat down on his mobile phone and dialled my number by accident. This was another of the things he often did, forgetting to lock the screen and making international calls from a supermarket queue or phoning business contacts late at night from the tube. He must have shifted in the passenger seat; I could suddenly hear more clearly. When his voice echoed down the line, it was like being slapped and not quite believing it had happened.

"My family have always said she's not good for me," Chris was complaining. Robert, a gentleman to the end, offered no opinion. "My family worry that she's ..." and suddenly the background crackling ramped up a notch and the message abruptly cut off.

His words cut deep; I had thought Rose and I genuinely cared about each other. It wasn't Chris who had arranged and cooked Christmas dinner for her over the past three years; it was me. The same for birthdays and Mother's Day. Yet his family had been discussing me, deciding I was unworthy of him? What exactly had he been telling them? Well, that was it. They could get just what they wanted. He could go right back where he had come from.

My main source of energy these days seemed to be anger; now it propelled me from zombie-like inertia into a whirling dervish of fury. In an instant, I had snatched up two framed photos of us, smiling out from a bookshelf, and hurled them outside onto the patio. When Chris finally walked back up the driveway, the images were still lying there, as far apart as they obviously belonged.

He walked inside, wielding a dented frame.

"Why would you do this?" he demanded. "I've said I'm sorry for last night. I didn't mean to ruin your birthday, you know I never meant for any of it to happen."

Not only had I become a person who threw things, I had also become a person who shouted.

"I heard you! I heard you tell Robert that your family think I'm not good enough for you."

Chris looked stricken, confused, unable to work out how I had managed to overhear a private conversation in a moving vehicle.

"You very helpfully left me a message." I brandished my phone. "Would you like to hear it? Or shall I just tell you?

You were backstabbing me *again*. Well, you can all get stuffed. You can cook your own mother's Christmas dinner this year."

Chris was obviously panicked now.

"No!" he stressed. "No, none of this is right. Mum never said that about you. She'd never say anything like that about you – you know how much she thinks of you."

"Yes, and so does Robert. Thanks so much for that."

I had made up my mind. It didn't matter if I was throwing away our last chance to have a family; I was not going to stay with Chris, not this time. One of us would have to leave; eventually, it was Chris who reluctantly packed a sports bag before I drove him to the train station in steely silence.

He turned to me as we came to a halt in the parking lot.

"Please don't do this. Don't make me go."

"It's already done. Just go."

"But I don't want to go. I want to stay and work this out."

I checked the rear-vision mirror and prepared to back out of the parking space, not listening to the words he still urgently delivered. Then, finally, he was standing outside, his bag on the ground beside him; I drove off and didn't look back.

When I returned home and walked into the empty lounge, I was overtaken by the same sense of calm that had settled around me during the first night I had spent alone after our earlier break-up less than two months before. I had been blinded by infertility; I realised that now. I had wanted a family so badly that I would have made any compromise to achieve it. Unwittingly, I had already given away far too much. Was that why Chris had been so cavalier at times? Did he know? Was he banking on me being desperate to have children?

I picked up a notebook and walked outside to sit in the sun. Dudley and Duke instantly appeared, jostling for hugs as if intuiting that that was exactly what I needed. Dudley eventually stretched out on the grass at my feet, while Duke sat on his haunches and earnestly looked on as I began to write:

Action Plan (make sure you do it)
- Get a new job
- Find somewhere to live

At last, Chris was gone and I was moving on. Now that I was on my own again, I wasn't going to become a mother in my thirties, that much was clear. But rather than feeling bereft, it was as if some of the pressure had lifted with Chris's departure. Perhaps, if I got things right this time, I could still find a way. It might even be easier, now that there was no one holding me back at every stage.

"I know, I know," I said to Duke. "I'll have to stop chucking photo frames and yelling at people if I want to be someone's mother."

He harrumphed down to the ground, bored now with whatever it was that I was up to.

I shook my head, as if dazed. How had I become this frenzied person? Was it infertility, was it my relationship with Chris or was it infertility *and* the relationship? Maybe it was me. Maybe underneath I'd always been frenzied and just didn't realise it yet. I hadn't always dealt with work stress as well as I could have, I knew that much. I wasn't that fixated on fertility, though, was I? I'd tried without trying for more than two years, I'd given up temperature charting within months of discovering it and, even now, I still hadn't given in to constantly peeing on ovulation sticks or pregnancy tests. No, all things considered, I was not a pregnancy obsessive.

I wasn't yet ready to see that Chris might well have surveyed the past twenty-four hours and reached a vastly different conclusion. Fixations. They sneak up on you. And fixations of the biologically-driven kind are the most difficult to escape.

Unaware still of some of the most difficult lessons that infertility had to offer, I continued with my list:

- Streamline possessions

Hmm, what was the fourth thing I should do? It seemed to me that the challenges offered by points one and two were more than enough.

Just as I put down my pen and began to consider the reality of returning to singledom at the age of thirty-nine, Dudley and Duke sprang to their feet in a synchronised flash. The vine-workers must be arriving, I thought. Or Mary and Ian, back from lunch with friends. But when I looked up, I saw a lone figure at the end of the driveway, carrying a sports bag and trudging towards the house.

Oh no. How had he got back here so quickly?

Dudley and Duke galloped up to Chris, ears flapping and tails wagging to a demented beat. "Traitors," I muttered under my breath as he bent down to greet them and they nudged him so enthusiastically that he nearly lost his balance.

I wasn't ready for this unexpected reunion. I didn't know where to look or what to say.

"I need water," Chris announced when he reached the house. "I'm gasping."

"How on earth did you get back here so fast?" I asked, ignoring his request and visualising the series of hills and valleys that lay between us and the train station.

"I started walking home and, just up from the station, a lady stopped to pick me up," he explained.

"A lady?"

"Yes, English. In her fifties, I'd say. Anyway, she thought I looked a bit hot and bothered and that I might need some help." He was breathing heavily, wiping his forehead with the back of his hand and wearing the righteous expression of one who has just completed an ultra-marathon.

"I didn't have any water," he continued. "I was in all sorts of trouble in that heat. I think she felt a bit sorry for me, walking in the sun."

"Of course she did," I said. "Of course she bloody did."

Chris responded to the trouble he found himself in by booking another sperm test. "I want to show you I'm serious about this," he said. "I won't let you down this time."

The promise was enough to draw me back in. I looked on warily as he rifled through a random collection of items from the bottom of his work bag. Eventually, between a crumpled pile of receipts and a disintegrating pack of chewy mints, he triumphantly unearthed the details he was searching for. It was one useful piece of information provided by Janet Brown – how to arrange a new test at the laboratory used by her clinic. A little later, Chris emerged from the lounge to inform me that he would be taking the test the next time we were in London.

And so it played out later that week, the latest instalment in the ongoing saga of the sperm analysis. The scene this time was a four-star hotel we normally couldn't afford. However, we had managed to book a room at bargain rates, thanks to a renovation programme that had turned part of the usually grand resort into a building site. You couldn't tell that from within our room, though. It was opulently furnished, with mood lighting that delicately picked out the monogrammed stationery and the marble bathroom units.

"At least you've got romantic surroundings this time," I noted as the day of the test arrived and Chris prepared himself for the now familiar routine of providing bodily fluids for inspection. "Velvet curtains. What more do you want?"

"Let's hope it does the trick," he said nervously. "What time's the taxi coming again?"

"2.15pm, you've got a while yet. Better pace yourself, I suppose. Well, good luck! Let me know how you get on."

I kissed him on the cheek and picked up my bag, ready to leave for the office.

"Where are you going?" Chris enquired, looking stricken.

"Work, 2.30 start. Remember?"

"But what if I can't do it on my own? I thought you were going to stay to help."

"Huh?"

"I might need you. To go downstairs and keep the taxi waiting if … you know …"

He looked so alarmed that I rushed to reassure him. "Okay then. Okay. I can stay. But don't worry about it – it'll be fine. I'll just tell him you're in a meeting that's running over if worst comes to worst."

I could see Chris battling to keep all thoughts of that scenario at bay. "It won't, though," I added hurriedly. "You'll be fine. Look how well you did that first time we went to the hospital."

"Yes," he sighed. "But I'm older now, how do I know I've still got it in me?"

"For Pete's sake, if you're that worried about it, I'll go and buy you a magazine," I joked.

"No!" he insisted. "No. I feel much better now I know you're here."

I stole a glance at the clock. 1.45pm. I should have left for work ten minutes ago. Mentally, I was calculating how I could still get there on time. Maybe Chris's taxi could take me on to the office after the laboratory. Yes, maybe the taxi would do it. Although I'd still be late. It was a busy route; it could even be slower than the tube. Damn! I tried to appear unconcerned, light-hearted.

"Can I have a hug?" Chris asked forlornly. "I feel a bit funny."

"I know," I sympathised, sliding up next to him on the bed. "It'll be done soon, though. And at least you're here with me, not in some clinic with people walking up and down outside."

"Hmm." He rested his head on my shoulder. "Thanks for staying, sweetheart."

I remained silent, hoping he couldn't feel the tension mounting within my body. On some level, I had already begun to sense what was about to happen, or if not sensed it then feared it.

"Do you think it's too early to start now?" Chris asked suddenly. "Would it still be fresh enough? I mean, this is the problem – we can't be sure the taxi will turn up on time."

"It won't matter," I replied confidently. "The lab's just down the road. You've got quite a bit more leeway this time."

"Okay then," he said, heading to the bathroom with a plastic cup in hand. "Well, wish me luck."

Just as I reached into my bag to check for phone messages, he emerged again. "Where's my sample pot? Have we got my sample pot?"

I pointed to the desk on the far wall.

"Ah. Good. Okay. Good." And he disappeared back into the bathroom.

I watched each minute tick round on the digital clock next to the bed. As it moved closer and closer to the time I should have been starting work, I fought back the urge to run out to the lift and then all the way down the road to the tube station. Surely he must be done soon. Weren't men obsessed with this very thing? Didn't they do it all the time? The bathroom door swished open, genteel and serene like the furnishings in the room. Phew. Now we could get going. I scooped up my bag and strode to the desk to grab the sample pot.

"Sorry about this, Lou. I'm just a bit hot. Maybe it might work better if we tried it together."

I willed all evidence of frustration to leave my face. "Don't worry," I said, smiling. "I'm sure it'll just be a false start. Maybe take a break for a bit. You've got time …"

Time. Time. Time. The one thing I did not have right then was time, and neither did he, not after the past fifteen minutes.

"Would you lie with me for a bit? Could we try it together?" he appealed.

It was the least sensuous offer I had ever had and, by quite some measure, the least tempting. And it appeared Chris wasn't feeling any more convinced by this awkward assignation than I was.

"Huh, and I thought public school boys could wank for England." I laughed, trying to lighten the mood.

After that, I tried my best. I trawled my mind for any sex tip I'd ever read in *Cosmopolitan* magazine at the age of twenty. Of course, I didn't actually need any help then; in those days I had the opposite problem. It must have been the intervening nineteen years of gravity and its unfortunate effects, I thought wryly. Surely we wouldn't have this problem if he really fancied me?

I felt like a spectacularly inept paid escort – I had a certain timeframe within which to achieve results and I was failing miserably. He didn't find me attractive. Deep down, I'd known that all along. Not only was I infertile, I was also increasingly incapable of arousing a man to action. I bet he wouldn't have this problem if I was a scrawny blonde, I thought darkly. At one point, I was so desperate to succeed that I even whipped out my leather gloves and put them on, just in case it might make him feel that he was with someone else; it wasn't me there next to him, it was the type of woman he could actually get excited about. It didn't work.

2.15. Any minute, the phone on the desk would bleep to let us know the taxi had arrived.

"Look," I started, somehow feeling that I was alone in this all over again. "I've got to get going. We'll just have to leave it for now."

"But my test! The taxi. I really want to get this done. It's just a silly thing. I'll get over it, I don't know why I'm being so silly."

Chris registered the expression he had seen haunt my face so many times over the years. "It's not you, sweetheart. Please don't think it's you."

"I'm really late for work. Just do whatever you feel like doing. I've got to go."

"You take the taxi," he said as I headed for the door to do just that. "I'll ring them. Maybe I can do it—" And I let the door shut behind me and ran for the lift.

All of this and we still would not have a basic sperm test result. Maybe I'd just carry on anyway, without one. But wasn't that exactly what I'd tried to do with Janet Brown? And look how that had turned out. I felt stymied at every turn.

I wasn't going to have children and, obviously, no one was ever going to fancy me again either. Face it, I told myself. As a woman, you're pretty much done.

Eventually, I rushed into the office, still blinking back tears. I was thirty-seven minutes late.

"What's this?" one of my male colleagues enquired loudly as I tried to slip by unnoticed. "Still on Swiss time?"

"Nah," chimed in another. "She'd have been early if she was on Swiss time. They're an hour ahead."

"It's not a Swiss thing," chortled a third. "It's a woman thing. You know what they're like – bloody spare me!"

Their laughter rumbled through the open-plan office as I sat down and tried to think of anything but sperm tests and fertility. And men. All of the three who had just spoken had children. Naturally, in all senses.

About two hours later, Chris rang my mobile phone.

"It was hideous," he wailed as soon as I answered and began walking to the usually empty corridor outside the women's toilets. "Appalling! You won't believe what has just happened to me. It was outrageous."

He paused as if for dramatic effect.

"Someone walked in on me!"

"No," I exclaimed. "No way. Hang on, was it the hotel cleaners? I thought they'd been already."

"No! Not there. At the laboratory. I was trying to do my sample at the laboratory."

"Oh no. That's even worse." I grimaced into the phone. "Urgh, I feel embarrassed just thinking about it."

"Imagine how I felt," Chris replied indignantly.

It turned out that, after I left the hotel, he had walked to the laboratory anyway, and explained that he had arranged to drop off a sample for testing, but had run out of time to collect it.

"They said I could do it there," he said, "so I thought I'd better try. Some people always do it that way apparently."

He was shown to a small white room containing only a sink and a chair. "There was nothing on the walls, it was just a white box – not even any magazines. Nothing."

"How did it happen?" I asked, still feeling mortified on his behalf.

"It was appalling," he repeated. "I had my trousers down around my ankles and I was, you know, trying to get it done. Then the door opened and a man walked right in!"

"Oh geez."

"He was carrying a tool kit," Chris continued, sounding unintentionally comical. "He was a plumber, come to fix the sink."

I put a hand to my face as if trying to block the mental image. "Bloody hell. What did you do?"

"Well, he left straight away. He just said, 'Sorry mate, sorry about that.'" I was unable to stifle a groan. "Then I put my jeans back on properly, went out to reception and gave them a piece of my mind. I can't believe they would let someone walk in on a client like that."

"But wasn't there a lock on the door? Didn't you check to make sure?"

"Of course I did!" Chris's voice rose above the background clamour of a city street. "I don't tend to go round doing that sort of thing in public. The lock didn't work, but I thought there'd be some sort of procedure. I didn't expect someone to just come marching in."

"Poor you. That's unbelievable."

"You do understand, don't you?" he asked. "That I couldn't continue in the circumstances?"

"Of course I do. What a nightmare." But I was unable to stop myself from adding, "This is exactly why it would have been so much better to have just done it in the hotel room in the first place."

"I know," he said. "I know. I just got a bit jittery about it. I wish I hadn't now. Obviously. It's just the pressure some-times, you know what it's like."

"Well, look, don't worry about it anymore – you don't have to go back there and see any of them again. Besides, they don't know who you are. I doubt they'd even recognise you."

"Not with my pants on, anyway," Chris retorted wryly.

We ended our call and I returned to work, heavy in the knowledge that we were plainly not meant to have children. How much clearer could the message be? Every time we had sought conventional medical help – every time – something had gone wrong. How many more roadblocks could be thrown up in front of us? From performance anxiety to plumbers; it was as if the fertility Gods were conspiring to ensure that we did not, under any circumstances, become parents.

It appeared that someone, somewhere, certainly wanted to tell us something. We had been travelling this road for nearly five years and we were no closer to parenthood than when we had started out. Actually, I realised with a jolt, it was even worse than that – now that I was thirty-nine, parenthood was further away than it had ever been.

TWENTY-FOUR

For the first couple of Decembers, Christmas felt pretty much the same as it always did. Since we were trying to have a family, there was even an added poignancy – maybe next year, it would be us. We would be the ones with a swaddled infant of our own, taking extra pleasure from the Christmas story because now we knew how it felt to be mother, father and baby. We would have baby's first stocking, first Christmas tree ornament, first Santa hat ... I knew that neither of us would have the slightest need for gifts of our own – any one of those moments would have been enough. But then it didn't happen. And Christmas, instead of offering a glimpse of magic, began to expose everything we were missing. Our child, who we so wanted to share this family time with, had not arrived. Every year, Chris and I linked fingers around either branch of the turkey wishbone and silently made our invocations. There was no need to ask, "What did you wish for?" We both knew. And, as time passed, the wishes became more wistful, then more pleading, then more of a request for an actual miracle.

I had grown up with big, sprawling family Christmases. At the beginning of every December, my brother Ray and I followed Mum through the paddocks to the thicket of native bush where we each had tree-huts. Mum would select a branch from one of the towering Cypresses, climb a ladder and saw it off near the trunk. That was our Christmas tree, shouldered back across the fields by Mum and Ray. After it had been lifted into a bucket and packed in earth, two additions would be placed beneath it – a homemade wreath with four advent candles and a 'baby' in a manger; every year, Mum took one of my dolls, dressed it in white and placed it in a handmade wooden cradle, on a bed of straw from the barn. On Christmas Eve, I dragged a sunlounger inside and lay on it under a blanket while we watched *The Two Ronnies' Christmas Special*, then the time would finally come and we would drive into town for midnight mass with its flickering candles and carol singing.

On Christmas day, some of my elder brothers and sisters would always be there, as well as Dad's mother, who was the only grandparent we had left, and a couple of aunts and uncles. It was loud and funny and relaxed and, being summer in the southern hemisphere, the celebrations took place both indoors and out. Mum made her secret-recipe fried chicken and there was always a 'proper' Christmas pudding, filled with foil-wrapped coins. Ray and I battled every year to be the one who got the 50 cent. On Christmas night, long after we had finally gone to bed, still savouring the goodies that had arrived that morning in stocking legs on the end of our bunks, we could hear the adults laughing and joking and pretending to argue over the board games they played in opposing teams. When I lay in bed and listened, I felt part of something. It wasn't just Mum and me and Ray, which sometimes felt a bit scary without Dad; there were all these others, who brought presents every year and played endless cricket matches with us, who read us stories and hugged us warmly as our family filled the house.

This was the Christmas I wanted my children to have. Chris felt the same, even though we both knew that our 21st century children would no doubt prefer to spend the day in front of a PlayStation screen. Already, I wanted Christmas to mean more to them than that, these children who didn't exist yet.

At the end of our first year without using birth control, we enjoyed a warmly familiar southern hemisphere Christmas at home. It was 2003, a year since my sister Vanda had visited me in London and I had confided that we were ready to have children. I was still so relaxed about it that I didn't feel anything missing that Christmas; I thought 2004 would probably be our year. But when the holiday season rolled around again twelve months later, there was just myself, Chris and his mum Rose, now aged eighty-eight. I cooked Christmas dinner for the three of us in our London flat and, sometimes during the day, the silence that settled around felt slightly too heavy. By 2005, Rose could no longer travel and, from then on, we spent Christmas at her retirement flat, Chris and I sharing a single bed that filled the entire spare room. I was thirty-seven years old; was I not supposed to have a home of my own, children running through the open-plan rooms and Granny resting in an armchair in the corner of the lounge? Suddenly, these quiet Christmases began to whisper that I had failed in some way.

I hoped to escape that gnawing feeling in 2006, when I was sure it would be different. We had moved to Switzerland, we would enjoy Christmas in a home that was made for children; surely something would change now that our life was more family-friendly? And there was nothing like a change of scene, particularly one that offered the novelty of Christmas in another country, to take the pressure off.

However, in the end, family called in another way. No one in the UK was going to see Rose on Christmas day; she would be alone. So we drove back to her flat, where the three of us sat around the table and chatted before watching TV for the rest of the day, each taking it in turns to doze off. While the others were napping, I sat on our bed and silently stared at the wall. It felt like time had fast-forwarded over a huge chunk of my life. The bustling Christmases I thought I would enjoy during my thirties didn't exist; I had leapt straight from early thirties to pensionerhood.

And what if this was Rose's last Christmas? What if she never got to hold the grandchild I had imagined her cradling each Christmas for several years now? I just wanted the day to be over, a new year to begin.

By 2007, as we moved into our sixth year of infertility, Christmas was no longer Christmas. It had become the time of year when I struggled the most. I couldn't sit there again, like an eighty-year-old, when I should have been with my children, when there should have been noisy, messy chaos unfurling all around me. The emptiness was too much to take. The longing to be a proper part of this family festival was starting to overwhelm me; I wasn't even sure that I could stop myself from bursting into tears at the table, around which would be sitting two middle-aged people and a pensioner. It became clear that we had to find another way to approach Christmas. So we found ourselves weighing the burden of the family we had never had against the commitment we owed to our existing family.

"We're not leaving Rose on her own," I told Chris. "But there must be a way we can make Christmas better for all of us."

In the end, I found a solution by once again turning infertility on its head – what were people with children always complaining that they missed?

"Peace and quiet?" ventured Chris. "Money? Sanity?"

"But we're missing those last two ourselves." I laughed. "All thanks to *not* having children." He gave a knowing smile. "Anyway," I added, "they don't get too many romantic weekends away, do they? So we should make the most of it. Let's do a romantic Christmas."

"What?" asked Chris, looking incredulous. "In Mum's single bed?"

"No, not that. What about a nice B&B down the road and we drive over to see your mum each day, cook the dinner and all the rest of it?"

He was instantly enthusiastic; we found a suitable romantic getaway and made a booking, using the credit card that normally paid for fertility investigations or treatments. After all, this was just another brick wall that infertility had brought us up against. Before we left Switzerland, I ordered the Christmas food online and had it delivered to Rose's flat. Chris had talked her through our plan several times, but she seemed confused by it, and even more baffled when he asked her to check the expiry dates on the grocery delivery. We hoped it would all work out when we got there.

Throughout our fertility struggles, I seem to have developed the knack of ovulating at stressful times. Or maybe any time would be stressful after you've been trying to conceive for more than five years. Whatever the case, I was apparently ovulating at yet another difficult time when we left the farmhouse that Christmas and began the nine-hour drive to Calais. As the seemingly endless autoroute stretched out before us, I had plenty of time to consider how I would raise the subject. Maybe I would wait and see where we spent the night; it was likely to be in a cheap motel in the north of France, breaking up the journey before travelling across to England the following day.

It was 9pm before we slouched on either side of the double bed in a motel room and shared a pizza, our box of wrapped Christmas presents sitting on the floor beside us.

I tried a strategy that I thought might work. "I didn't want to mention it," I began cautiously, "because it's been such a long day. But I seem to be a bit ovulatory."

"Oh," Chris said sharply, unable to disguise his anxiety.

"But I was thinking," I continued, "since we're so knackered, what do you reckon about leaving it 'til the morning?"

"Yes," he answered a little too quickly. "Yes, that sounds good. But I'm happy to try now as well, if you are."

I didn't call his bluff; I could read the relief all over his face now that he had been let off the hook, for this night at least. And there was that word, the one he had used so often over the years when he spoke about making love to me: try. He would try. I wished he would find another way of describing it; I hated knowing that it took such a very great level of effort to procreate with me. What did that say about me as a woman? Infertile and unattractive, that's what I was. Apparently, there was no limit to the amount of times I could hit myself over the head with that thought.

Nevertheless, the next morning we set about 'trying' on both levels to make a baby as year five of our quest for conception dissolved into year six. I attempted to keep things as bright and relaxed as I could; I needed this last little bit of hope that we might be spared another year of this. I needed to know that, however slim, there was a chance that this could be the month.

Ominously, it was taking a while and I could tell Chris was making a great effort to concentrate on the task he faced; in the absence of a natural connection, he was forcing it, willing it to happen. Then we heard a trolley rattling along the path outside, loud rapping on the door next to ours.

"Allo! Monsieur? Allo!" The room cleaners were ready to start their work.

"For goodness' sake," Chris barked.

It was the way someone might react if interrupted during an urgent, supremely stressful task in the office. Clearly agitated, Chris kept trying. But he was overheated now, and sweaty, and I knew it was time to give up.

"It was the cleaners," he said. "How are you supposed to relax with that racket going on?"

Half an hour later, we packed the car and continued driving north, ever closer to the romantic Christmas break we had planned. I was silent, gazing out at the passing shapes that morphed out of the frozen, foggy landscape.

"Sweetheart," said Chris, reaching across to hold my hand. "It wasn't you. It was the cleaners. Nobody could make love with them outside."

I said nothing, just continued to stare out, as numb as if I had been standing there in the icy mist. I wondered if any other women felt as pained about ovulation as I did. I welcomed it, almost in reverence, whenever it appeared; my poor old body was thirty-nine and yet, here it was, still trying to perform this miracle most months. But I dreaded it, too. It was heart-wrenching to see it wasted, this biological gift that could be taken away at any moment. And it was becoming impossible not to resent Chris, not because he had a problem but because he refused to do anything about it. He still couldn't admit to it, even if his denial meant we didn't have children, such was the power of the hold it had over him. It was the room cleaners, it was the heat, it was the alignment of the moon; it was anything except his own mind.

This ovulation stress was yet another challenge I hadn't anticipated once infertility took hold. I thought I would perhaps have a little cry once a month when my period arrived and I realised that we still had not managed to conceive. I didn't foresee all the private tears I would shed at ovulation. I often didn't need to wait two weeks; I knew already that there was no point hoping. It was over before it had even begun. I was starting to realise that sometimes hope is the only thing that keeps you going. What is there, without it, but emptiness?

Perhaps that was why my mind persisted in seeking out hope in the most ridiculous of places. He had entered me, hadn't he? Perhaps a drop of pre-ejaculatory fluid had been emitted, perhaps that would be enough to get me pregnant. I was conceived in a similar way, wasn't I, to two people who hadn't *actually* had sex? I ignored the fact that they were sixteen and seventeen and still managed to convince myself each month that a miracle had occurred within me. My breasts tingled, I felt nauseous, I was more tired than usual, I had suddenly gone off a favourite food. Was that a funny taste in my mouth?

I thought it was real, all of it, but I see now that it was only my mind seeking out enough hope to keep me afloat. It wasn't just wishful thinking, it was more than that – it was a survival instinct of sorts.

᪔ ᪔ ᪔

The B&B could have been set in one of those Christmas cards where the snow falls in symmetrical twinkles upon the perfect house in the perfect neighbourhood. It was a sixteenth century home, set on a steep cobbled lane lined with one historic building after another; the nearest pub, a thirty-second walk up the cobbles, dated back to 1420, its cellars to 1156. Not far beyond the brow of the lane, at the highest point of the ancient town, was a Tudor castle overlooking the distant sea and, below that, a looming town gate that still spoke of musket-fire and smugglers. Inside the B&B, there were squishy leather chairs and couches, beamed ceilings, a log-fire that seemed always to be burning brightly and a Christmas tree that stretched from the ground floor to the mezzanine above.

The mezzanine landing, partly illuminated by the lights of the tree, creaked and shifted as we made our way along it to our room. The centrepiece was a four-poster bed, we saw that straight away. Further investigation revealed a plate of Christmas mince pies on the antique sideboard, a view of the garden through the window and a cavernous bathroom, instantly memorable for its claw-foot bath, basket of luxury spa products and quaintly sloping floor. We'd certainly got the brief right – this was exactly the place for the child-free.

The next day was Christmas Eve and at breakfast, beneath the towering tree, I noted that none of the other guests had children with them either. They were all much older than us or much younger; they had either had their family Christmases

292

or were yet to have them. Back upstairs, the four-poster bed did not make any difference to our attempts at lovemaking. We didn't have any syringes with us, no Plan B.

"I thought it would be okay," said Chris. "I mean, we don't *really* need to use those."

Afterwards, I could feel my throat closing over with emotion, but it seemed ungrateful to cry, even in private. How could I be in tears when I was surrounded by all of this? Still, later that morning while we were getting ready to go out and explore, I told Chris to go ahead without me. It was a relief when he left, puzzled as to why he was being sent on alone, and I immediately slumped down on the edge of the bath and cried, hurt and angry thoughts propelling the tears down my cheeks. *I should have chosen someone else. Why, oh why, did I end up with a man like this? He's stopping me from trying to have children and he doesn't even care. Romantic break? What a joke.*

The feelings of rejection that, as an adopted child, I had battled all my life were rising once again to join the fear and pain and confusion about not having children of my own. It was Chris. Him and his ego and his wretched issues had caused all of this. *Damn egotistical man.*

The door to our room swished open. "Sweetheart? Is everything all right? I've been waiting for you. It's not the same on my own."

I wiped my dripping nose with a tissue. "Sorry!" I called from behind the bathroom door. "My hair went wrong. Why don't you go down to that teashop we saw yesterday and I'll meet you there in ten minutes?"

"Are you sure everything's okay?" he asked tentatively.

"Fine. Honestly, I'll see you there."

"Can't I just wait here with you?" the voice implored from the other side of the door. "Normally we do everything together, it's not like you to send me away."

I sighed heavily. "Whatever."

293

After I had camouflaged all signs of tears and bitter thoughts, we spent the day discovering one character-filled wonder after another. This is how I would cope, I thought, if I never had children. I would travel. Permanently. It was the only thing that seemed capable of distracting me from the gnawing pain of infertility.

I began to brighten, to enjoy the day for what it was. I would not think of the children I didn't have, I would not.

Later in the afternoon, when darkness had fallen, we heard carols echoing out of the stone church in the centre of the town. It reminded me, instantly, of my childhood, when we had gone to midnight mass on Christmas Eve.

"Shall we go?" I asked Chris expectantly.

"Only if I can sing really loudly," he said with a laugh. Chris was still secretly upset that he had not become a modern-day Frank Sinatra, and he also secretly thought that perhaps it wasn't too late.

We crossed the courtyard, lit by lanterns, and entered the church through a spectacular arched wooden door that would have dwarfed even the most rotund of Father Christmases. We took a carol list from a smiling volunteer in a Santa hat and made our way to a pew at the back of the church.

"It's empty!" I said. "Do you think we're early – or do people just not go to church at Christmas anymore?"

"Probably not," Chris replied. "When was the last time you went?"

"Um. Maybe 1994?"

He chuckled. "There you are then."

We held hands and huddled closely together to keep warm, the flagstone floor like a frozen tomb beneath our feet. The recorded carols kept playing and slowly, eventually, the expanse of empty pews before us began to fill up.

I didn't notice it at first. We were almost surrounded on all sides before it began to sink in. A hundred excited faces bounced happily in the seats and a hundred high-pitched voices competed with the sound of the carols. Suddenly I realised: this was the children's nativity service. As far as I could see, we were the only two childless people in the church. Every other adult was accompanied by a mini-version, or several mini-versions, of themselves, sometimes with grandparents in tow, perfectly completing the picture of natural progression. Buggies lined up along the sides of the church, too many to count. They had all had children, every single one of these people had had children, just like that. How did they do it? *How* did they get to have children? Something must be seriously wrong with us if we couldn't manage this simple thing that had filled a church on Christmas Eve.

"I've got to get out of here," I whispered urgently to Chris. "All these toddlers, all these babies."

I was gone before he could answer, weaving between buggies down the central aisle and almost running by the time I reached the outsized door. I was seized by a type of panic, not dissimilar to the way I felt whenever I sat down in an aeroplane seat. I ran out of the church yard and down onto the high street, where Chris finally managed to catch up with me.

"Lou!" he gasped. "What happened? One minute you were there, then—"

I suddenly began to cry, there in the street. Chris instantly pulled me close. "Oh sweetheart," he spoke into the top of my head. "We'd never have gone if we'd known it was for children. We didn't know."

"I'm sorry," I hiccupped eventually. "I think I must be going mad. I'm sorry."

"It's okay," he said quietly. "I felt it too. It's just so easy for all of them, isn't it?"

"You don't mind?" I asked. "Missing the carols?"

"Not at all. For one thing, that little boy in front of us had an enormous length of snot dangling from his nostril. I wasn't sure how much longer I could take it. It was revolting! For God's sake, don't these smug parents have tissues?"

We erupted into laughter. "I thought the same," I confessed. "No wonder we're not parents – we're both freaked out by a bit of snot." I was quiet for a moment. "Do you think it's right," I asked, "that you don't mind your own kid's snot?"

"I'd like to think it is," said Chris. "Come on, don't give up – by next Christmas we might know for ourselves."

Please, I thought, let that be true.

༂ ༂ ༂

Santa Claus arrived at breakfast on Christmas Day and handed out presents to each of the B&B's adult guests; there were no children there. Afterwards, Chris and I lay back on our four-poster bed and giggled while he did impressions of the establishment's proprietress, issuing Santa with his Order of Proceedings, like a determinedly proper courtier at Buckingham Palace. The talk fell away and we began to drift in each other's arms. It was warm, we were full, content. Suddenly, I snapped to.

"Yikes! We've got to get going."

I packed Rose's Christmas presents into a carrier bag and we made our way back across the mezzanine floor, taking one last look at the twinkling lights of the tree, down the stairs and out into a foggy day. The hour-long drive to Rose's retirement flat followed the contours of the coast as we dipped in and out of swirling patches of sea mist. We eventually arrived just before 11.30am.

"Lovely," exclaimed Rose. "It's about time for a drink, isn't it?"

Chris poured her a glass of sparkling wine, which she savoured with gusto and downed in several gulps.

We exchanged presents and I left mother and son talking at the table while I checked the fridge for our online grocery order and began making a plate of Christmas nibbles. Uh-oh! I caught Chris's eye from the doorway of the tiny kitchen and tilted my head, gesturing for him to join me.

"What?" he asked when he appeared before the open fridge door. "What is it?"

I kept my voice low. "That special chicken roast? With the cranberry stuffing? It's five days out of date."

"I knew Mum hadn't checked the dates," he said. "She came back to the phone far too quickly."

"Well, don't tell her whatever you do. We'll just have to improvise. I'd cook it if it was just us, but I'm not poisoning a ninety-year-old."

Throughout the afternoon, I made a succession of cold dishes and presented them at the table, hoping it would disguise the fact that I wasn't cooking Christmas dinner.

I was foraging in the fridge for some ham when my cellphone rang and an Australian number flashed up. "Loulou!" bellowed a voice from ten thousand miles away.

It was my old friend Dean, who had been single and childless when Chris and I first began trying to have a family; now he was married with two daughters, aged two-and-a-half and nine months.

"Merry Christmas!" he continued, sounding very merry indeed.

"Dean! Merry Christmas yourself. What have you been up to?"

"I'm done in," he laughed. "The girls had us up at 5am."

"Aw, I bet they're cute. Hey, is it Ellie's first Christmas?"

"Yep," he replied. "She didn't really know what was going on but it was awesome. And Mia's at the age now where she loves it. They piled into bed with us first thing, it was a great day. Total chaos, but you've gotta love it."

After Dean's phone call, I thought of Jai, who now had two sons, and of all our old friends – I couldn't think of one who hadn't had children over the past seven or eight years. *They've left me behind. This whole world has left me behind.*

Rose was telling Chris about Captain Bing, a famous spitfire pilot during World War II, who was also an old flame of hers. Rumour had it, he intended to marry her when the war was over.

I emerged from the kitchen with my plate of ham and cheese and took my seat at the table next to Chris. Rose had another slug of her drink, launched back into Captain Bing, then segued away to look over and enquire, "Nothing to do with me, but don't you think it's time to turn the oven on?"

"Ahh. Yes," I began, still wondering what I could use to replace the expired chicken roast.

"I don't know about you," Chris interjected, "but I'm really full. What if we had something light, then a gap, then Christmas pudding?"

"I couldn't eat another thing myself," Rose declared. "I say, is there any more of that wine?"

Eventually, we moved the few steps across to the lounge area and watched TV as the afternoon faded into darkness. It was like any other retirement flat, crammed with furniture that Rose used to lean on when she walked, one door blocked by two Zimmer frames that she refused to lean on at all. Instead of an overhead light, there was a progression of fringed lamps dotted around the room. Rose always sat in her high-backed armchair and we sat next to her on a two-seater couch. It was warm and safe, but all I could think was that it felt like the end of life rather than the beginning. There was no wishbone to pull this year, but I still wished: 'Please let 2008 be the year we get our new beginning.'

After the Christmas pudding and the crackers that we pulled with a series of pops rather than bangs – I was the only one who wore the paper hat within – Chris told Rose we would probably leave a bit after 9pm.

"Leave?" she asked, nonplussed. "You're not staying? I thought you were staying."

A stab of guilt caught me in the pit of my stomach; just because I couldn't cope with not having children, we were leaving an old lady on her own on Christmas night.

"No," Chris replied. "Remember I told you we're having a little break away for a few days? We're coming back to see you again before New Year, we can stay then if that's okay."

"Oh," said Rose. "I thought you were staying tonight. You're not driving all the way back there, are you? How exhausting! Are you sure you ought to do that?"

I was berating myself; I knew I should have written all of this down and posted it in a letter from Switzerland.

Later on, after we'd had tea and Christmas cake, I went into the bathroom while Chris smuggled the suspect chicken down to the car, where it couldn't do any damage. On the other side of the corridor, I could hear Rose in her bedroom, painfully lowering herself to the edge of her bed before reaching for the telephone and calling Chris's sister, Caroline.

"Yes," she said, her beautiful accent still crisp and clear, "yes, they're here. They've come and gone in the most extraordinary manner."

It was another of my infertility-inspired plans that had not worked. Rose was unhappy and, although our stay in the perfect, ancient town had lifted our spirits, the supposed romance of it had also underlined one thing: I had ovulated in a four-poster bed and we had still not managed to make love. The window of opportunity had closed; it would be at least 2008 before I became pregnant. Unless Christmas had bestowed an immaculate conception of biblical proportions.

TWENTY-FIVE

NEW YEAR 2008 TOOK us right back to the start in a way that I hadn't expected. Much like the first New Year in 2003, when we still felt a frisson at the seemingly daring decision to dispense with birth control, we suddenly had a Very Romantic Time. I couldn't keep up with these switches and about-turns – how could I be so frightening in December and yet so desirable in January? I didn't know, and there were far too many other questions taking up space in my head; there was no room left to untangle that one. All I knew was that, out of nowhere, we had now attempted to reproduce three times in one day. That wasn't even my first thought when I considered this unexpected renaissance – above all, babies included, I was just relieved to be 'wanted' again, to feel a little bit normal.

Now that I could temporarily stop worrying about being undesirable as well as infertile, I found I had enough energy to make a New Year List. Hence, I celebrated the happy turn of events by noting down All The Things That Might Be Wrong With Me. I thought it should probably stretch to 'pretty much everything except ovulation', which both conventional and complementary medicine had determined was actually happening. I sat down, ready to make a long and detailed list, but found myself repeatedly underlining the first words I wrote: blocked fallopian tubes. This was the fear that played on my mind the most. There might have been myriad reasons why I couldn't get pregnant but this was the one I routinely chose to fret over.

I juggled it round in my head, together with implantation problems and autoimmune issues, the top three on my list of concerns. I didn't even know how or why they had reached the top of the anxiety charts; they just had. It bothered me so much that I had long ago questioned our GP about having an HSG test to rule out blocked tubes, but she had waved away the inquiry.

"Oh well," she said, "you won't need that if you're having IVF – that would bypass tubal issues altogether."

I had been too slow to realise that we were still, relentlessly, trying to conceive naturally and it would all be a Big Fat Waste of Time if my tubes were impenetrable. Besides, I didn't even know if we would be having IVF – our GP had just assumed we would, since it had been more than two years, and at fertility clinics people called you 'Ms Together' before you could even ask the question.

The other thing I had been told about an HSG was that there was no point undergoing the procedure unnecessarily; I should wait for comprehensive sperm test results first, on the grounds that it would become irrelevant if any serious male factor issues were uncovered and assisted conception was therefore required. Again, why didn't I see that this made sense only if we progressed to fertility treatment? Even then, wouldn't it be worth knowing, for those times when we would inevitably continue to try naturally?

I had got sidetracked, somehow, and become caught up in waiting for the results of Chris's sperm test before taking the next step. It was such a simple, non-invasive test and it could tell us so much. Why hadn't he taken another one? Didn't he understand? I was running out of patience.

Inevitably, my New Year List led to a New Year Argument. Chris was affronted by my frustration over the length of time it had taken him to have The Test. He had done everything he could to help with fertility! How could I suggest he had let me down after everything he had done for us? I was acting highly unfairly and I made him feel bad about himself. Look how upset I had made him. Look what I was doing to him. He didn't deserve this. Hadn't he just recently been trying to take a test and a plumber had walked right in on him? What more could he do? Really! It was beyond the pale, this suggestion that he had been anything less than supportive. Why did I have to make him feel so useless? *Why?*

I just wanted him to take a sperm test; how had it tipped over into this?

I knew by now that it would be a day or so before he was ready to consider whether I had a relevant point. I might as well go for a walk while I waited it out. Also, I could alternately swear and snivel while stumbling along a deserted Swiss road, safe in the knowledge that there were only vines and donkeys to hear it. I set off alone and, when the time came to wander reluctantly homewards, opened the front door as quietly as I could. I didn't want to encounter Chris, not yet. I hoped he was upstairs listening to music or downstairs in our bedroom with the door shut. But as I tiptoed through the lounge, I heard his voice wafting down from above in urgent bursts. I knew immediately what it was – he was on the phone to Rose. This was what he did when things went wrong between us, rang his mother.

Suddenly, led only by instinct, I had to know what he was saying. So I did it; I moved in slow-motion to the first landing on the stairs then crouched down, climbing upwards on my hands and knees towards what I now saw was the closed door above me. Still on all-fours, I stopped on the final two steps and craned forward, as close to the door as I could get without advertising my arrival. He must have been using his mobile phone because every time he stopped speaking, I could hear Rose's voice, as clear and concise as ever.

The problem with eavesdropping on other people's conversations is that you think you're going to hear one thing, as if tuning in to a scheduled radio broadcast, but you end up hearing something else altogether, something that you would never have tuned in to if you had known.

Chris's voice conveyed his agitation. "She thinks I'm stopping her from having children, I can tell. That I've hampered her efforts. Honestly, I've done my best to take this test, I *am* going to take the test, I've told her that. It's not as if I've refused to take it – there are men out there who would do that you know – but still I seem to get the blame."

Chris was cut off mid-flow by Rose's swift retort. "You are *not* to blame if Louise does not have children. If she wanted children so badly, she should have had them with her husband. I do not see for a minute how this can be your fault."

I recoiled quickly, stung to realise that I had no allies here. I wondered how many other people believed I should have had a family with Jai. I would have been a terrible mother in my twenties, I thought angrily, but how could they know that? And in my thirties? They could also never know that, in moments like this, I would have traded anything to go back to another time, to try again to get it right. Jai was self sufficient, like me – he didn't rush off to lean on someone else when things went wrong, he didn't share secrets like this. I crawled backwards down the stairs and retreated to the silence of our bed. I was yet to realise that all the secrets I was keeping would soon make me very ill indeed.

❦ ❦ ❦

Joy to the world. The Great Sperm Test Wait was finally over. In early January 2008, Chris went to London and managed to provide a sample for analysis at the laboratory that Janet Brown had referred him to. It was two-and-a-half years since his first, inconclusive, test in 2005. "I know there's something wrong," he fretted as we travelled back home to Switzerland, where we would receive the results. "Something dastardly."

"Everyone thinks that," I reassured him, trying not to smile at his choice of words. "But this test is probably just going to prove that we seriously need to work out what's wrong with me. It's only a matter of ruling you out once and for all really." I stroked his arm as we sat nudged up together in our train seats. "Anyway, at least it's done now – that's the main thing."

Chris eyed me warily. "You wouldn't be angry, would you? If, you know, there was something drastically wrong?"

"Angry?"

"Well, you might think—"

"Why would anyone be angry about that? Would you be angry if I've got no eggs left soon? Or there's something wrong with my womb, or …?"

"Of course not, it's just …"

"I've only been annoyed because you've been dragging your feet about the test. It's nothing to do with the results – it's hardly like you can do anything about it, is it?"

"I know," Chris said quickly. "I know you're not made that way. It's just, well, I know how much you want to have children."

"C'mon," I cajoled. "Let's not worry about it anymore. It'll be fine."

After our foray into the real world, we were relieved to eventually turn into our driveway and retreat to the safety of the farmhouse, Dudley and Duke rushing up to greet us before we had even managed to exit the car. We were home again. Even better, there was a new closeness between us now that the issue of the test was not simmering in the background. We both instantly relaxed, neither of us realising for a minute what was about to transpire.

The phone call that would inform us of Chris's test results came through from London on a Monday afternoon. 2pm. We had each tried to pretend otherwise, but it was the only thought we could focus on all day. 2pm, we'll know at 2pm.

Down the phone line came a woman's voice, matter of fact, no emotion. All I knew about the voice was that it belonged to a specialist in male fertility from Janet Brown's clinic. Chris sat forward in an armchair, phone clasped to his ear, and I balanced on the arm, leaning in against the receiver to hear what she said.

I snatched a notebook and pen from the coffee table as she began explaining the parameters of a healthy semen analysis, the figures and percentages that a fertile sample should reach. Then she said it: the test had uncovered several serious issues that would explain the length of time it was taking us to conceive. My gut twisted and tightened, sending a spasm of apprehension upwards to fill my throat. I squeezed Chris's shoulder, in what I hoped was a reassuring gesture, as she continued.

The news travelled down the wires like a poisoned arrow piercing our protective bubble. The voice was now telling us that the analysis showed a sub-optimal count; craning to hear the figures, I scrawled *12.4 million/ideally 20.*

There was also sub-optimal motility. Was that what she was saying? I couldn't hear; I squashed my ear tighter against the phone. Two motility parameters? There were two? I missed the first, something to do with rapid progression which sounded quite important, but wrote down *31 per cent motility.* Before I could add that the ideal was more than 50 per cent, we had moved on to morphology. As the voice delivered the result in a monotone that betrayed no hint of feeling, my stomach crashed to the floor, joined a split second later by my heart and then my mouth.

"Your sperm shape shows only one per cent normal," she said. "The reference value should ideally be 15 per cent or more normally shaped sperm. These parameters may well be a major contributory factor to the length of time it is taking you to conceive."

In the split second it took to process all of this, Chris was speaking into his side of the receiver. "But some of my sperm's in fine form," he announced brightly.

There was an extra beat before the voice replied.

"No," she said, "I'm afraid the sample wasn't in fine form, unfortunately."

However, she explained, there were ways of improving the situation. For instance, there were lots of coiled tails in the sample, which could suggest that length of abstinence might be a problem; Chris had also mentioned that his sperm appeared yellowish at times and that pointed to the same issue. In short, he might improve his sample quality if he ejaculated more often. She suggested increasing frequency to every three to four days. Another layer of tension swept in; how on earth was he going to force himself to make love to me every three or four days? No. It wasn't going to happen. He'd have to do it himself. If I was there, he'd never achieve it. Wasn't that what had caused all these lengthy periods of abstinence in the first place?

The voice had moved on to other lifestyle factors that could be tweaked to improve sperm quality. Chris should decrease his alcohol intake to an occasional glass of red wine and he might also benefit from consulting one of the clinic's nutritionists, who could explain how to maximise sperm quality through diet.

She suggested he make all of these changes and repeat the test in three months' time. If there was an improvement, natural conception might be an option but realistically – especially given the fact that I would turn forty later in the year – assisted conception might be more appropriate.

And if there was no improvement?

"Should your sperm parameters remain the same, assisted conception may be the only realistic option for you both if you want to seriously give yourselves a good chance of conceiving."

The voice went on to describe ICSI (Intracytoplasmic Sperm Injection), one of the most invasive procedures available. It involved the injection of a single sperm directly into the egg in order to fertilise it. I was now so anxious that I struggled to hold the pen still when I wrote, but I scribbled *£4,500, 12% chance of success.*

We ended the call and stared at each other, like two strangers watching a fatal accident unfold in front of us.

"I knew it," Chris said, his left leg jiggling frantically as he sat there. "Didn't I say so? I've had an inkling all my life that my sperm might not be up to it. I must have known, somewhere inside."

I hugged him tightly, only moving away because his bouncing leg was jarring me up and down, an uncomfortable physical manifestation of the jolt we had just received.

"She said there's stuff you can do," I offered, still perched on the arm of the chair. "Anyway, who knows what's wrong with me as well – we're probably a right pair."

Chris was still for a moment. "It's nice of you to say that, even though we know it's not true."

"C'mon, we don't know. It could easily be true. My thyroid for instance."

He ignored me, staring sadly at the floor in silence before delivering his next thought in the sombre, earnest tone of a mourner at a funeral.

"I'd understand if you left me," he said. "You've still got time to meet someone else."

Determined not to cry in front of him, I blinked back the tears that were lined up ready to fall.

"Don't be stupid, as if I'd do that. Anyway, sperm results can fluctuate one day to the next – it could be a different story if you try again in three months. Especially if you follow her suggestions."

"I wouldn't blame you," he said. "If you did leave."

"If you say that again, I'm going to dong you with that damn phone," I joked. Finally, he smiled. "And it's not as if you've got no sperm at all. You've got millions."

"It's just a shame they're nearly all decrepit." He grinned ruefully. "I wonder how many decent ones I had in my twenties. It would have been vastly better then, wouldn't it? I probably could have become a father in my twenties."

The phone consultation from London cost another £120; it had proved the most telling £120 we had spent in more than five years of infertility. For the first time, we had a specific mountain to climb rather than just blundering around in the wilderness hoping we'd one day scale the right peak.

We must have known, after five years, that something had to be wrong, but somehow it still came as a shock. I realised with another unsettling lurch that I had actually believed, deep down, the issue was as simple as lack of regular sex; it was a diversion that had thrown me off course, consistently demanded attention and soaked up energy. Like the red herring in a crime drama, it had sucked me in.

I told Chris I needed to have a shower, even though I'd already had one; it was just a place to hide because I couldn't maintain the sanguine front for much longer. I did not want to make it worse by breaking down in front of him.

As the water fell, I rested my forehead against the tiles on the wall and sobbed as quietly as I could. I was nearly forty. I would never become a mother, not now. The blow struck at a jagged void deep in my stomach, the exact place I used to feel the pain of separation from my birth parents, and sometimes still did. I never thought it would happen, that I could lose this umbilical connection twice in my life. I doubled over; only my forehead on the tiles was holding me up.

❦ ❦ ❦

After I had reluctantly turned off the shower, I dotted concealer around my eyes and breezed into the lounge. I spent the rest of the afternoon trying to appear unshaken, suggesting that we could research acupuncture for male fertility and joking about Chris being prescribed his jollies every three to four days.

"You'll have to keep a wank diary," I said with a snort. "It'll be like high school all over again." Brazil nuts. She'd also said he should eat a lot of Brazil nuts.

Early in the evening, Chris disappeared upstairs to listen to music and I wandered outside, searching the sky for help. I found myself at the side of the house, from where grapevines stretched all the way to the stone spires of the village in the distance. I flopped down on the grass and watched the sun set; finally, I could let go. My eyes were open but I was soon unable to see through the tears that seemed to have a life of their own, that rolled constantly, involuntarily, without any conscious input from me.

I don't know how long it was before I sensed movement at the corner of the house. I turned slowly, expecting to see Chris. But it was Duke, padding towards me. He then did something he'd never done before – he sat down right beside me, almost on top of me, so that we were resting hip to hip and shoulder to shoulder, each staring ahead at the sunset. With his warmth against my side, I finally had someone to lean on.

As the last vestiges of the day's sun became burnt orange slashes in the sky, I put an arm around big, strong, gentle Duke and nestled my cheek into his neck. Somehow I had stopped crying, partly because I felt comforted and partly because I didn't want to depress Duke, who wore the soulful expression of one who feels things deeply. I huddled into him, my stinging eyes soothed on the silky tufts of fur behind his ears and it was as if he *knew*. We stayed there, hugged up side by side in the silence, until the light faded completely.

309

Over the preceding five years, I had increasingly felt that I was falling and I just wanted someone to catch me, to make it stop before I hit rock bottom. But the experts I consulted didn't do it and my own partner didn't do it. How is it that a Labrador instinctively knew what was needed but my own species couldn't fathom it? I didn't want that moment with Duke to end; when I think about it now, I realise it was the only time in ten years that I ever felt truly comforted.

⁂ ⁂ ⁂

I must have caught a virus. There were bound to be lots of bugs on all the trains we travelled back and forth on. That had to be what it was. A couple of weeks after receiving the sperm test results, I managed to travel to London and to complete my work there, much as I always had. Except now, I could go for entire days in the office without speaking to anyone; it seemed too draining, too much trouble, to get up from my desk and chat about something. What would I even chat about? I couldn't think of anything that mattered, except that I would never be a mother.

It was as if I was so exhausted that my body was shutting down unnecessary functions in order to keep the vital ones running. Social niceties were the first to go. I still managed a low wattage smile in the general direction of other people, but I didn't want to talk to them; I wanted to lie down, preferably in the dark. Back in Switzerland, I went to bed as soon as we returned from London and found it increasingly difficult to order my body to get up again. I was back to counting ceiling tiles. *Two, four, six, eight, ten, twelve.* Sometimes I just stared at the ceiling, too tired even to count, and felt tears trickle down the sides of my face and onto the pillow. I didn't wipe them away; I didn't move. It was like being covered from head to toe in a leaden shroud. I would say the words in my head: Get up! Move. Get out of bed. But my body ignored the commands. I wanted to lift an arm or a leg, or even just my head, but nothing would respond. Was this virus affecting my central nervous system? Why wasn't my body working? I wanted to move, but I was covered in lead.

Chris would come bustling in sometime after midday and do his best to help me. "Why don't I make you some breakfast? You just need a good meal then you'll feel better."

"I can't get up," I would say wanly.

"I know, I know," he soothed. "You never did like the cold, did you? I don't blame you, it's absolutely freezing. But why don't you come through to the lounge? I've put the heating on in the lounge …"

"Okay, I'm coming."

Half an hour later, he would be back. "Lou? What's happening? I've been waiting for you. Do you need another cup of tea? Would that help? I'll make you tea in your favourite mug."

I would haul myself up in bed, slow-motion, as if sixty years had passed overnight, and sip the tea. Then, when I had finished, I remained motionless in this new position, slumped against the headboard. *Move. Get up. For God's sake, move.*

The way it worked on those days is that Chris would come back in and worry that I was ill, that maybe I should stay in bed until I felt better.

"No!" I responded. "It's not that bad. I can't stay here all day. I've got to get up, I'm getting up."

Finally, I would ask for his help. "Could you bring my clothes over? It's so cold. Maybe I just need to get dressed in bed."

He would rifle through the pile of clothes on my bedroom chair, holding up jeans and jogging pants, t-shirts and sweatshirts while I nodded my assent or pointed to which ones I planned to wear. Then he tucked them in under the duvet to warm them up and another half hour passed while I did nothing.

Eventually, I would smile like a shy child and ask Chris to help me get dressed. We normally made a joke of it; he thought I was teasing him, he didn't know that my limbs would not respond when I asked them to move. He thought I was just being playful, like when we had water fights, or silly, like when I lobbed spinach balls at his head during *Question Time*.

Or maybe, deep down, he did know because he was so gentle when he lifted me, forwards to thread each arm through a sleeve, or backwards to manoeuvre a foot into a trouser leg. Even fully dressed, I still floundered like a marooned jellyfish on the shore. "Do you want your moon boots?" he asked then, referring to the last present Jai had ever given me, a pair of wool-lined boots from home.

"Yes please." And he would juggle first one foot and then the other as he tried to pull them on and upwards over my ankles. As he laughed about getting the clumsy accessories stuck, each one on the wrong foot, I thought, 'What a shame. What a shame he never got to dress his children like this. He would have been a really patient dad.' Then I thought, 'Oh no! I wanted to have children and now I've become one.'

"Okay," Chris would announce. "You're ready to go."

"Um. Can you get me up?"

And he would lean over the bed, wrap my hands around his neck and, taking my full weight, haul me upwards and on to my feet, like a drunk being steadied and guided. It was perhaps twenty paces from the bedroom to the lounge but I would walk them as if they were the final twenty paces of a marathon, then I would flop down, exhausted, onto the couch.

I always gained enough momentum by evening to cook dinner and I would start to enjoy it and think, 'Great, I'm getting better. Tomorrow it will be different.'

But then there I would be again the next morning, too heavy and tired even to count ceiling tiles. If Chris had not pulled me to my feet on those days, I wonder what would have happened. Would I ever have got up at all? I am embarrassed admitting this. I can hear my mother, and all the strong, self-sufficient women she grew up with, sighing and tutting. *You're indulged, spoilt, lazy. We just had to get on with things, we didn't have the luxury of lying around all day.* Or perhaps they might say, *problems! You don't know what problems are. You don't know you're born.*

But I did know problems and nearly every one of them, I had kept secret. *I* was a secret myself, for that matter. No one knew who I really was, who my parents were, just like they didn't know the secrets of our infertility or of our impotence. They start to weigh a lot these secrets, when you begin to add one on top of the other. I was indeed suffering a type of malaise, just not the kind I thought.

⁊⁊ ⁊⁊ ⁊⁊

Until I became infertile, synchronicity was one of my favourite words. Whenever I sensed its presence, through the arrival of an apparently meaningful coincidence, I felt as if I had been sent a special, private little sign. *You're on the right track. This is meant to be. You're in the flow, in the zone. Help will turn up just when you need it.*

It took nearly a full ten years of infertility to realise that synchronicity had abandoned me altogether. When I tried to have children, nothing fell my way. There were no signs, no cosmic nudges, no fortuitous meetings when I found myself in just the right place at just the right time. In fact, the exact opposite happened: barriers appeared in the most unexpected of places.

I've thought about it often but I can barely see a single time when synchronicity guided me during infertility. For a full ten years, I just bumbled around on my own, mostly in the dark. I could have done with an illuminated signpost now and then, or even a cryptic hint, but there was nothing, no predetermined route to pregnancy. However, there was one other synchronicity, or coincidence, or whatever you want to call it, that turned up right on cue. It didn't help me conceive, but it did ensure that I actually survived infertility. Without it, I'm not sure I would have made it through.

Once the results of the sperm test began to sink in, there was an odd mix of relief that we finally knew what to target and anxiety about whether we could succeed in doing so. Was it too late? Did we still have a chance?

In the aftermath, there was a sort of shockwave effect as one new realisation gave rise to another. It didn't take long for the collateral damage to show up. It taunted and haunted me: what if we had known this in 2005? What if Chris had taken his repeat test, like he was supposed to, and this information had come to light more than two years ago? How much further along could we be now if we'd just have known?

Resentment began to seethe, unseen, to the surface. It had infiltrated our relationship before I even knew it was there. I would make a comment, not quite coming out and accusing Chris of slowing us down, but letting it be known that I had noted it. And so our weeks would become punctuated with rows about Chris dragging his feet, delaying the diagnosis until I was nearly forty years old.

Still, I didn't confide in anyone. I had been bred to keep secrets and, besides, look what had happened when I spilled the hidden side of me at a fertility clinic. It was just another thing to accommodate within, this rancour that now piled up on top of the sadness and the secrets. Meanwhile, I was still having trouble getting up in the morning, or even in the afternoon; it seemed a long time for a virus to last. I guess, though, that I knew by now it wasn't a virus. It was more familiar than I wanted to admit, this thing that shrouded me. I had felt this way before, sometimes, when I was in my twenties but it had never been so prolonged and it normally coincided with something painful; a relationship break-up, excessive stress at work or the distress that crept up sometimes about being adopted, 'unwanted'. But it was one day in bed, maybe two. It didn't drag on and on, not like this.

"You should get some counselling." Had Jai said that once? I remembered my mother marching me to the doctor when I was seventeen years old and regularly stopped eating for five days at a time. "I think she's depressed," I heard her say. I was surprised, not because she thought that but because I hadn't realised Mum knew what depression was, or rather that she would acknowledge it as an actual, credible thing.

"Louise is over-sensitive." That was the way my family usually summed it up.

All of this accumulated detritus finally came tumbling down one Tuesday night when I was supposed to be packing for London. Chris was upstairs, trying to foresee which clothes he would need for the next week at work. I could hear the floorboards expanding and contracting as he crossed back and forth to a full-length mirror in one of the spare bedrooms. I should have been up there, too, but I lay on the couch, again unable to move.

On that night, it felt as if my entire body had been overtaken with grief. I rocked slightly with the pain, but there was not enough momentum to propel me upwards, back into normal life. And then I was thinking it: *I just want to go to sleep*. It was different to any thought I had had before. Once, when I was a teenager, I had concocted a dramatic plan to end my life in a car crash. *Then they'll see, then they'll want me!* But all along, I knew I wouldn't really do it. This was nothing like that. It was not a dramatic declaration of anything, it was just a deep, overwhelming desire to go to sleep. I was walking quietly towards it, for me, not because of anyone else. *There's two packets of tramadol in the bedroom, you still have some tramadol.*

According to drugs.com, tramadol is a narcotic-like pain reliever, used to treat moderate to severe pain. I had been prescribed it for a neck injury several years before, but had never bothered taking it. I didn't take prescription drugs, not if I could help it. It surprised me then to realise that if I got up off the couch, I would walk to the bedroom and take the tramadol. All of it. Until I was asleep.

Part of me was still shocked by that. It was as if something that normally lay in the shadows of my mind had reared up and seized control, leading me to the bedroom, despite the tiny, rational voice that ordered: *do not leave this couch!* I was going to do it, I was going to sleep. I would not turn forty, fifty, sixty, seventy and maybe even eighty without having children or grandchildren. I would not have to endure this pointless, childless life. How lovely it would be to sleep through the emptiness. *No! Hold on. Just hold on. Keep holding on.* I gripped the sides of the sofa to ensure I did not get up. Having spent weeks ordering myself to move, I was now pleading with myself not to. *Hold on, hold on, hold on.* If I stood up, I knew I would do it. It was a terrible, quiet, certain knowing. *Hold on, hold on.*

I was lying there, grasping both sides of the sofa cushion, and only just holding on in all senses, when something briefly broke through. The television, which had blurred into the background when I stopped watching it an hour ago, was still broadcasting to no one in particular from the corner of the room. Usually I would have switched channels by now, or turned it off altogether, but I had just left it, transmitting a late-night schedule that I was not currently hearing and would normally never see. I was suddenly aware of a voice filling the room: "Can a book really cure depression?" Those few words, although delivered via such a prosaic medium, had the same effect as if I had just received a celestial slap. The timing of it, the synchronicity, jolted me instantly back to my senses.

I turned my head towards the TV and began to listen. It was Alan Yentob, a BBC executive and presenter, who was outlining the premise of this latest documentary in his series, *Imagine*. He would be putting the self-help industry to the test, examining the success of self-help books and courses in particular. There was one book, he said, that had been credited with curing depression in two-thirds of people who read it. I let go of the couch and laughed out loud. Whatever the reality, it felt like I was somehow *meant* to see this programme. The rustic voices of my childhood again: *Can you credit it? First she's going to kill herself then she's receiving messages from the bloody TV! I've heard it all now.*

I realised how it might sound, but how can you describe the intuitive *yes!* that you feel in a moment of synchronicity? A sceptical Alan Yentob was now discussing the cult of positive thinking. "Can reading *The Secret* really change your life?" I might buy something like that, I thought; that's all I need because I'm not *really* depressed, just a bit blue at the moment, down in the dumps. No, he concluded. There was no evidence that it would change your life. Oh.

He went through a roll call of books with familiar names, like *Feel the Fear and Do It Anyway*, or *Awaken the Giant Within*. I knew them all; in bookshops, the self-help section was generally right next to health, where I had spent hours of my life reading about how to get pregnant. And, though I hid them from view when my family came to stay, I was also the guilty keeper of a collection of self-help titles myself.

It turned out that, of all the self-help offerings on the market, there was one that came out on top in study after study; there was a body of evidence that it actually worked. Uncharacteristically energised, I dashed into the kitchen to grab pen and paper. I returned to the couch in time to scribble: *Feeling Good: The New Mood Therapy. David D Burns (M.D).* There it was, the helping hand I needed. Apparently, it was the original cognitive behavioural therapy tome, prescribed by some doctors instead of antidepressants and curing depression in two-thirds of readers.

It doesn't matter that this discovery was, in all probability, a random event like any other. It was the way it made me feel: that I was not necessarily alone. The possibility was enough to keep me going, to ensure I held on after all. It silenced all thoughts of finding relief in a packet of painkillers.

I ordered the book online the next day and it wasn't until it arrived and I began reading it that I understood how crucial it was that those few words – can a book cure depression? – had echoed through the lounge at exactly the time they did.

I still thought of depression as being a bit of a 'heavy' word for what I was experiencing. If a doctor had asked me about it, I would have said, "Oh, you know, I feel a bit *bleurgh* sometimes, but who wouldn't after more than five years of this?" Then I would have laughed, like I generally did in such situations, and said something to brighten the mood – "they're not joking when they say infertility stinks."

So, early in the book, when I went through the Burns Depression Checklist, created by the doctor who had written *Feeling Good*, I expected to record a mild level of depression, at worst. After I had answered all the questions, rating how often I had experienced a wide range of symptoms during the past week, I tallied up my score. When I turned the page to read how to interpret the outcome, it was like falling too fast in a lift.

According to the Burns Depression Checklist, I was suffering from severe depression; not only that, I was at the very upper end of it and one more point would have tipped me over into an extreme level of depression. My score was seventy-five out of a possible 100; a note below the table of scores suggested that anyone with a persistent score above ten might benefit from professional treatment. Ten! Things were obviously much worse than I had realised. And next to it was another word of caution: anyone with suicidal feelings should seek an immediate consultation with a mental health professional.

So this was what was wrong with me? I must have known already – how could you miss it? – but I had been brought up to tough it out. Normally, I would think, 'Well, that's just another thing you've failed at – toughing it out.' However, I devoured the rest of the book in a matter of days and I learnt the most obvious, amazing thing: you can talk back to thoughts like that. All this time I had been believing them, taking them at face value, and letting them roam unchallenged to do their damage. Now I was being given a list of "ten cognitive distortions that form the basis of all your depressions". They ranged from 'All-or-Nothing Thinking' and 'Overgeneralisation' to 'Emotional Reasoning' and 'Should Statements'. Once you understood which of the toxic ten had come out to play in any given situation, it became much easier to realise why you were feeling so bad, and to turn the thoughts around. Apparently, it was thinking, not emotions that lay at the core of the problem.

The first page of *Feeling Good* reiterated some of the facts from the BBC documentary – the book was rated the most helpful on depression from a list of more than 1,000 self-help titles; five controlled studies published in scientific journals over a decade indicated that 70 per cent of depressed people who read *Feeling Good* improved within four weeks even though they received no other treatment. It added that Dr Burns did not recommend any self-help book as a substitute for professional therapy. I knew he was right, but only if you made the right choice of therapist, if you thoroughly checked their credentials before handing over to them the most vulnerable aspects of yourself.

So far, during this battle with infertility, I had paid £200 to talk to someone who looked at his watch when I was about to confide my most shameful secret and another £165 to someone who admonished me for the way I felt. Those consultations represented some of the most expensive entries in my notional fertility accounts register. The cheapest was the £5.99 I had paid for this book. It didn't take away the pain of infertility – nothing did – but it ensured that I kept my head above water even though the tide was surging all around me. It also cleared out some of the flotsam and jetsam of the past, leaving a bit more breathing space to deal with the fact that it had been more than five years and I still was not pregnant.

I had hit rock bottom, but now synchronicity had thrown me a lifeline; I might continue to struggle but I knew that I would never sink so far again.

TWENTY-SIX

A SILVER ENVELOPE WAS waiting for us on the kitchen table in Switzerland. I had known about its contents since the New Year, but now I had it in my hand – an invitation to Mum's eightieth birthday in April, two months away. Vanda, my sister, had included a note: "I know you probably can't come all this way but I thought you'd like to see the invites." Mum's face smiled out from the front of the card, eyes still sparkling like a much younger woman. The party would be at one of my favourite venues, overlooking the ocean. More than anything, I wanted to be there. I hadn't been home since Christmas 2003; the gap was much longer than I ever thought it would be but I'd been sidetracked – bushwhacked really – by infertility and somehow it had happened – I had not seen my family for more than four years.

In much earlier daydreams, I had pictured Chris and me moving back to the southern hemisphere for good around 2008, this very year. Our child would be two or three years old; it would be the right time, particularly if we were now trying for a little brother or sister. I saw the scene at the airport so clearly that I could almost feel it unfolding – grandmother and grandchild meeting for the first time, aunts and uncles, cousins; tears of happiness and shrieks of laughter in the arrivals lounge. I welled up a bit just thinking about it. Our child would know they were part of an enormous, warm, extended family; they would never have to worry about being alone. Then there was the lifestyle; as much as I loved Europe, I still thought the southern hemisphere was the best place in the world to be a kid. We should have been home permanently by now, living our 'real' life, Chris, me and our child.

I longingly read the details on the invitation. "Look," I showed Chris. "Vanda's done an amazing job."

"You should go," he said instantly. "Why don't you go? They'd be over the moon to see you."

"Let's think about it. I mean, I want to, but I don't know. Maybe if I could get there by train!"

"You could get sedatives," Chris offered, "for the flight."

I wistfully stroked Mum's photo with my index finger, as if it would somehow let her know I was thinking of her. "I just don't know if I should spend the money – we might need it for treatment and stuff. And it would be a really bad time to muck up my cycle. You know, with the stress and the long-haul flight and everything." I paused. "But I do really want to go. Oh well, maybe something will come up."

I didn't say it out loud – I must have realised how stupid it sounded after such prolonged infertility – but I was also thinking, 'What if that's the month I'm actually pregnant? What if I've got pregnant and I ruin it by taking a long-haul flight?'

The part of me that still hoped I would become a mother never seemed to give up. It appeared there was nothing you could say or do to stop that tiny, expectant voice popping up each month, spotting symptoms that weren't there and painting scenarios that would never be. I put the card up on the mantelpiece in the lounge and studied the stamp on the envelope; mountains and lakes, an image of home.

Two days later, Chris came down to the kitchen after speaking to Rose on the phone upstairs.

"Guess what?" he called from halfway down the stairs. "Mum wants to give you £1,000. She wants you to be able to go home, she doesn't want you to miss your mum's birthday."

"Wow, that's amazing. I can't believe anyone would do that. But I can't take money off a pensioner."

"I told her that's what you'd say, but she's adamant. She thinks the world of you, you know. She wouldn't make an

322

offer like that to just anyone." Chris gave me a hug. "By the way, she wants to know if there's anything she can do with the fertility issue. Maybe if she can help to pay for treatment or something."

"That's amazing," I said again, the words catching in my throat a little.

Rose was nearly ninety-one years old; she lived in a modest flat with very few luxuries and barely spent anything on herself. Her offer was one of the most supportive, generous things anyone had done for me.

Chris caught my eye, suddenly serious. "I hope you believe me now about what you heard me say to Robert that day. When we'd had that row? It genuinely wasn't true. You know how it is when you're upset – you say things you don't mean. Mum's always been incredibly fond of you."

We flopped onto the couch, limbs entwined, and I confided in Chris about worrying that there might be complications if I took a long-haul flight and it turned out I was only just pregnant. "I feel like I can't afford to take any risks at my age," I explained.

"I thought about that, too," he said. "It would be just our luck, wouldn't it, that it would happen that month?"

It might have been more than five years, but it seemed it wasn't only me who was finding it hard to let go of hope. Although I had gradually drifted away from acupuncture with Maggie after we moved to Switzerland, we had made renewed efforts to tackle our infertility since receiving Chris's test results. They had come through on a Monday in January – by the following Monday Chris was at a clinic in London, having his first consultation with David Taylor, the excellent acupuncturist who had treated me in the early days of our quest to conceive.

They had 'clicked' instantly, as I thought they might, and had made immediate progress.

"It takes some men months to feel comfortable about opening up and telling me what you've just told me in one session," David said. "It makes it much easier to know what treatment would best suit you."

As with most things, Chris was diagnosed as being the polar opposite to me. According to Traditional Chinese Medicine, he had an overabundance of yang energy, which, amongst other things, showed itself as excess heat throughout the body. He would be undergoing acupuncture to help balance this out, as well as taking Chinese herbs.

Chris was buoyed up when he returned after his first appointment. "He's so down to earth," he said of David. "I liked him straight away. He said he could tell I was a hot person the minute I walked in – he could see it in my face and feel it in my handshake."

"Did he check your pulses and look at your tongue and draw diagrams to explain what was happening?" I asked.

"Oh yes, all of that. He was very thorough. I've had my first lot of acupuncture, too."

"He thinks he can do something then?"

Chris grinned. "He was very upfront about it. He said there are no guarantees, but he has had success treating men with fertility issues. Particularly with this excess heat, it's dire for sperm. So he thinks we might see quite different results if he can cool me down a bit."

Suddenly, I was not the only one doing everything I could to improve my fertility. "No drinking for me," Chris continued. "None at all. Alcohol is one of the worst things for heating you up. And I've got to take nine herbal tablets a day – nine – plus a male multivitamin supplement."

"Welcome to the club," I said. "And don't forget the wank diary and the Brazil nuts."

Chris laughed. "David's in favour of both of those, by the way. He thinks they could help."

I thought about how we had first moved to Switzerland, believing that a less stressful lifestyle might be enough to help us conceive. That was nearly two years ago; now we knew it wasn't quite so simple. We had talked often about what we should do and where we should live – that had never stopped – and over the preceding few months we had been leaning towards a permanent move to Switzerland. No more commuting to London, the final piece of stress removed. We'd even been to see a mortgage advisor during one of our work trips; we wanted to know if we could afford to buy a home of our own in Switzerland. "We can lend you £160,000 to £200,000," he told Chris. "No trouble. More if you want to add Louise to the mortgage."

I was astounded. We were each carrying fairly heavy debt already, due both to infertility and one of its offbeat by-products, the relocation to mainland Europe. However, we began looking at property in the price range the mortgage advisor suggested. We had seen four houses so far, none of them quite right, and been just too late for a converted windmill that seemed perfect for us. We thought it was what we wanted, but now it felt like the ground was shifting again.

I began scrawling out budgets on spare pieces of paper, calculating the cost of staying in Switzerland versus the cost of living in the UK. Suddenly, it was all about money – we hadn't made any decisions about fertility treatment, but it seemed that subconsciously we were already preparing the ground, wondering how we could stretch to paying £4,500 for ICSI, or whatever else we stumbled upon that might help. We already knew that we would try at least three months' treatment with David, a cost that hadn't been factored in when we first became long-distance commuters to London.

By March, we had come to a decision that would have been unthinkable two months previously: we would have to leave Switzerland.

"Do you really want to go?" Chris asked, as we strolled the empty rural lanes surrounding the farmhouse.

"No. Do you?"

"No."

We each burst into laughter.

"This is just typical of us," I said, "doing everything upside down and back-to-front."

"Oh well." Chris chuckled. "Keeps life interesting. Think how boring it would be…"

"What? If we were organised and competent?"

"Actually, I think we're vastly more organised and competent than a lot of people."

"You would!" I laughed.

We stopped to pat the donkeys who roamed the valley below the farmhouse, their winter coats shedding in our hands.

"I could have lived here forever," I said, overlooking my long-held daydreams about moving back home. "Imagine if we'd had a family – the farmhouse is perfect for it, the kitchen, the bedrooms, the lawn, everything."

"I know," said Chris. "I wouldn't have wanted any more out of life either."

I wistfully looked around, at the rows of vines in the distance and back to the donkeys and their crooked stone stable. "I still can't believe it didn't happen. Shows how naive I am, thinking Switzerland was going to magic up a baby."

"I thought it would happen, too," Chris mused sadly as we linked hands and turned to meander up the winding road to the top of the hill.

By late April, we were saying goodbye. Mary and Ian had kindly offered to store our possessions in the farmhouse loft, in case we could find a way to return. All of our larger furniture was already in storage in the UK, having been packed away when we left for Switzerland in 2006. Somewhere in the southern hemisphere, I still had even more furniture in long-term storage – all these fragmented pieces of my life scattered across three countries; it aptly summed up my failed attempts at settling down, creating a family base. Without a family, it was easy to become rootless.

On the morning we left Switzerland, I dropped to my knees to say goodbye to Dudley and Duke, wrapping my arms around their necks as they jostled for position on either side of me. While Chris chatted to Mary and Ian at the car, I doubled back and hugged the two Labradors all over again.

"Thank you, boys," I whispered to them. "I'll always love you, wherever I am." Dudley slammed a paw into my lap and slobbered on my jacket.

As we drove off, waving well beyond the time anyone could see us, I blinked away the tears and summoned the spirit of my indomitable mother.

"Needs must," she would have said. "Needs must."

A week earlier, she had turned eighty on the other side of the world and I wasn't there.

"I'll go at Christmas instead," I told myself. "Give this new treatment time to work. Unless I'm pregnant at Christmas, of course … what if I'm pregnant?"

TWENTY-SEVEN

DURING MY TIME IN the Ten-Year Club, about one billion three hundred million babies have been born around the world. 1,300,000,000 – all those zeros, all those new lives. Of the almost unimaginable number of babies who have arrived throughout the past ten years, nine have been born into my immediate family and several hundred to friends, colleagues and acquaintances. Some of them have made it seem more difficult to cope with infertility than others. However, none had the same profound effect as seven births that sparked global headlines in 2008.

At about the time we were moving back to the UK, it emerged that an Austrian man called Josef Fritzl had imprisoned his own daughter in a cellar for twenty-four years and, against her will, fathered seven children with her. One, a twin boy, died shortly after birth; Fritzl disposed of his body in an incinerator.

Like everyone else, our first thoughts were for his victims; how could such a thing be endured, how could you ever recover? However, as the story, with all its twisted machinations, unfolded before us on the TV news, it gave rise to another bitter question: how did a man like that get to become a father? *Why* did a man like that get to become a father?

"I don't bloody believe it," said Chris, as he watched the rolling footage, and I knew exactly what he didn't believe because I was thinking the same thing.

In that moment, I looked across at Chris, who would have been a good, decent and kind father, and I looked at the face of Fritzl on the TV screen and I thought, *That proves it. There really is no God. There is no reason or meaning to anything –*

it's all just random. If I had any faith at all left over from my childhood at a Catholic school, that was the moment I lost it.

It wasn't as if, before that point, I thought all children were delivered into the arms of loving families or that babies were not born into terrible circumstances every day. Maybe my world view had become too small, maybe these people and these situations were just blurred images at the very periphery of my vision. However, there was something about the events that occurred in the cellar in Austria – perhaps even as simple as the timing of the news – that brought all of those images into sharp relief.

In the face of such human suffering, it's ultimately self-interested to relate it back to your own situation but infertility doesn't always allow you to grasp that perspective. So in 2008, still mired in infertility, what I honestly thought was: That monster of a man can have *seven* children in those circumstances, yet we can't even have *one.* Seven. How can that possibly be? I was yet to understand that such a thought was as futile as wondering why a tsunami claimed one man but not his neighbour. For the time being, I had lost my faith. Infertility, like any painful challenge, had shaken up my cosy, complacent world view.

I was never a natural church-goer; I didn't know the word for it in my childhood, but if I was anything then, I was probably pagan. We went to church now and then, Mum, Dad, me and Ray, and I could never understand why God would want to spend his time in such a stale, lifeless building when he could be outdoors enjoying the wonders people said he had created.

I felt like jumping up sometimes and letting everyone know: "You won't find God here! He's outside in the paddocks and trees." I sat on my hands in church to stop myself doing anything I might regret.

After Dad died when I was seven, God loomed larger in our lives. Mum joined the Catholic Church and suddenly we had to say the Rosary every night, even when it was still light outside and I could have been out there with my animals and tree-huts and hiding places. We took it in turns: ten Hail Marys followed by one Glory Be, one decade after another for what felt like forever. Ray and I soon worked out that it would be over sooner if we just talked faster; he became particularly adept at delivering ten Hail Marys in the manner of a racing commentator. His galloping rosary whipped past at such speed that he often got away with saying only nine instead of ten. We both considered that a huge victory.

At our new school, where we were taught mostly by nuns, we also had to confess our sins once a month. Unfortunately, confession was taken by Father Bruce, a kind and jovial man who had become a friend of the family. I felt I knew him too well to disappoint him with what I really got up to so I devised a system where I told him about three small sins that I hadn't committed for every really big one that I thought I probably had. When he handed down my penance afterwards, I added an extra five Hail Marys to make up for the fact that I had lied at confession. Overall, I wasn't a very successful Catholic but, even so, it never occurred to me to question whether God was actually there. I had always just assumed he was.

By my late teens, I had stopped going to mass altogether, except on Christmas Eve; it wasn't that I had stopped believing in God, it was that I still believed he was not to be found in a building. Those days, I was a 'just-in-case' believer, delivering desperate pleas and prayers when I was in trouble, and keeping quiet the rest of the time – a bit like taking out religious insurance.

During my twenties, I discovered Oprah, which in turn led to the discovery of self-help books and a subtle change in the terms I used to describe faith in a higher power. Now it was all about 'the universe', spirituality, synchronicity and 'uncommon sense'. However, it didn't matter whether you called it 'God' or 'The Universe', the underlying belief was still the same: someone, or something, was ultimately in charge of it all. Things happened *for a reason*.

Through every challenge I faced, I still thought this – right up until the time I began to realise that I really might not have children. I had always seen infertility as just another challenge, albeit the toughest yet, that I would overcome. I could emerge a better person for it, sagely share with others the lessons I had learned through infertility, how it was necessary for my development and had, in the end, made me a better person – and a better parent. I was just being tested, that's all that was happening; the universe would not abandon me completely, it wouldn't leave me with nothing at the end of this. Hadn't I even realised after four years that my prayers were all wrong? It was no good single-mindedly praying for a baby, demanding a child just like that. I began praying for people to help me along the way, for me to receive the information I needed, for the wisdom to know which path to take. See. I had learned something. I was having my character built. But then no answers seemed to come. One billion, three hundred million babies, but none of them born to me. I felt abandoned all right, as well as full to the brim with grief, palpably bitter and more than just a little angry. If the universe and I had once been friends, there had been a spectacular falling-out and we were no longer on speaking terms.

This is where I would like to stop discussing faith because I don't know, not fully, what I believe in now. Infertility has shaken every belief loose and dropped each one from a great height, leaving a broken, haphazard pile of ideas on the floor. I'm still working out how to put them all back together.

After ten years, I have reached only a handful of conclusions and none of them exactly represent great philosophical breakthroughs. Other, wiser people have known these things all along. At the top of the list: we live in a random world. The most irritating phrase I can hear now is, 'It was meant to be'. This was summed up by an exchange I heard on a tube train in central London while travelling to yet another appointment to find out why I couldn't get pregnant:

Woman 1: "Wow. You're brave to have a third. Congratulations."

Woman 2: "Well, we were undecided about it, to be honest. Three children! What a handful. But we just thought 'if it's meant to be, it will be'."

Woman 1: "Oh yes, that's the thing – if it's meant to be, it *will* be. You're so right. We had exactly that with Katelyn. We weren't planning a third at all."

Woman 2, laughing: "We must be way too fertile."

Woman 1: "Well, if it's meant to be, what can you do about it?"

Before infertility, I can't say I got the urge to shout at strangers in public. But I wanted, more than anything, to leap up and say, "Hang on a minute! How come your six children are *all meant to be*? Does that mean the children I've never had were *never meant to be*?"

I wanted to whip out a diagram of healthy sperm meeting healthy egg, to show them it was nature that caused pregnancy not some benevolent being in the sky that selected them from the billions of people on earth and decreed, "Yes, you! You are the one."

I wanted to tell them that nature is random, indifferent – it doesn't care whether you'd be a good parent or the worst parent who ever walked; all it needs is the appropriate biological circumstances and boom! You have created new life. Why does it make us feel so much better to take these random, indifferent events and attach meaning to them? Why am I so important that the good things that happen to me are *meant to be?*

It was a thought I used to beat myself up with, earlier in this wrangle with infertility: *you are not meant to be a mother.* But nothing that happens in the natural world is designed to match these thought patterns. If the conditions are right, a tsunami will be a tsunami regardless of who lies in its path at the time. It's how you respond to the random event, what you choose to do with it, that counts. I was a bit slow on the uptake with infertility; I didn't run to higher ground fast enough. It's hardly surprising I nearly drowned.

When I was flailing around in 2008, it came as a shock to realise, suddenly, that I didn't believe in anything. Nothing at all. It was just another way in which I was cut adrift, except this time I was cut adrift not just from others but from my former self. Who was this strange woman who had no faith? It was as alien to me as the urge to shout at people on trains. The way it felt was … like nothing. It just felt numb and empty, like if you took the word 'pointless' and made it into a person. Bland nothingness is what you get.

The supposedly ordinary challenge of trying to get pregnant had morphed into a much bigger existential battle: if I never conceived, would I ever again believe that there was a deeper point to life? Not that I could see the question that clearly; it was more a matter of learning to survive when you've cashed in all your insurance policies. For a while, there was nothing to fall back on.

This loss of faith, this wondering what you can now believe in, is the type of thing no one mentions at fertility clinics. No one tells you: Oh, by the way, when infertility's done with you, don't expect to recognise who the heck you were beforehand. I didn't imagine, when I set out to have a family, that I would spend several years sitting on the floor trying to piece back together the broken shards of my faith. It could take a lifetime – after all, I'm hardly the first person in history to wonder whether it's possible to reconcile the random events of the natural world with the existence of a positive higher power. But I think I am reconciling it, slowly. And here's a little confession to sum up the confusion: even when I really believed that I no longer believed, I still said a silent 'Hail Mary' for those in distress if an emergency siren screamed past on the road outside. Just in case.

TWENTY-EIGHT

OUR NEW HOME IN London was a one-room studio flat, the type of place you rent when your life is in limbo. It was the sixth property we had shared in six years, quite a tally for a couple who said they wanted to settle down. Despite all that we had left behind in Switzerland, I enjoyed living in one room. It reminded me of the anticipation that had fizzed through every day when I first moved to the northern hemisphere and discovered the art of studio living. Sometimes it still felt like an adventure, this return to where I had started out in London. And besides, there were no empty spaces in a studio flat, no gaps where a family should be. At least living here, there were no reminders of the state we were striving for, but never reaching.

Chris was less convinced. "I never thought I'd live in one room," he said, taking in the bed at one end of our flat and the kitchen sink at the other. "I haven't lived in one room since I was eighteen."

But he adapted. There was no space for a couch, so he bought a bean bag, lounged on the floor and thought that perhaps he should have become a hippie all along.

"Anyway," I reassured him, "it's just for a while. Just to save a bit of money while we pay for this fertility stuff."

We each increased our hours at work and I set my focus on ICSI, since that seemed to be what we were headed for. Chris was still having regular treatment with David and, in a couple more months, he would take another test and then we'd decide. I, too, had gone back to acupuncture with David; I wanted to be in good shape for whatever treatment lay ahead.

The funny thing was, Chris and I got along better living in one room in London than we did sharing a rambling farm-house in Switzerland. And then it dawned on me: we hadn't missed one month. Ever since Chris received his diagnosis, there had been no blips at ovulation or elsewhere, no arguments about the blips, nothing. We had just attempted natural conception each month as if it were, well, the most natural thing in the world.

'Huh', I thought, 'that's a coincidence.'

Suddenly it felt like Chris was *involved* in our efforts to have a family. He had bottles of Chinese herbs lined up on the bench and swallowed three tablets at every meal, he stockpiled male fertility vitamins, bought three for the price of two at Boots. He went to acupuncture, he ate Brazil nuts every day, he got teased at work for not drinking, he ensured his sperm was regularly 'moved along' – and he wanted to make love every second day throughout ovulation, as recommended in our situation. Was David Taylor hypnotising him as well? So this was what it felt like, to have two people pulling together in the same direction. It was an almost physical relief, this sharing of the burden.

Despite the lack of space, books about fertility and conception continued to mount an assault on my side of the bed. I had moved on now to learning more about enhancing fertility through diet. I read *The Fertility Diet: How to Maximize Your Chances of Having a Baby at Any Age* and quickly improved the contents of our fridge. I banned peas, soya and rhubarb and made sure Chris understood that aspartame, often found in diet drinks and foods, was the very work of the devil. We drank carrot juice and pomegranate, cut back on white carbohydrates and began getting more exercise.

It was encouraging to read a book written by someone who had intensively researched the topic and believed I could still do it, still become a mother, even though I was now closing in on forty. It provided a mental and emotional lift; infertility had nearly beaten me, but I would make a fresh start and try again. I wasn't done just yet, thank you very much. And then I stumbled upon the thing I had been hoping for all along: 'natural' IVF.

It was a newspaper article, again, that alerted me to this option. Apparently there was a fertility clinic in London where you could undergo assisted conception minus the high dosage of drugs. It was achieving success by taking a more mild, natural approach; there were fewer side effects from this type of treatment and it also cost less due to the lesser reliance on expensive fertility medications. So it happened again. Hope sprung anew. *This* would be the key. This would be the vital piece of information that led to me getting pregnant!

There had always been three barriers to assisted conception for me: money, anxiety caused by the earlier incidence of sexual abuse and concern about how I would respond to the drug protocols. I didn't want to invest money that I didn't have into fertility treatment that scared the hell out of me, only to find that it was all a waste of time because an adverse reaction derailed the whole thing. If only I could have stated it so plainly then. But I was overcome by so many competing emotions and it was enough to cope with them all, let alone explain it to anyone else. For some reason, at the time I just didn't have the words to pitch up at a fertility clinic and say, 'Hello, here I am and these are my concerns.' I was also still extremely guarded after our damaging experience at Janet Brown's clinic; we couldn't risk a repeat of that. This time I would be much more circumspect before I told someone at one of these clinics what was really on my mind.

Nevertheless, in mid-summer Chris and I took the day off work and caught a train to southwest London for a consultation about natural IVF. In three days' time, it would be one year since I had last set foot in a fertility clinic.

"This time, I'm hardly going to say anything," I decided as we crossed the River Thames at Richmond, craning forward to take in the soothing view.

"No Lou," Chris replied firmly. "You must be free to say what you want. This time, I won't interfere, I won't say a thing – I give you my word. I'll just sit there and listen."

I smiled at him. "Well, it might be handy if you spoke now and then."

"I just want you to know I won't be taking over," he said. "I promise you that."

The clinic was in a suburban setting, much less salubrious than the one we had visited a year earlier. There was a rail bridge, a garage, a pub with breakfast for £2.99, several small bakeries and a sprinkling of charity shops. We almost missed our destination, set back slightly from the congested road. I liked the clinic as soon as I stepped inside, precisely because it had not dressed itself up as one big glossy advert for the fertility industry. That self-promotional approach was starting to feel as appropriate to me as showing off your range of celebrity-endorsed gold-plated coffins at a funeral.

Thankfully, at this clinic there were no framed magazine covers boasting on the walls, no own-brand vitamins and minerals; it was functional and understated. A reception desk, some chairs and a water cooler. There was one other couple sitting there and I felt my heart twist when I saw them. They were so quiet and polite, speaking in feather-soft voices and looking as if they were sorry for taking up any room at all; the deep sorrow on their faces was also gently etched but it hit you all the harder for it. I suddenly wondered if I might be experiencing a menopausal surge of hormones because I wanted to cry for them, and almost did. Even though I still didn't believe anyone was listening, I prayed that they got their family. They looked too fragile, I thought, to be going through this.

In the waiting area, I picked up a magazine and read the same paragraph several times while, in my peripheral vision, Chris's right leg bucked violently up and down.

"Don't jiggle," I whispered.

He stopped momentarily, looking pained at the effort involved in sitting still. I had my own private theory that all this jiggling was frying his sperm. No wonder he was always overheated; his legs were constantly on the run somewhere. He did it as unconsciously as breathing and had been unable to quit the habit, even though it might have improved his test results if his sperm got a break from being routinely shaken up. You start to look for any way of gaining an advantage when infertility has dragged on for so long.

Chris stood up and walked back and forth to the water cooler, filling and refilling his plastic beaker, checking and rechecking whether I wanted one.

"I need a wee," he hissed after the third or fourth cup. He was on his way back down the corridor from the bathroom when we were called through for our appointment.

I remember three separate consultations with various doctors or nurses in three separate rooms. I can't remember the order of the first two because it's the final one that made the lasting impression; sure enough, it was the procedure I'd rather overlook that staked its claim on my memory.

I do remember that I was glad to have found the clinic; the staff were thorough and friendly and it felt like we were finally making progress, moving things along. We saw a nurse for blood tests and to answer the familiar set of questions about our health and fertility history. Our main consultation was with the clinic director, the one I had read about in the newspaper article. I concentrated on not saying too much, sticking to the facts; we couldn't afford to mess up another of these appointments. However, it soon became clear that wasn't going to happen with this doctor. She was very obviously an expert in her field, professional and efficient but still warm; I felt at ease with her. In retrospect, I didn't say enough. It was safe to speak up this time, but I didn't. We discussed the tests that Chris and I would each undergo before a treatment plan was confirmed, although it appeared that – if his sperm analysis remained unchanged and I was still capable of providing my own eggs – ICSI would be the most suitable option.

The front I kept up in these situations was too effective. I didn't blink as the doctor explained the process of egg retrieval, when a needle would be attached to an internal ultrasound probe and inserted into my vagina while I was under sedation. I nodded in an interested manner, hoping that I appeared poised and calm, even though pangs of fear were ricocheting off the sides of my stomach.

I said nothing, gave nothing away. I had been raised to be strong and self-sufficient. Where I came from, you did not ask for special treatment just because there had been an 'incident' when you were a child. You did not tell a stranger that you had been sexually abused at the age of eleven; the code of silence was so entrenched that I hadn't even known the vocabulary for it. What did I call it? How did I describe it, this thing that had happened? No one ever talked about it on a farm in the southern hemisphere. And if I did manage to say the words, to tell someone why I was too afraid to be sedated while in such a vulnerable position? The thought of everyone whispering and making a fuss and treating me differently was worse than the thought of just going ahead with this procedure that would carry me right back to the past, when I had no control over what happened to me and I couldn't make it stop. I didn't want to be the one who was different, not again.

We were talking now about the medication involved in the treatment. There was some medication, still, with 'soft' IVF; I hadn't realised that. I thought I could avoid it altogether. I barely questioned the information; my mind was whizzing, whirling and freefalling, trying to run away from an egg retrieval. It didn't matter about the drugs. I didn't care what she said I had to take. I wouldn't be doing this. *I can't do it.* I started panicking and fretting about whether Chris could even manage to provide a sample for treatment, supposing I did go through with this thing. What if I endured all that and he said it was too much pressure to produce a sample to order? I worried that I couldn't be sure of him.

"Do you have any questions or anything you'd like to discuss?" the doctor asked after thoroughly explaining the procedure.

"No." I smiled. "No, that all sounds fine. Excellent."

Chris looked as if he wanted to say something, but had thought better of it.

"Well," she said. "We can get some of the tests under way today, if you'd like. I'll just check with the nurses but I think we might have a scan slot available."

As soon as she left the room, Chris turned to me, eyes full of sympathy and concern. "You won't be able to do it," he said instantly. "Will you?"

I blew out my cheeks as if trying to stop myself being sick.

"It's okay," he offered, squeezing my hand. "You don't have to do it. I don't blame you. It sounds appalling."

"Plenty of other women manage far worse," I observed.

"Is it the needle? That's what would get to me."

"The whole thing," I muttered. "The being sedated while they do it. Oh no, I'd probably be in stirrups. And what if it's a man? What if—"

"It's okay," Chris soothed again. "Let's not even think about it at the moment."

"We'd better have these tests though," I added, forcing myself back on track.

"That's the other thing," Chris said. "My sperm might be swimming like champions now, for all we know. We might not need to do this at all if that's the case."

341

"Yeah, but what about me? I'm nearly forty – who knows what's going on inside me. Hell! Did she just say I'm having a scan?"

When the doctor returned and it sank in that I was indeed about to have a scan, I found that my curiosity about the results, especially now that I was so much older, outweighed my usual anxieties about the procedure.

The nurse who would be doing the scan seemed warm and sympathetic, vastly different from the monosyllabic girl who had carried out my original scan in 2005, when I was still only thirty-six. Hadn't our GP already commented on my age then? What would she say now? I braced myself to appear calm and centred if the nurse looked at the screen and said my reproductive life was over.

This time, Chris was allowed into the room while I had the scan. He sat on the other side of a curtain next to the bed, almost a silhouette in the dimly-lit atmosphere. At first, I was more relaxed than for the original scan; perhaps I appeared too relaxed because it seemed that, as it went on, there were more and more people in the room. The first time, there had been just the two of us. Now there was the nurse doing the scan, another two nurses talking in the far corner, Chris behind the curtain and, halfway through, the doctor herself opened the door and breezed in. She studied the screen, tallied up follicles and discussed her findings with the nurse.

"I thought so," she said, looking over at me with a smile. "This is all very positive."

Apparently, everything was normal and it appeared there would be some eggs left to retrieve after all. I liked the doctor even more for appearing genuinely pleased on our behalf. If I was going to tell anyone, I should have told her. At the time, I was too busy dealing with the adrenaline that had surged up unbidden. This had gone on long enough now, I needed to get out of there, I needed to run. *Too many people. Too many people looking*. I felt exposed and embarrassed, as unsettled and disconcerted as if I had started the day fully dressed but then somehow found myself naked in the street.

My right ovary was causing difficulties; the scan took a bit longer because it was tricky to locate. The nurse apologised as she manipulated the probe deeper to the right. It was uncomfortable but that wasn't the problem. I had to get out of there. I couldn't have been more jumpy if I was being pursued by a clawed predator in the jungle. Still I smiled and nodded and chatted, as if discussing moisturiser, or interior decorating, over a cup of tea.

Finally, I could put my clothes back on again, keeping up the act so well that I almost convinced myself everything was fine. It was good news, they said. Now we would just wait for Chris's next test and take it from there.

On the way home, I felt a deep ache in my right side, the same as after the first scan. My hidden ovary.

"See," said Chris. "I told you there was nothing to worry about. You never listen to me when I say you don't look anywhere near your age."

"I don't think fertility cares what you look like," I snapped.

For some reason, I was overcome with irritation and anger, like I didn't want Chris anywhere near me. Back at the flat, I rejected his offer of a hug and suggested he went out for a walk.

"I'm going to have a quick nap," I said, wishing he would stop stalling and just go. Why the bloody hell wouldn't he shut up and leave me alone?

Finally, I got rid of him – because that's what it amounted to – and curled up in a tight ball on the bed. I began to cry and started frantically rubbing at my arms as if manically flicking dust off my shirt. I didn't seem able to stop, even though there was nothing to rub away.

It was Chris's fault. He had done this to me. All his problems and his fussing – yes, that's what it was, fussing – his wavering and his refusal to take tests, dragging everything out, letting it go on and on. *And fucking on.* Now I was facing this. If I had chosen someone more ... more ... more *reliable*, I would never have been in this position. Why? Why had I even gone out with him in the first place? I was stupid, that's what I was. Why did we even have to meet? Surely if I had met the 'right' person, they wouldn't have done this to me and I wouldn't feel this way. He'd taken control of me and my future, that's what he'd done.

The problem is that infertility is an invisible adversary. It's difficult to blame something you can't really see, or even picture as an actual 'thing', so when you need to hit out, you aim at something more tangible – like the person you see before you every single day. There it is right there, a visible target. When I stewed and churned and brooded on the painful situation I found myself in, it was Chris it kept coming back to. If only he had taken his test earlier, like he promised he would. If only he had addressed his performance anxiety, like he said he would. If only the appointment with Janet Brown had been used to help me, like he pledged it would. If only he hadn't derailed it, just because someone laughed at him once at school. Big deal! Nothing had even *happened* to him. And now he just got to sit there behind a curtain, without a concern in the world, while I was stripped bare on the other side of it. Because of him. He made me feel like this. Rub, rub, rubbing at my arms.

Perhaps it was too painful to make it a story about past damage, or even about infertility, but without realising it, I turned it into a story about Chris. It seemed to make sense, that it would be about him. Wasn't he the other half of this wretched failing enterprise? And wasn't it obvious that he hadn't worked as hard as I had, to become a parent?

I didn't know then, what a trigger was, or that infertility had just landed a king-hit on the worst of mine. It would be four years after that day's appointment until I saw the concept mentioned on an online forum. It linked through to this excerpt on a psychologist's blog: *A trigger is something that sets off a memory transporting a person back to the event of the original trauma.*

I had known, of course, that it was there in the background, but I hadn't realised it was having such a devastating effect on the present day. I had always preferred to minimise it, in every way. At the time, I was like a fish hooked on a line, with no awareness of being so manipulated. I thought it was infertility that I was fighting. And Chris. But this is what infertility does – it's not content with causing wounds of its own; it likes to stab at old wounds too. The anger that surged through me after these new events was not fresh anger – it was anger that had never been allowed out. It should have been aimed at another man in another time. But for several years yet it would be aimed firmly at Chris whenever infertility pulled the trigger. It's one of the saddest by-products of not being able to have children, yet it's not something that people could even imagine when they sympathise with you about your lack of fertility. They just think of the babies you haven't had; the rest of the damage, like infertility itself, is invisible.

෧ ෧ ෧

Once again, we were carrying a pot of sperm across London, this time on a train. Eager to know if his results had improved, Chris had not delayed on this test. The sample container was tucked into the front left pocket of his jeans, with a protective hand placed over the top, while his right leg continued its endless sprint to nowhere, jiggling up and down next to me.

"Did you think it looked better?" Chris asked. "Than last time? I'm sure it looked better."

345

"Oh yes," I said, despite not having a clue if there was any difference or not. "Definitely. It was definitely better."

We arrived back at the natural IVF clinic well within the all-important hour, handed over the pot and began another anxious wait. The following day, we were having lunch in a café that seemed to be serving half of London at once when Chris's phone rang. He leapt up from his seat, nodding decisively to let me know 'this is it' when he heard the voice on the other end of the line. He disappeared outside at a speed his jiggling leg would have approved of, and was lost to my view by a dozen queuing backs. Within minutes, he returned just as quickly, smiling widely.

"Good news," he announced before he had even sat back down. "It's improved. You won't believe the difference." Before I could burst with delight, he added, "They still say we'll need treatment, though."

The improvement was such that morphology was no longer being pinpointed as an issue. The sample showed an increase from one per cent normal forms to 15 per cent. It was motility that the clinic had zeroed in on as a contributory cause to the length of time it was taking us to conceive (15 per cent, compared to the norm of more than 50 per cent). However, there had been a vast turnaround in general since the last test and Chris returned to his healthy sperm regimen with renewed vigour.

He came home even more buoyed up after his next consultation with David. "It's one of the biggest improvements he's seen with male fertility," Chris reported. "Natural conception's back on the table now. That's what he said – it's a possibility."

David had also changed the ingredients in Chris's herbal tablets, tweaking them to focus more specifically on motility. I hoped more than ever that it could make a difference. My interest in these more natural approaches to health had been boosted further by something that happened at the scan I had just undertaken. Before I was overcome by the chain reaction it set off, the nurse had made a comment that stopped me in my tracks. I think I might even have laughed in disbelief.

"You've got one small fibroid here," she said. "On the left side. But it's okay – it's out of the way and not causing any trouble."

It was almost word for word what Samuel, the French osteopath, had told me when I had consulted him. Left side. Small fibroid. Not causing any problems. But he did not have an ultrasound scanner, or any other equipment, to help him peer beneath the surface. He had done nothing more than lay his hands on my stomach while manipulating my injured back. How could he have known, and in such specific detail? At the time, I toyed with the idea of his comments being true but ultimately dismissed them, unable to see how such knowledge could be possible. However, it seemed I had just been proven wrong. And the situation occurred exactly when I needed it to.

Having decided that all events were random and that there was no great mystery or meaning to life, I was finding that my days had taken on a bland, beige hue. Regardless of what my mortal soul thought about it, my imagination was getting bored with this sterile way of living – it needed a bit of intrigue to liven things up. Through the riddle of Samuel and my left fibroid, that part of me was reawakened and I began to edge slowly back towards believing in something. I just wasn't sure what it would be yet. As I should have known with fertility and us, there were plenty of challenges still ahead to help me decide.

Twenty-nine

THERE ARE MOMENTS WHEN something new or exciting or even just pleasant happens and, for that fleeting passage of time, you are free of infertility. It is hard to describe the relief provided by these brief escapes. A sort of lightness descended whenever I forgot, for a blessed beat or two, that I was not able to have children. It was too much to hope that the ceasefire could last an entire day – even if there have been no other reminders, infertility always waits when you rest your head on the pillow at night – but any distraction, any happy 'normal' event, might provide a minute, or an hour, or an afternoon, of welcome respite.

A week after we had received the latest of Chris's test results, I was looking forward to one of these valuable days off from infertility. My cousin and her husband were visiting London from the southern hemisphere and I was going to meet them and become a tourist again. Nothing could make me happier – even the longest queue at the most clichéd of holiday attractions is a source of delight for me. It was still what I thought I would do if I never had a family: travel the world, queuing up at one historic monument after another. On that day, our destination was of a more natural bent – we planned to explore Hampstead Heath, followed by afternoon tea alongside Kenwood House on the north side of the park.

Although Bev and I were cousins, the age difference between us meant that she had always been more like an aunt to me. She and her husband, Morrie, were now in their sixties and this was their first overseas trip; their earlier lives had been dedicated to raising a family of four. Bev was another of my family's hyper-fertile women – like my sister Jane, she had conceived each of her children on the first month of trying. I knew this because she was one of the few people I had briefly confided in about our struggle to conceive. She said things like: "I'm sure that if you don't have a family, you will find another purpose for your life."

We met outside the tube station at Hampstead and strolled down the hill, past cafés and bookshops and boutiques, to the Heath.

"Geez," Morrie exclaimed as we passed a delicatessen. "Eight pounds for a handful of olives. Eight quid! Do you know how many Australian dollars that is? For about six damn olives. Did they grow those things on the bloomin' tree of life itself – is that what it is?"

Bev and I left him to his wry calculations and chatted about home, as well as each of the countries in Asia that they had visited en route. By the time we reached the top of Parliament Hill, with one of my favourite views in the world stretched out before us, I couldn't have been more relaxed. I scanned the London cityscape, as I always did, for St Paul's Cathedral and couldn't help smiling down at it.

"You really love it here, don't you?" Bev observed. "Mind you, I can see why."

"I'm surprised they don't charge us ten quid a pop for this flamin' view," Morrie piped up. "It's 50p just to blow your own nose in this city."

We all laughed, knowing that secretly he was having the time of his life.

When we finally sat down for afternoon tea an hour later, it was one of those rare moments when infertility did not sit with me. With Bev and Morrie, I was just who I always had been before all this started – carefree, laidback, enjoying my surroundings. I took a sip of tea and savoured the idea that here I was: on Hampstead Heath, in London, where I had always wanted to be.

349

"So," said Bev from the other side of the table. "What are you doing about the fertility issue at the moment?"

A fertile person might not understand this but, to me, such a query at such a time was the equivalent of pulling my chair out from under me as I went to sit down. I thought frantically about how to keep it brief, how to get off this subject that I did not want to discuss. Not today. But I was caught off-guard and I hadn't yet realised that the key to survival as an infertile person is to have a stock response prepared ahead of time.

"Um. Well. Yeah," I stuttered while Bev eyed me expectantly. "We've had more tests," I managed in a rush. "We're just … um … thinking about what to do about Chris's … um … test," I finished lamely.

"What test?" Morrie enquired, swallowing a scone in one bite.

Oh God. I did not want to discuss my partner's sperm with anyone, let alone a sixty-year-old man.

Two sets of eyes bored into me.

"Sperm test," I muttered, putting on my usual outwardly calm act to disguise my discomfort.

"Ah." Morrie's eyebrows shot upwards.

Bev had more questions, so many more questions that soon they knew Chris's morphology had improved from one per cent to 15 per cent, the clinic recommended ICSI and I was still considered a 'viable' candidate for this.

I began to ramble about acupuncture, and its many benefits, just so we could stop talking about sperm.

Bev was suddenly earnest. "You do realise," she said, looking straight into my eyes, "that you will soon be too old for this?"

I scrabbled around for the appropriate response as adrenaline seized my stomach in the wake of her pronouncement.

"Well, my egg reserve's okay at the moment. I know there could be all sorts of other issues – around implantation, say, but that's not necessarily anything to do with age."

"I read that a woman is infertile for the ten years before menopause," Bev persisted. "So if your mother went through the menopause at fifty-one, then that means you're nearly at the cut-off point. Are you satisfied you'll know when the time has come to stop?"

I nodded slowly, wondering yet again what the hell to say. For one thing, I was 99 per cent sure her statistics were wrong.

"Well," I repeated. "I think I'll just listen to my body. It will let me know when it's had enough and I'll listen to it."

"I'm happy with that," Bev concluded with a satisfied nod.

Unfortunately, that day on Hampstead Heath was far from the only time I regretted mentioning our fertility problems to other people.

ᘒᘒ ᘒᘒ ᘒᘒ

It starts with 'just relax and it will happen', surely the personal favourite of the infertile everywhere. This is what fertile people counsel you to do during the first year or so of 'trying'. Apparently, malfunctioning reproductive organs can be whipped back into shape by taking a holiday and forgetting about conception altogether. Buy an airline ticket for your flight to family life.

I wish I had been bold enough in the early days to provide, in great detail, evidence of exactly how relaxed Chris and I had been. For the first year, at least, I was in no hurry to conceive; in my naivety, I remained the polar opposite of uptight. How I wish I had informed any would-be fertility experts: "Well, actually we were very relaxed three times in one day in a hotel room in Melbourne, another few times on the floor at home and – ooh yes – supremely relaxed at the naturist beach in Corsica."

The point is that, for at least a couple of years, I *was* relaxed about conception and it wasn't happening. As if that's not annoying enough, there must be few things less relaxing than being told to relax by people who have conceived children so easily that some of them didn't even mean to. Why do people think that when you've been trying to conceive for three years, it would be helpful to tell you about their sister's friend who was trying for a baby for five months, then took a holiday and – what do you know? – it happened?

It's also supremely baffling to find that, when you admit to infertility, other women will immediately respond by telling you how exceptionally fertile they are. Years ago, when I was still stupid enough to mention it, I told an old school friend about our efforts to have a family. "Oh you poor thing," she said. "I just have to think 'baby' and I get pregnant."

I genuinely don't understand it, the number of women who can't wait to tell an infertile person that they conceived on the first month of trying. To me, it's the equivalent of doing star-jumps in front of a cardiac patient while shouting, "Poor you, lying in your hospital bed. Look how strong my heart is – I can do stair-running too. No heart attacks for me!" Of course, most people would never contemplate doing such a thing yet, without a second thought, they will be equally as crass when discussing fertility.

I have come to realise over the years that it's not unlike bereavement – until you actually lose someone you love dearly, you can never really know what it feels like. Those who do not know grief act as if normal life resumes once the last hymn has faded out at the funeral. "Time heals all," they'll say by way of comfort for the grieving. But when you've lost your father, or your wife or your brother, you know different. You know that normal life will never resume. You know that the pain can still catch you unawares twenty years later and that your life is forever changed. It seems a strange human foible that we are so eager to pass on advice about things we've never experienced and certainly never felt.

It's one of the worst things about being infertile, this realisation that so few people really understand it. The baseless advice and the unhelpful comments just underline the isolation you already feel when you are trying to have a family like everyone else, but failing.

When we lived in Switzerland, part of the reason I loved Dudley and Duke so much was that they provided warmth and comfort, minus the unhelpful human clichés. They didn't say: "It will happen the minute you stop trying." Or: "How are the baby plans coming along? Any news? No? Well, Joe's going to be a dad, happened straight away." And they didn't say: "You won't be able to lie around all day if you have a baby you know." They just laid a head on my lap or my shoulder and let me know that they were there. In the midst of it all, a human friend – a fertile one, who had a family of their own – turned up at the farmhouse and informed me, "You don't want to have children."

It hurts when you're battling along in year five or year six, the things people say. Then you get closer to year ten and some of the comments start to seem ridiculously funny. I know better than to discuss fertility with anyone now, but imagine if I did. What would they say to a person who has been copulating on demand for ten years and still can't produce an embryo? Is there even a cliché out there for someone like me?

I find that those who knew about it are lost for words now, or perhaps they are just taking their cues from my silence. The last really amusing piece of advice I received came in 2009, when an aunt learned that we had been advised to have fertility treatment, due to a male factor issue with motility.

"Oh," she said. "You need reflexology. I read a magazine article about a woman who had been trying for a baby for years – then she had reflexology and she was pregnant within weeks."

"Reflexology's probably quite good," I conceded. "Only thing is, it won't improve the motility issue."

"Oh no dear," she continued, unfazed. "Don't worry about that – you take yourself off for some reflexology and, mark my words, you'll be pregnant before you know it."

My mind boggled with images of reflexology magically turning my ageing eggs into biological surf-lifesavers, running down my fallopian tubes and throwing a flotation ring to any non-swimming sperm, or perhaps providing mouth-to-mouth resuscitation for the stragglers that had already gone belly-up along the way. As silly as it seems, fertility will forever remain solely a woman's preserve as far as some people are concerned.

At least my mother, practical as always, had some relatively sensible advice, on finally hearing the truth about why we had missed her eightieth birthday.

"A cold flannel round the crown jewels might do the trick," she noted. "You want to keep 'em cool – a man's equipment is outside the body for a reason."

Meanwhile, of all the comments over all the years, it was left to a person with experience of infertility to get it 100 per cent right. My sister Vanda, who took two years to conceive her first son, was the only one who instinctively knew how to handle it.

She emailed me in 2008: "Sorry to hear about the pregnancy troubles – I have a small inkling of how you must be feeling as that was us for two years before Daniel came along, so I can only imagine how it must be after five years! As you know I am not a person who asks questions about stuff – I believe that if people want me to know something then they will tell me. But I hope you also know that if you want to talk about anything I am always here. Hope you will get a positive outcome before too long."

Nothing else needed to be said. Vanda has never raised it with me since, and that's just the way I like it.

❧ ❧ ❧

Two months after my cousin Bev informed me that I was approaching fertility Armageddon, I turned forty. And a funny thing happened – I stopped panicking about my age. Maybe it seemed that the worst had already occurred now I was no longer in my thirties, or maybe I had just grown into a deep understanding of my body. I found that I trusted it implicitly to know what it was doing. Other people were welcome to their opinions, but I was the one who knew my own biological functions. Both mentally and physically, I had never been healthier. In a perverse sort of way, I had infertility to thank for this – it had caused me to stop treating my body as a display case for make-up and clothes and to start providing real support for the vital functions being carried out beneath.

The type of people who formerly advise to 'just relax and it will happen' have an awful lot to say about a woman's age when she hits forty. Of course, there is a wealth of data about ageing and its effect on reproduction, but too many people seem to overlook the fact that we don't all age en masse; we age separately and uniquely. Dr Christiane Northrup, the highly-respected author of *Women's Bodies, Women's Wisdom*, phrased it like this: "If you are over forty and trying to get pregnant, examine your programming about being 'too old'."

She wrote, "While statistics show that in general, women's fertility declines as they age, most women don't realise that such statistics do not predict whether any individual woman will have difficulty conceiving." She noted that, "A lot of women over forty may not realise how fertile they are ..."

In fact, one of the painful paradoxes about being a forty-year-old woman who wants to have a baby is this: armchair experts will routinely inform you that you are 'too old', yet statistics reflect an increase in the number of women over forty who are undergoing pregnancy terminations. The rise in these figures recently led to a warning from UK fertility experts that women over forty should not assume they could safely abandon contraception.

As if to underline these comments, I had increasingly felt that my body was revving up during the monthly cycle, rather than applying the brakes. My instincts were further put into words by an obstetrician I later saw on a documentary about multiple births. She explained that a woman's chances of naturally conceiving multiples increased as she aged.

"As women get older, they're more likely to release an egg from each ovary at the same time," she said. "It's about nature getting the last bit of reproductive potential out of you. So you're at the point where your ovaries are likely to fail and it's almost like, if there are any good eggs there, your body wants to make sure they're used."

I had already sensed that my body was starting to do this, almost as if it was staging one last stand, but had dismissed my instincts as fanciful. It didn't chime with what other people said about women like me.

Interestingly, and frustratingly, these same people never mentioned Chris's age, even though he was nearly fifteen years older than me. Scientific studies also pinpointed a decline in male fertility over the age of forty, as well as linking older fathers to an increased risk of genetic disorders, but no one had ever sat him down and asked whether he realised he was now "too old for this".

When I turned forty, there was only one candle on my birthday cake. It signalled a change of attitude: this was year one of a new, stronger approach. I would no longer be knocked off my stride by other people's opinions about my body; it was mine and mine alone to know. For now at least, my monthly cycle was operating smoothly and reliably, with signs of ovulation most months. I realised of course that, so far, this had not been enough to get me pregnant. But we were edging towards treatment at the natural fertility clinic. I had enough of a credit buffer left on one of my cards for one cycle of treatment; Chris had asked about remortgaging his house to turn that into two, or even three. I was steeling myself to go through with it, mentally preparing and trying to toughen up, which is what I still thought was needed.

There were always questions, of course, the biggest of all: is it worth it? All of this for a 15 per cent chance of success.

"I'd do it in a heartbeat if there was a 100 per cent guarantee," I told Chris.

He gave a wry laugh. "If there was a 100 per cent guarantee, it would cost a lot more than a few thousand pounds."

We both knew it was time to answer the questions once and for all. At least we had a lot more information now, at least we had found a way to get the money, at least we knew where we were heading. I should have known better by then. This was fertility and us after all. It was odd how the ground seemed to shift every time we thought we had found a solution. Yet again, we were making plans and infertility was laughing.

THIRTY

Two days after I turned forty, we both lost our jobs. At one stroke, the company we worked for wiped all contract positions from its books. Perhaps it said something about what my career had become that this turn of events felt a lot more liberating than it should have. If I didn't have fertility costs in the back of my mind, I would have felt like a prisoner awarded parole. Chris and I were each offered new roles on what equated to half-pay; we declined, confident that we could find work elsewhere. I knew what I had to do now and, for once, it didn't have any connection with fertility: it was time to go home and see my family. I rang Mum and told her we would be there for Christmas, arriving in the southern hemisphere in late November and returning to the UK in late January. I had not seen Mum since January 2003 – all of the time between, certainly the latter years, seemed to have been eaten up with my efforts to have children of my own. I feared more than anything that I would devote all this time and effort to parenthood, only to find that I ended up without children and without seeing my own mother again too. I dreaded hearing the news that she was gone; I couldn't get that phone call and know that it was nearly five years since I had last seen her. This time, fertility could wait.

"Anyway," said Chris, ever optimistic. "I've got great faith in the southern hemisphere sun – and all that light. You're much more likely to get pregnant down there than you are living this lifestyle."

I packed my beach gear, along with a box of fertility-friendly lubricant that would supposedly help Chris's sperm on its journey. Once again, our belongings went into storage and we left our studio flat after only six months. By now, I was juggling three credit cards to cover costs like airline flights or fertility expenses – just when I thought I had run out of credit, the limit magically increased and, as a result, I still had £6,000 on one card earmarked for prospective IVF. Having a baby? Priceless, as the advert might say.

On the flight to San Francisco, I again observed that palms really can sweat – not just a little clamminess, but enough moisture to require constant mopping up with a succession of tissues. I had not been on a plane since the abandoned landing on our way back from Switzerland; what I really needed was to be drunk or, even better, tranquilised. However, I didn't want to risk any further disruption to my cycle; these long-haul flights across the time zones were enough on their own. For the first hour, I managed some semblance of calm, reading a magazine, staring at a crossword, watching the beginning of a romcom. Then I ran out of energy to fool myself that I was a 'normal' traveller and reverted to panic mode for the remaining nine-and-a-half hours, tetchy and jumpy and sweaty and unable to speak.

Maybe my nervy appearance was what alerted customs officials after we landed in the United States; for whatever reason I found myself being asked to open my luggage and to pull the fertility-friendly lubricant from its packet and place it on a display table in the arrivals hall. It's possible that I have never been so annoyed about not being able to conceive naturally. In my heightened state, I wanted to shout, "Ask me! Go on. Ask me how many years I've been trying to have a baby." It's the type of hysteria you can normally keep under control in everyday life, assuming your nerves have not just spent eleven hours being fed through a shredder.

I had two days to get over it before repeating the exercise with a thirteen-hour flight to the southern hemisphere. Helpfully, the next plane began shaking and shivering the instant we took off, then bucked and jolted its way through the night for an entire twelve hours. I had accepted, long before we reached the Pacific Islands, that I was going to die half a flight short of seeing my mother again. Chris held me tight and urged me to focus on the welcome that awaited at the other end. When the landing gear finally came to rest on home ground, it was one of the happiest moments of my life.

२६ २६ २६

This time, Christmas was not the most difficult period of the year. I didn't notice the gaping hole where a family should be, or not so much at least, now that I was back in the midst of one. Mum, at the head of the clan, still had more energy at eighty than I did at forty. She cooked roast dinners, made a 'proper' Christmas cake and the traditional pudding, bursting with foil-wrapped coins – and, having baked all morning, drove off to play table tennis afterwards. Worrying about her on the other side of the world, I had overlooked my own mantra – we don't all age at the same rate. Mum came back from table tennis and proceeded to challenge Chris to a game of badminton in her hallway, laughing raucously when she sideswiped the pictures on the wall with her racket. If I ever managed to make her a grandmother again – she already was one thirteen times over – then my children were still guaranteed a good time if they went to stay with Granny.

There were twelve of us on Christmas day, and many more over the holiday season as a whole – brothers, sisters, nieces, nephews, aunts, uncles and cousins. We welcomed the New Year with arms linked in a sprawling circle of relatives, all singing *Auld Lang Syne* outside on the lawn at the top of our voices. No one else in the rowdy circle knew, but even before the chime of midnight we had already moved into our seventh year of trying to conceive. It was now 2009 – was it really New

Year's Day 2003 when Vanda and Amy had interrupted us, giggling and carefree as we let reproduction take its course? Or at least thought that's what we were doing.

My sister Jane asked about our fertility issues while we were sitting together on the beach one day in early January. "Well," she said with a smile, "perhaps you'll make a little southern hemisphere baby while you're here."

We did our very best to try. It had been nearly a year since the receipt of Chris's test results in Switzerland and, in that entire time, there had been no glitches at all. It was such a relief to know we could actually try for a baby each month that I felt physically lighter, as if my age had suddenly reversed by five or ten years. I could cope so much better with failing if I knew I had least turned up and given it a go. "How very romantic of you," Chris laughed when I told him as much.

There was now just one other problem: I did not want to leave the southern hemisphere. I wanted to stay at home with my family. Something had changed since the last time I was here. Was it just that I would have been permanently at home by now anyway, if I'd had children? I wanted this life for them so much, even though they didn't even exist. I lay in bed at night, running through scenario after scenario in my head as I tried to work out a way that we could stay. What if I was pregnant? Imagine that. We'd have no choice – I couldn't possibly fly then.

Of course, there was no southern hemisphere baby – why did I still hope after all this time? – and in the end we had to settle for delaying our flight back to the UK by a week. It was the first time that neither of us had wanted to return and the family seemed to sense it. Mum, my two sisters, three of my nieces, one nephew and a brother-in-law gathered to wave us off at the airport; it seemed counterintuitive to be leaving them behind in favour of Heathrow, where there would be no one to greet us. Vanda sat next to me in a departure hall café and wrapped her hands around my index fingers, holding tight and pulling a face that said, 'Don't go.'

It was the fourth time I had departed for the UK from that same airport, but it was the first time I had shed any tears over it. There were many reasons we couldn't stay, from finances to visa status to employment, and of course there was Rose, waiting alone for us to come back. But, in truth, the call of home was stronger than all of those factors. The main reason I really left again, even though not a part of me wanted to go, was that I didn't have children. No one in London would care or even notice, but if I stayed at home I would be the only person I knew of my generation who did not have a family. It was that type of place – you went there for the lifestyle and to settle down. Many of my peers from high school, the ones who had never left the area, now had nineteen- and twenty-year-old sons and daughters. The others, who had moved away to pursue careers or travel, had since migrated back and were raising younger families. I had noticed over the past two months that it didn't matter how many friends of the family we met or how many barbecues and dinners we went to, there was no one at any of them who was like us.

"I'd be the only childless woman in the village," I joked to Chris, trying to make light of it. It was uncomfortable, though, the feeling that I would again be the odd one out. I'd felt it in various ways all my life through being adopted, then through being part of a single-parent family in an era when it was still unusual, and I wasn't prepared to be the 'different' one this time. That's why I loved London; it allowed me to hide, to be just another face on the street, childless or not. I liked the fact that fellow travellers on the tube couldn't care less about my parental status. If, as I was starting to suspect, I really was a person who would forever fall through the cracks, then London was the right place to do it. I hugged my family close and said goodbye.

If a miracle had happened and the seed of a southern hemisphere baby really had been planted in my womb, it would have taken a second miracle for it to stay there. The flight back to San Francisco did not just buck and jolt for twelve hours, it plummeted and plunged, up and down, side to side, for the entire trip. It was like riding a malevolent rollercoaster that never followed the same track twice. I downed four herbal sedatives, which I had never tested before, and two Panadol on an empty stomach and lolled, incoherent, in my seat. My airways felt a bit blocked, but it was probably just the altitude. I came around to find an oxygen mask attached to my face and a flight attendant from my home country poised anxiously above me. It was a long time since I had felt either so ill or so embarrassed. As she squatted beside my seat to offer a cup of lemonade, the plane shot upwards with such force that the contents of the glass arced a foot in the air and splashed down all around, like an in-flight water feature. Somewhere behind me, someone was throwing up.

"It can be even worse than this over the Pacific at this time of year," she assured me. "Last week the turbulence was so bad, we had flight crew being thrown out of their bunks."

She gave up her break and worked through the night, swaying up and down the aisles with dry toast and flat lemonade, to ensure her growing group of ill passengers arrived in one piece. As dawn broke not far out of San Francisco, I began to recover.

"Thank goodness," she smiled. "You've got some colour back in your cheeks – you had us all worried there for a while."

I thanked her for looking after me all night. "Oh," she said. "I barely needed to. You've got a good one there – he didn't take his eyes off you, not once."

I looked across at Chris, still clasping one of my hands. "He's been getting you to take fluids all through the night," she added, "when you weren't quite with us. Mopping you down with a cold flannel, everything. He's been an absolute star."

It was one of those moments when you realise that, after six years of infertility, there is still something left of the relationship you started out with. We had raged and sulked and shouted and blamed, yet here it was amongst all the damage – a little shard of unbroken care for each other. It was about to be tested even further, but at least it had survived the turbulence so far, both on the plane and off it. Chris leaned over and kissed me on the nose, like he always had. "It's okay," he whispered. "Nearly there."

❧ ❧ ❧

Since being infertile, I've made some really stupid decisions. Perhaps it's because the emotions involved become so pervasive that they leach into everything. My rational brain didn't have a chance sometimes, not when infertility had seized the controls. How else to explain what I decided to do next?

We returned to find the UK mired in recession; a year earlier it would have seemed improbable to say the least that a long-standing brand like Woolworths would be wiped from every high street but, in our absence, it had happened. Along with a lot more besides. The mood could not have been more different from the southern hemisphere, where it was still summer and everyone I knew was still in work. Home felt further away than ever. Chris and I were holed up in Rose's spare room, huddled together at night in the single bed, wondering where we were going to live. Despite the fact that neither of us had a job, we went flat hunting in London.

When we first met, before any thought of trying to conceive had taken hold, Chris had lived in the terraced house that he owned in the country, twenty minutes down the road from Rose's flat. He still owned it, with the same tenants in residence since 2003. "I think we're going to have to go back there, you know," Chris said after another day of viewing cramped flats in London that would cost £1,500 a month to rent.

The idea filled me with dread, although I couldn't fully explain why.

"I don't think I can live with you there," I said, "stuck together in the middle of nowhere like that."

"Is it always going to be like this?" Chris retorted, stung by my words. "Are you always going to hold it against me, what happened with Janet Brown, what happened in Switzerland? Because if you are, then there's not much point going on, is there?"

"I don't know," I snapped. "I don't know what it is. I just can't live there with you, all right."

"You're so angry with me," he said. "Deep down, you can't stand me, not really, I can feel it."

The stand-off had its origins two days earlier, when I was cooking dinner and Rose and Chris were sitting at the table. I had heard Chris's mother say, "I know Louise can be difficult, but I'm terribly fond of her, you know."

He had rushed to shush her before she said any more; he could see by my face that I felt betrayed all over again, because if he hadn't told her that I was difficult, then who had? I had never been anything but obliging and polite in her presence. I wanted to scream: "I'll tell you what difficult is. Difficult is refusing to take a sperm test. Difficult is holding back your partner when they're doing everything they bloody can to have a family."

He was right; I was beginning to hold it all against him, deep down. But there wasn't time to dwell on that, not if I wanted to become a mother. I was starting to realise just how far I'd fallen through the cracks, forty years old with no job and sleeping in a single bed, and that was only thanks to the hospitality of a very elderly lady.

"Look at us," I said to Chris. "What the hell have we got to offer a kid? It's probably just as well it's never worked out."

I was talking about our financial situation and about employment; I should really have been talking about our relationship because the first two things could be remedied – the depth of resentment that was lying camouflaged between us might be a bit more difficult to shift. I ignored it, swallowed down the anger that flared now and then, and continued marching onwards, refusing to deviate from my path, still hoping it would lead to pregnancy.

It was my fault that we moved to London, into a flat that we couldn't afford. I needed to be in the city that had always sheltered me when times were tough. There were lots of hiding places in London and lots of distractions. There was also the 'natural' fertility clinic and I still had £6,000 available on one credit card. Like I said, I've made some really stupid decisions since being infertile.

THIRTY-ONE

OUR NEW NEIGHBOUR IN London was a former belly dancer who referred to herself as a retired actress because she once had a non-speaking role in a movie made for television. She was given to stopping us in the street and delivering monologues about the life she had lived on the edge of show business during the 1970s. She was now sixty-two years old but kept the same hours as when she had danced in nightclubs all over Europe. She rose at 2.30pm, stayed up drinking until 5am and spent the time in between chain-smoking in her lounge and writing letters in cod legalese to most of our other neighbours, with whom she was permanently enraged.

Sometimes it was drains that set her off, sometimes it was trees or foxes; any of these issues could spark a midnight rant, delivered in a shriek that should have cracked the windows and followed with a flurry of apoplectic door slamming. Lorna was the reason we had no internet connection for the first few months of our tenancy. She owned the downstairs flat and the garden – "I own the freehold to the front path" was one of the first things she ever said to me – and we rented the two-bedroom flat upstairs. In an expletive-ridden series of shrieks, she made it abundantly clear that she would not be allowing our broadband provider to bury a shallow cable down one side of her front garden; it would shake the building's foundations and bring down the whole house. It would also 'ruin' her garden, which consisted of a few dead shrubs, some cracked paving tiles and assorted bin-bags of rubbish.

However, none of these eccentricities was the most interesting thing about Lorna as far as I was concerned. The one thing I really wanted to hear a monologue about was how she had managed to have a baby at the age of forty-four. For Lorna did not live alone – she shared her flat with her eighteen-year-old son, born just before her forty-fifth birthday. Not only that, but her pregnancy came soon after a doctor had informed her that her fertile days were over and she needed a hysterectomy. The same man was surprised to encounter her on a hospital ward two days after she had given birth to her son. Pointing out the healthy baby asleep in her arms, she told the astonished medic: "You can tell me I need a hysterectomy when *you've* grown a fucking vagina!"

Since I was still 'only' forty, Lorna gave me hope that I could yet become a mother. I couldn't fling one leg up the wall behind my ears as Lorna was wont to do mid-monologue, but surely if she could produce a baby in her forties, then I might have a chance to do so, too. I didn't smoke or drink for one thing although, given the number of my acquaintances who conceived while regularly doing both, I was beginning to wonder if I should start. I put the unhelpful thought out of my head and had another glass of carrot juice.

We moved in above Lorna in mid-March and in mid-April left her conducting her series of dramatic performances to no one in particular while we returned to Switzerland to collect our belongings. The furniture we previously had in storage had arrived from the north of England and our flat was taking on the appearance of a home belonging to two settled adults.

Mary and Ian, our former landlords in Switzerland, e-mailed to say we should stay one last night on the vineyard before driving back to England. As we trundled south in a hired van, Chris and I talked animatedly about seeing Dudley and Duke again and sleeping for one last time in the farmhouse we had never wanted to leave. We finally arrived mid-afternoon and pulled into our familiar parking space at the side of the house, wondering who owned the car that was already sitting there. The Labradors, wagging not just their tails but their entire bodies, immediately arrived to frisk us from top to toe, followed shortly by Mary who settled for a kiss on each cheek by way of welcome. I couldn't wait to open the farmhouse door and revisit our old home. But as we stood talking beside the van, the door opened from the inside and the tall figure of a man in his late thirties strode out.

"Hey there," he called in an American accent. "You must be our predecessors." My stomach and face dropped in unison.

"This is Alan," Mary explained. "He and his family are our new tenants." On cue, his wife and two daughters, aged about six and eight, emerged over the threshold. Of course. Time had moved on. Why wouldn't it? It just seemed that, more and more often, it was moving on and leaving us behind.

Chris and I carried our bags across to Mary and Ian's converted barn at the other end of the lawn and set off for a walk through the surrounding grapevines. As we strolled up the gentle hill on the edge of the village, we looked back and saw Alan's daughters in the distance, playing a game of chase on the farmhouse lawn. Since moving out of earshot, we had spoken of nothing but the new tenants.

"They're living our life," I said sadly. "That's what I thought our life would be."

"I know," Chris replied. "I can't stand seeing someone else living there. It still feels like home. It feels like we've just got back from London and we should be having tea in that kitchen now."

"They had to have children," I added cynically. "Of course they did."

"Oh well," said Chris. "At least we'll get to say goodbye properly when we go in to collect our things."

Later in the afternoon, we knocked on the farmhouse door and went up to the loft to start transferring our possessions to the van. Alan's wife Georgia was in the kitchen cooking dinner, their daughters were doing homework in the lounge, 'our' bedroom door was shut and so was the one opposite, now shared by the two girls. We contented ourselves with one last look around the upstairs lounge as we hauled bags of bedding and boxes of books out of the storage cupboard and downstairs to the driveway. The opportunity of starting a family of our own in the farmhouse was well and truly lost to us.

That night, Mary and Ian were as hospitable as ever, plying us with an endless supply of food and drinks, but afterwards I lay crestfallen in their upstairs bedroom, eyes wide open in the darkness.

Alan and Georgia came out to wave goodbye when we drove away early the next day. We were barely ten minutes down the road when the argument started.

"That should have been me," I muttered darkly. "It was supposed to be us there, having a family. But it's always got to be these perfect people, doesn't it?"

"It was hard for me to see, too," said Chris. "But we did our best, sweetheart. That's all we can do."

"No we didn't," I protested. "Maybe if we had done our best, we might have had a child by now, you never know. We might have had the chance to live there like they are if—"

"Oh, not this again," Chris snapped. "I'm doing my best, you must see that. How can it all be my fault?"

"Well, I wasn't the one who took years to have a sperm test, was I? If we'd got those results sooner, who knows what could have happened."

"This is ridiculous!" Chris slammed the van into fifth gear. "I don't deserve this. We're having a nice drive through Switzerland and now you've turned it into this."

"Oh sorry. Have I upset you? Well, how do you think I felt when you hijacked my appointment with Janet Brown? Or when you—"

"I didn't hijack it. Really, this is silly. Why must you always treat me like the enemy?"

I stared, unblinking, out of the passenger side window. "Because you've acted like one, that's why."

"I can't believe you could say that after all I've done for you – all I've done for us."

Back and forth it went for more than 200 miles of the B roads in both Switzerland and France, the row that never ran out of fuel but never travelled anywhere decent either. When we pulled into a budget motel for the night, there were no words left for either of us to say. In the silence of our white-washed room, I realised that, with particularly cruel timing, my period had arrived. I took some Panadol for the cramps that gripped my midriff and lay down forlornly on the bunk bed.

"I'm really sorry, Lou," Chris said softly, realising what had happened.

"I bet Georgia doesn't even get stomach cramps," I growled.

⁊⅙ ⁊⅙ ⁊⅙

The call from MBNA, one of my credit card providers, flashed up on my phone the week after we returned from Switzerland. It was a woman who demanded to know why I had missed a scheduled monthly payment when we were still in the southern hemisphere.

"That can't be right," I said, instantly worried and confused. "I paid everything online – and well within time. Can I just get my diary?" I returned to the call to confirm that I had paid £185 that month, as usual.

"It was £10 short," the crisp voice replied. "That counts as a missed payment."

"But it's always £185."

"Your interest rate was adjusted in January. The minimum monthly payment is now £195."

"Oh, I didn't realise. I was out of the country for a couple of months."

The voice did not comment on this. "As a result of your missed payment, we have conducted a review on your account. I see that you have a total of £15,000 outstanding with three different providers."

"Yes."

"What have you spent that much money on?"

"Pardon?"

"That's a very high level of debt to be carrying. How have you accrued it?"

I just knew the owner of that voice had children and that she'd had them instantly and easily, while she progressed through life ticking off each milestone at precisely the prescribed moment.

"Trying to have a family mostly," I replied as evenly as I could. "For more than six years. I haven't spent it on shoes and handbags, if that's what you're asking."

There was a momentary pause, a change of tone when she resumed speaking.

"I see. Well. We have taken the decision, as a result of our investigations, to reduce your credit limit by £6,000. It might be possible to review it again in the future once your overall level of debt has decreased. If you could work on bringing it down, that would be beneficial."

I hung up and cursed infertility for the thousandth time. It wasn't the only issue that had got me into this situation, but it seemed there wasn't an area of my life where it couldn't knock me off course.

Now, for the sake of £10, I had lost the buffer I had earmarked for treatment at the 'natural' IVF clinic. It really did seem that every time we made plans regarding fertility, an unforeseen U-turn would follow.

I overlooked the fact that I no longer believed in anything except randomness and told Chris, "I'm not meant to be a mother! Could it be any more clear?"

"That's not true," he retorted. "And that woman had no right asking what you've spent your money on. It's none of her business. Why should you have to tell her we can't have a family?"

"Well, technically, I suppose it's her money though, isn't it. And some of it pre-dates the fertility thing—"

"It's no more hers than yours. Anyway, forget about them and their exorbitant interest rates, I'm going to ring Mark Mayes."

Mark was the account manager who had offered to loan us up to £200,000 the previous year when we were considering buying a property in Switzerland.

"I must be able to get some sort of loan or mortgage extension," Chris said. "There's plenty of equity in my house still."

He returned from his call wearing an expression that did not require translation.

"It's a 'no' then," I ventured.

"They won't loan us a penny," Chris confirmed. "Even £4,000 added to my mortgage is out of the question. They've tightened all the rules since the crash. They're not lending a bean if they can help it. Mark says it's not even worth trying an application."

As usual, our timing was out. The previous year, banks and credit card companies had been throwing money at us, to the point where I regularly opened statements to find my credit limit had magically increased by several thousand pounds. Now, if we wanted to fund fertility treatment before I got much older, there was only one way of doing it – selling Chris's house.

"At least we've got that option," he said, forehead creasing up as he considered it.

"No!" I replied, adamant. "You are not ending up without a family *and* without a house. It's the only thing you've got – you need to hold onto it."

Without realising it, I was increasingly taking a more defensive position when confronted with infertility, shoring up protection in case the worst happened and our family really never arrived. I was prepared to risk almost anything, including my personal credit rating, for a baby who might never come, but to sell Chris's house in a recession? If we did so and the resultant fertility treatment was not successful – we were being quoted a hit rate of less than 20 per cent – then we really would emerge at the other end of this challenge with nothing. There were times still, under the ongoing pressure, when we wondered if we'd even have each other.

We agreed not to sell the house. We'd either have to save the money or find another way around it. I was forty years old, we had been trying to conceive for nearly six-and-a-half years and fertility treatment was out of reach. We were both technically unemployed and a global recession had taken hold. My response to all of this was to spend a large chunk of my time in the park, walking barefoot on the grass and savouring the feel of the earth beneath my toes. It was an unorthodox reaction, to say the least.

In 2009, I thought it was because I was momentarily free, having spent nearly twenty-five years in offices, where I could see nothing of the outside world. But it wasn't just that. It turned out that if I was going to make the biggest compromise of all – never becoming a mother – then I wasn't prepared to accept other, smaller compromises. They all had to go. It might have been more helpful if I had realised that at the time. Perhaps it was too painful for my mind to accept what my instincts already knew – I probably was not going to become a parent and, if so, it was time to start improving the parts of my life that would be left behind in the wake of infertility.

❦ ❦ ❦

It seeped in slowly, this sea change, and swept first across my career. I would not be returning to the profession that had dominated my life since the age of seventeen. I had known from the beginning that it was the wrong place for me. If my profession was a person, then we were polar opposites – it was bolshie and argumentative, I was shy and peace-loving; it was a show-off, I shunned the limelight; it wanted to compete aggressively, I wanted to quietly run my own race. Every day when I went to work, it was as if I put my soul in a box and left it there. If that's what my children had needed me to do to support them, then I would have done it, despite the fact that I had planned a career break when I had my family. But what was I doing it for now? The sorrow of infertility was enough; there wasn't the room somehow for another draining situation.

I ignored several job offers and informed Chris that I wanted to start my own business. From now on, I would work for myself. As I knew he would be, he was instantly supportive, not once mentioning the recession or the pitfalls of striking out on my own in such treacherous times. Despite all our heated rows about fertility, one thing was clear: he still had faith in me. Sometimes, being with Chris was like having your own personal cheerleader. As far as he was concerned, there was nothing I couldn't do. Perhaps he also understood the other reason I was reluctant to return to office life. Another tidal shift had crept in over the years – the increasingly obvious need for isolation. I could no longer face sitting in offices listening to colleagues talk about their children, the births of their babies, the pregnancies of their wives. I wanted to shut the door and block it all out.

So, in the midst of the worst global recession since the Great Depression, I started a business. It consisted of a laptop, a desk and a broken chair – propped up, I hoped, by the twenty-three years of knowledge I had gleaned throughout my career. Chris returned to the type of office where we used to work together and said he would support me through the start-up. Now working from home, I was able to return to nature with a vengeance in my ongoing quest to conceive. I continued to walk barefoot on the grass every day, made sure I got sun on my skin for vitamin D and plenty of daylight for a healthy circadian rhythm. I downed a glass of sludgy green liquid every lunchtime, hoping that the organically-grown grasses, grains and vegetables within would infuse my body with more than 125 vitamins, minerals and amino acids, as promised on the bottle. I had been taking preconception vitamins for nearly seven years; to these I added high-strength acidophilus and a rotating mixture of supplements that included L-Tyrosine for thyroid support and blue green algae because the woman in the health food shop said it worked wonders.

I stopped cooking anything in plastic containers, for fear of chemicals leaching into our food, and no longer bought drinking water housed in plastic. My body, sustained for much of its life on either nothing at all or red meat and junk food, must have thought my mind had been hijacked by an intruder.

I was not the only one attempting to invite fertility in via the health-food route. Chris kept up his daily male vitamins and David's herbal tablets, as well as experimenting with high-dose vitamin C for sperm motility and eating packet after packet of Brazil nuts for all-round reproductive health.

We also managed something that had sometimes proved a step too far during my thirties – we had sex every month at ovulation and beyond, sometimes spontaneously. This is it, I thought, even at the age of forty years, eight months. I really will get pregnant this time! Forty-one was a lot later than I expected to become a mother, but I would welcome it all the more because of the prolonged wait for my much-wanted child.

I finally bought a copy of *The Secret* and began visualising myself holding my son or daughter in my arms. I'd pictured this, over and over, as long ago as 2004 – my baby had seemed so real, it was almost as if I could reach out and touch him. I thought I actually saw him once, chuckling. Then he never arrived and I stopped visualising. Now, encouraged by what I read, I acted 'as if' it was going to happen.

I went shopping and bought baby socks, size zero to three months, three pairs in soft stripy blue. I placed the doll-sized accessories in my underwear drawer and tenderly stroked them every day when I opened it. Whenever we made love, I reverted to that old trick afterwards, doing awkward shoulder-stands with legs propped up against the wall; something else I'd long given up on. Without researching whether it was safe, I took eggs – British Blacktail, free-range, from Waitrose – and separated the whites before inserting them via syringe, a magic river that was going to carry Chris's sperm, finally, to its long-awaited destination.

This is how infertility rattles your foundations – it's hard to feel stable when, on the one hand, you are making changes 'in case' you don't become a parent and, on the other, you still hope endlessly that this might be the month it finally happens. The two mind-sets do not sit comfortably with each other; it is as if they belong in two different heads but you have to find space for them in just the one. Sometimes you wonder what has happened to your own mind, and if it hasn't gotten away from you, just a little. But it's natural that it would be destabilising, trying to balance two opposing forces that wax and wane, often in synch with your own cycle. Up, down, back and forth – it didn't matter. I still wasn't pregnant. My skin, however, was glowing; a small consolation but one that could sometimes cheer me for a few minutes at a time. You learn to seize on these little pleasures when prolonged infertility sets about dismantling your life.

❧ ❧ ❧

Eight days after my forty-first birthday, we got the early-morning phone call from the southern hemisphere that I had long dreaded. I was half-asleep still when Chris sat down gently on my side of the bed and placed a reassuring hand on my shoulder. I knew him well enough to sense, even in my groggy state, that something terrible had happened. My eyes flew open.

"What's happened? Is it Mum? Is Mum okay?"

"Sweetheart," Chris said quietly. "It's not your mum. Don't worry, she's fine. But Vanda's just phoned and I'm afraid she had some very bad news about George."

George was the middle of my three brothers, the gentle music-loving, sports-mad scholar who had accepted my arrival into his life when he was thirteen with exceptionally good humour.

"He's had a massive heart attack at home." Chris enveloped me in a hug as his words sank in. "He's in hospital now, but I'm really sorry – Vanda said it doesn't look good."

The following morning, the phone rang again. George had died in hospital, surrounded by his extended family and close friends. He was fifty-four years old.

I couldn't afford to fly home at short notice – the best fare I could find cost several thousand pounds – so Chris and I held our own 'memorial' for George at 2am the next Tuesday, coinciding exactly with his funeral in the southern hemisphere. George was a teacher and when I read his obituary and saw the tributes to him, I realised that my modest brother, who never told us of his achievements, had transformed the lives of scores of children. It brought me up short to remember that this was what other people were doing to enhance the world around them. Thanks to infertility, I had just spent nearly seven years of my life giving very little of myself to anyone. In the weeks after George's death, I realised it had to stop. I had to turn it around.

"I've got to do something meaningful," I told Chris. "Look at George and all he gave to the world. I can't keep sitting here doing nothing because all my energy's going into having children. I've got to find something to *do*. Something that matters."

And despite the inspiration I took from George, there it was in the back of my mind, the small hopeful thought that refused to be silenced: *Now would be a really good time to get pregnant. Our family needs some good news.*

As the seventh year of our quest to conceive came to a close, it seemed I didn't know who I was – a woman who accepted it was time to move on or a woman forever beguiled by the whispered incantation: *mother*. Could there be any word worthy enough to replace that one?

THIRTY-TWO

IF TIME HAD LEFT us behind, 2010 made a great job of pointing that out. For one thing, this wasn't just another year turning over – the eighth as it happened – it was a new decade. The switch from 09 to 10 seemed to underline just how long we had stagnated in the area of life that meant the most to us. I tried to inject some forward momentum by throwing my energy into the new business; perhaps the change in my career would trigger long overdue movement in other quarters. However, in mid-February the initial message brought by 2010 was hammered home even further. I realised that I had not only been overtaken by a new decade, I had been overtaken by the next generation of my own family.

I opened an e-mail from my sister Vanda and instantly noted that she seemed to have written much more than usual. When I reached the middle of the message, I understood why. It was one of those e-mails where the writer needs to pass on something that might be upsetting so they bury it in the centre – opening with the news would be too insensitive and ending with it too obvious (I didn't know how to say this so I've left it 'til last); it inevitably gets plonked in the middle to make it appear casual, no bigger deal than anything else that has been mentioned. Vanda was such a natural soother of troubled waters that she had unwittingly written exactly three paragraphs before the big news and three paragraphs after it.

"On to other news," she wrote mid-e-mail, "...we are getting an addition to the family in June kind courtesy of Jules!"

Jules? My brother Ray's eldest daughter? I didn't know she had a boyfriend.

I had already braced myself for when my nieces began having children of their own, but – even though Jules was in her mid-twenties and would make a wonderful mother – this was not the niece I had expected. I had been sure the first announcement would come from one of her older cousins. But, continued Vanda, a scan had just confirmed that Jules would be having a daughter at the beginning of June; everyone was surprised and delighted.

I had been trying to bring a new addition into the family for more than seven years; I didn't want to be the sort of person who was hurt by someone else's happy news, but that didn't stop the shot of pain at gut level. It's one of the hardest things to explain when you're infertile, the way it feels to hear someone else announce the precious news that you had long hoped to announce yourself.

It's not that I wasn't happy for the niece I loved dearly – it's more that joy at her news somehow shone a light on my own profound sadness. Vanda had taken such care, of course, because she knew how difficult it was to assimilate. How could it be so easy for others, this thing that had taken me more than seven long, hard, painful years and still I hadn't managed it?

The truth of being infertile is this ugly: when I told Chris about Jules, his first words were, "Oh, I'm sorry sweetheart." Someone is having a new baby and we are sorry, albeit not that this conception has happened, just that ours never did.

We both made sure to add that Jules was a born mother and the baby was a lucky little girl, but there can be something about the initial reaction that makes you feel a bit sullied afterwards, that you've let yourself down, been a smaller, more selfish person than you wanted to be.

Sadly, there is sometimes no controlling it. As ever with me, it took a while to sink in. That night, I phoned Mum and tried not to notice the accidental change in her voice when she mentioned Jules. I bluffed my way through the conversation, saying, "Good on her for surprising us all." I wondered, was Mum, from the other side of the world, noticing any subtle change in my own voice when I said that? I hoped I was a pretty good bluffer, by now.

But the following day – a Sunday – I went to bed and did not get up again until Tuesday. I slept and cried and lay motionless, back to staring at the ceiling again; it seemed that infertility would never lose the power to knock me flat on my back.

As ever, the old adversary waited until I got back on my feet then returned to take another shot a couple of weeks later. There was another e-mail from Vanda, who, due to her easy manner, had obviously been appointed as our family's Imparter of News That May be Difficult. It seemed that Jules's announcement had given her younger brother the courage to deliver some news of his own. At the age of seventeen and still living at home, he was about to become a dad; the baby was due in exactly the same month as Jules's daughter.

"Tom?" said Chris, increasingly incredulous about the contents of my e-mails. "But he was just a kid last time I saw him. Isn't he still at school?"

"No," I said. "He's seventeen and taller than you."

"Blimey," Chris noted. "I could easily be his father. I could be becoming a grandfather now."

"Actually, you could even be *Tom's* grandfather," I pointed out. "If you'd had a child at twenty and then they had a child at twenty."

"I'm not even going to think about that!" Chris replied, frantically smooth-smooth-smoothing the sides of his hair in the mirror.

"I'd have been so proud if I'd had a son like Tom," I said wistfully.

At the end of 2003 – our first year of trying to conceive – we had gone home to the southern hemisphere for Christmas and sometimes we'd taken Tom out with us, to play cricket or to buy pies and sweets; he was ten years old. By 2010, I was already surrounded by friends and colleagues who had met their partners, begun dating, got married and had several children in the time that we had been treading water trying to have a family. Now someone who was ten years old when this first started was about to become a parent. It would have been funny if it wasn't so sad.

I managed to make a joke of it when I discussed it with Mum on the phone – "Gosh, I hope their younger sister isn't going to get in on the act" – but it was difficult to see it as anything but a harsh reminder about all that had gotten away from us. I wondered if the rest of my family had already decided that it was obvious: Chris and I would not be having children. Well! Defiance surged up, unbidden. They could think that but I was damned if I was giving up. So much for accepting that it was time to move on. In fact, these latest developments went on to have the opposite effect – they galvanised me into action all over again. I was going to do something, I just wasn't sure what yet.

Then, in March, a glossy magazine about our local area fell through the letterbox, and there it was – the latest article to inspire a new approach in my battle with infertility. It was Traditional Chinese Medicine again, but this was different; the article didn't even mention fertility, it said something much more striking – a veteran practitioner from China had used acupuncture, massage and herbs to help a teenager, who had previously been confined to a wheelchair, regain the use of his legs. The boy who had been told he would never walk again was now walking. I read it then put the magazine aside, telling myself that we had had enough acupuncture and Chinese herbs to produce a family three times over. Chris's treatment with David Taylor had been reluctantly put on hold several months earlier, due to lack of funds. But the bit of me that Would

Not Give Up had quietly noted the address of the Chinese practitioner's clinic. It was two train stops away. A couple of days later, I sidled up to the magazine, flicked through it until I found the article then wrote the clinic phone number in my diary. Just in case. It was two train stops away in the cheaper direction; surely it wouldn't cost *too* much, this suburban clinic? Still, I let it lie a bit longer. It was a bigger step than I realised, hoping and trying again.

In the end, it was anger that propelled me through the door of Li Wei's clinic, situated just across from Poundland on a traffic-polluted high street where banks of steel shutters crashed down on the shop fronts at night. I had left the house because Chris and I had had another row – probably about sperm tests he didn't take or possibly about performance anxiety that he ignored; those were still the hotly-contested topics, each argument morphing into the other like some sort of toxic Groundhog Day. But through the murkiness of it all, I was persistently returning to an increasingly clear thought: I would have moved forward a lot faster these past seven years if I had been moving alone.

"I don't need you," I thought as my feet carried me to the train station and my fingers tapped out Li Wei's destination on the ticket machine. "I'll do this on my own. Plenty of women do it that way."

When I got there, I went to a bookshop, then a coffee shop, then along the river for a bit. Back on the high street, I walked slowly past the clinic in one direction, then back in the other. It looked just like all the other Traditional Chinese Medicine clinics you see on high streets, although perhaps even a little more basic than some. On the third sortie past, I finally pushed open the door and went in. There were several plastic chairs against the wall on the left, with laminated press clippings blu-tacked above them. A couple of paces opposite, on the right, was a small consultation desk. I stood between both, facing the counter at the back and taking in the vast multitude of dried herbs that lined the shelves on the rear wall. A diminutive woman in a white coat appeared from a tight corridor beyond the counter. Li Wei had appointments for the next two hours, she said, but he could see me for an initial consultation at 4.15 that afternoon. I gave her my name and booked in.

When I returned, after another tour of the book shop, the coffee shop and the river, augmented with forty-five minutes in Poundland, I found Li Wei himself sitting at the consultation desk. He was a slim, wiry man with a carpet of black hair and when we began to discuss the reason for my visit, he spoke in fast, quiet bursts. The difference between Li Wei and some of the practitioners I had seen in central London was that he was as matter-of-fact about the consultation as any GP in a doctors' surgery; he was missing that air of 'woo, I'm performing exotic miracles' that was evident in some western practitioners. In his small suburban clinic, there was no need to contrive an eastern influence by placing giant brass buddhas and arty shots of lotus flowers around the room; this was not a fancy 'alternative' form of treatment to him, it was just the healthcare he had grown up with in China and later went on to practice. Just as David Taylor's down-to-earth approach had suited me, so did Li Wei's.

However, when he asked about the reasons for my consultation, something inside me balked at mentioning infertility. I was afraid, at first, that he might laugh – "Forty-one! You've left it a bit late" – or that I might actually start crying right there on the plastic chair if I told him what I'd been doing for the past seven years. So I started out tentatively, outlining the pain I was increasingly feeling from old sports injuries; as well as having a creaking back, I had recently been getting sharp pains in the ends of my fingers and toes. A bit of numbness, too, sometimes.

Li Wei noted all of this down before beginning his examination. After checking several different pulse points and studying my tongue, eyes and face, he gazed across the desk and told me all about myself.

"You feel cold easily when others do not?" I nodded. A solid five minutes or more of nodding followed as he asked about my sluggish digestion, queried whether I sometimes felt depressed or perhaps 'stuck' and frustrated, wondered if I found it particularly hard to lose weight, if my energy levels were low compared to others. Did I need a lot of sleep but, even after nine or ten hours, still felt more tired when I woke up than when I went to bed? He asked me to describe my menstrual flow and wondered if I had suffered from fibroids or menstrual clots. I told him that a small fibroid had shown up on a scan eighteen months earlier and that, over the past few months, I had been occasionally troubled by the appearance of large clots during my period.

He did not look in the least surprised that all of this was spot-on, returning my incessant nods with an inflection of his own as I confirmed the existence of every issue he raised. The list was long and specific.

"This caused by liver chi stagnation," he went on to say, explaining how my sluggish pulse and pale white tongue, along with other observations, had led him to this diagnosis. I had previously seen four different acupuncturists; none of them had mentioned my liver (although David's assessment of the type of treatment necessary was a perfect match).

Li Wei asked more about the size and siting of the fibroid; gaining in confidence, I saw my moment and seized it. "It was at a fertility clinic," I explained. "The scan where it showed up. I spent a really long time trying to have a family and now … well … I'll be forty-two this year so time's kind of run out."

Li Wei shook his head vigorously. "This is western belief. I treat you, not age. I treat person! In Chinese medicine, this not old, not when all systems of body brought into balance."

And so I was off again, testing out yet another new way to conceive. It was unlikely that we were going to save enough for fertility treatment within the next year, so this type of approach seemed the only option. I found that I still wanted to actually *do* something rather than just sitting around watching time pass.

Embarrassingly, even though I was forty-one years old and had never fallen pregnant despite seven-plus years of trying, I still felt the same as ever when I began a new approach. It happened again: hope sprung anew. *This* would be the key. This would be the vital piece of information that led to me getting pregnant!

I wonder if it's not actually hope that I've been hitting myself over the head with all these years. Perhaps it's the hope that's more damaging than the infertility itself – or perhaps the hope *is* the infertility, just as much as the despair. That's what makes it so insidious; whatever choice you make – keep trying or give up – there will be a demon to wrestle down either path. For now, I chose the path marked 'hope'; it's a subjective thing, when to give up, and I wasn't ready to surrender, not yet. I went home and told Chris about Li Wei; several days later he joined me in the suburban clinic for a consultation of his own. Latest row over, it seemed that we were back to trying to resolve this together.

Again Li Wei examined the pulses, tongue, eyes and face then issued a list of characteristics that perfectly summed up Chris – from his 'hot' body temperature and temperament to his weak bladder, constant fidgeting and tendency to dive into a situation before stopping to weigh up the facts.

"Kidney chi out of balance," Li Wei concluded.

When another client, who had been sitting on one of the plastic chairs behind us, was called through to the treatment rooms, Chris told Li Wei about his sperm test results and how he believed acupuncture and herbs had helped to vastly improve the morphology reading. Li Wei was confident that he could also improve the sperm motility problem, as long as Chris stuck to the treatment he prescribed over the next few months.

After booking in to begin acupuncture the following week, we stood side by side at the counter and watched as Li Wei studiously selected and weighed a range of dried herbs from the extensive assortment on the shelves behind, concocting a different recipe for each of us. We paid about £80 each by credit card – overlooking the fact that it was much more expensive than the herbs we had bought from David – and left clutching personalised white plastic pots, joking as we walked down the street about magic ingredients for getting people up the duff.

As soon as we got home, I tentatively placed three spoons of my light brown herbal mixture in a mug and added boiling water, bracing myself to drink the resulting murk, which had the appearance of tea filtered through cattle dung. Surprisingly, it both smelt and tasted of coffee, with a liquorishy after-kick that could have been tailor-made for my taste buds. I felt instantly warmed and soothed.

Unfortunately, Chris was not so lucky. His mixture was black, with large granules floating on the surface of the water and it gave off the distinct whiff of fermented silage. He approached the mug as if it were poison, holding it at arm's length before reluctantly bringing it to his mouth with one hand while theatrically blocking his nose with the other.

"This is the most appallingly disgusting thing I've ever drunk," he complained after ingesting a mouthful. "How come you get a nice cup of coffee and I get this? Heaven knows what's in here." He shook his head, laughing.

"Well, that's what you get for being a hot person," I replied, pleased for once to be cold and sluggish.

"Rank, despicable, disgusting, foul, ghastly, horrible …"
Then he took another couple of sips, followed by a slightly
bigger glug. "Actually."

"What? All that fuss and you like it now?"

"It's got rather a nice aftertaste, once it's gone down. I think
I might get on okay with this after all." He paused. "By the
way, you know how yours is like coffee?"

"Yes."

"I was just wondering when I'll be allowed a proper cup of
coffee again?"

I laughed into my mug of herbs. "When you get me pregnant.
After that, you can eat and drink whatever you like. Well, as
long as it won't kill you – you've got to stick around for a long
time if you're going to have a family."

So, throughout the summer and early autumn, we downed
the hot herbal drinks twice a day and saw Li Wei for regular
acupuncture treatments, Chris having two sessions for every
one of mine, as prescribed.

I also underwent violent back massages that felt like
someone was repeatedly trying to chop through my spine with
a mallet and Chris returned home with a series of large, angry
red circles across his back, where Li Wei had augmented the
acupuncture with cupping therapy. I wondered if my own
back wasn't going to break in two and Chris sometimes looked
like he should have been quarantined with an infectious rash.
Despite this, neither of us had ever felt better.

"It's as if I can feel tension surging out and energy surging
in," Chris declared.

We both had glowing skin and, once again, I was relieved
of any pre-menstrual symptoms and stomach cramps. The
clots that had begun to worry me disappeared entirely.
Even better, we still never missed the chance to target ovulation.

"I feel like a new man in every way," Chris announced, and
it appeared that he did.

At the beginning of October, I turned forty-two, still hoping that later in the month I would discover I was pregnant, that there might be a happy ending, a last-gasp reprieve.

We had followed advice about male factor issues and had timed sex for every second day throughout ovulation – even with Li Wei's intervention, every second day throughout the entire month was still a bridge too far – and all signs indicated that I had indeed ovulated. Then I awoke on day twenty-four of my cycle and felt somehow different; my pulse, usually slow, low and difficult to find, had speeded up and was as active and obvious as a jumping bean. Apart from just feeling 'different' in general, I was hit by unexpected waves of nausea on and off throughout the day. I told myself not to get too excited; I would wait to see what happened.

Day twenty-five and day twenty-six brought exactly the same developments. I said nothing to Chris – we had tasted enough false hope over the past seven-and-a-half years – but privately dared to think that, at last, perhaps … here was a breakthrough. Although I was already tip-toeing towards optimism, even I was taken aback by what happened when I began to cook dinner on day twenty-seven. I was making an old standby, a Thai chicken curry that filled the kitchen with the aroma of lemongrass and coconut milk. As I stood stirring the pungent mixture in the pan, something hit me in an instant with no prior warning: I was about to throw up. I dropped the spoon I was holding and shot out of the room to escape the smell that had suddenly turned my stomach. I returned again and it kept happening – every time I got a whiff of it, this flavour I had always loved inhaling, the gag reflex would kick in again.

I stood stock-still in the bathroom to check my pulse: still jumping. It never felt like this; I knew that because I'd been trying to read it for the past five years, ever since Maggie had shown me how to during our early acupuncture sessions. A jolt of adrenaline-fuelled realisation streaked from head to toe in a nano-second. It had happened! It must have.

I served up our meals but was unable to eat mine. I couldn't be anywhere near that smell. I couldn't help thinking of my sister Vanda, who had always suffered morning sickness almost from the moment of conception.

"Are you okay sweetheart?" Chris enquired. "You don't quite seem yourself."

I broke all the promises I had made about waiting to see what happened and told him what was going on.

"Maybe it's just a bug," I added, trying to play it down. "But it doesn't feel like a bug and I just feel … different." There was no other way of explaining it, the odd sensation that had enveloped me for the past three days.

Chris's face was instantly transformed as it dawned on him that maybe he had something to hope for.

"Let's wait a bit," I said quickly. "It's only day twenty-seven. But if I still feel like this in a couple of days, maybe I'll take a test."

I wish I had taken an early response test right there and then. But there were still none in the house and I refused to be so hopeful that I bought one on a whim. I wanted a bit more evidence before I risked another result window with its one lonely line that seemed to laugh at me for even looking.

We went to bed happy, tucked in against each other as we dreamed our private dreams about what might happen next. Then I awoke on day twenty-eight and every symptom had dropped away. I took my pulse soon after opening my eyes and, for the first time in several days, struggled to locate it. Whatever it was, it was over. I knew it straight away.

"Don't give up," Chris said when I told him. "You don't know for sure. It could still be happening."

"No," I said flatly. "It's not happening – it's all just stopped. I can tell."

I felt embarrassed, as if I was some sort of sad cliché – the woman who imagines pregnancy symptoms because she is so desperate for them to be real. But I had been monitoring my cycles for seven years; I knew what was normal for me and what wasn't. One of the upsides of being forty-two was that I knew my own body in a way that I never had when I was younger. And now I knew that something different had happened this cycle and, sometime overnight, whatever it was had just drifted away. It sounds pathetic to say *'I felt different'* – it would hardly form the basis of a scientific study – but how can you explain an inner knowing that something was there and then it wasn't?

Sure enough, two days later, on the anniversary of my brother George's death, my period arrived. It was a Sunday. I went to the park and lay on the grass in the sun, staring up at the clouds and wishing they would form their wispy white tails into letters that clearly spelt out what I should do.

"I thought today would be the day," I said to Chris. "I didn't tell you, but I was going to take a test. I thought it might happen, like a little parting gift from George … why do I have to be such an idiot?"

"You're not an idiot," Chris said, reaching across the grass to take my hand. "Everyone would have thought of George straight away if you'd found out you were pregnant today."

"Well, maybe not. But the timing just felt really significant. It would have been so special to finally get there today. Urgh! Why do I have these *stupid* daydreams?"

"Because you're you," Chris answered. "And I wouldn't have it any other way. Anyway, I thought the same as you were thinking, if it's any consolation."

"Sorry," I whispered. "That it didn't happen."

"Me too," Chris said quietly. Then he instantly brightened. "But don't give up. It's still a step forward, coming that close. Li Wei's obviously had a wonderful effect on both of us. Who knows what next month could bring?"

The next day, I pulled out all of my fertility books and read everything I could about herbs, vitamins and minerals to support natural conception. Then I went to the supermarket and bought some radish because one of my books said it was an ancient remedy for thyroid support. It tasted like rancid dirt, but I ate it daily for the next few weeks. It had no discernible effect except to ruin the flavour of my meals. I gave it up and continued the search for the Next Big Thing. If I didn't get pregnant by January 2011, I would be forty-three years old before I became a mother. No one had to tell me what the odds were about that.

⁂ ⁂ ⁂

In the end, there were three additions to our family in 2010, all of them girls. Tom's daughter arrived first, in May, closely followed by Jules's in June. The third was born to another of my nieces – Poppy, one of my sister Jane's three married daughters. Her little girl arrived two days before my forty-second birthday and I was thrilled because everyone knew that Poppy and her husband would make the nicest parents on earth. But their perfectly-planned entrance to parenthood was also a reminder of how I should have lived my life, if only I had realised that it might take eight years to conceive. Ruefully, I mused that I might have got going in my twenties, too, if I knew what lay ahead.

"But you said it yourself," Chris interjected. "You would have been a lousy mother in your twenties. You did the right thing, waiting 'til you knew you'd be a decent parent."

"I'd have been *useless* in my twenties," I confirmed. "I thought thirty-three or thirty-four was a good compromise – not too old, not too young."

What I had also thought was that, by the time I became a great-aunt, I would have school-age children of my own.

Now, I was not only forty-two and childless, I would soon find myself being called Great Aunty Louise whenever I went home. That conjured an image of a woman as old and doddery as everyone said my ovaries had surely become. Great Aunty Louise sounded soft and cuddly, but also like she might have long white hairs protruding from her chin, wafting above the 1950s-style glasses she wore slung around her neck on a silver chain. Wasn't it only yesterday that I was twenty-five years old and had no idea that it could take eight years *not* to conceive? I asked myself the same thing all over again: how had this happened?

If the younger generation of my family was giving me pause for thought, the older generation of Chris's family was simultaneously doing the same. While we had been so fixated on having children, we hadn't paid enough attention to the changes we noticed in Rose. She was increasingly suspicious of the carers who arrived twice daily to do her shopping, cleaning and cooking, since she was no longer able to leave the house. The phone calls she regularly made to Chris became more desperate and confused; unfortunately, it was easy to play that down because those worrying chats were interspersed with conversations as witty and lucid as ever.

"I tell everyone you're trying to pack me off to a home," she teased when Chris yet again raised the subject of full-time residential care.

However, around the time I turned forty-two, Rose was admitted to a retirement home for respite care after contracting a leg infection; she had refused to take the antibiotics prescribed for it, on the grounds that her carers were trying to poison her. When I visited her one Friday, it was the first time I had set foot inside an old people's home in the UK. I was horrified. Rose was also horrified, but additionally furious; she remained a feisty character who knew her own mind and clearly did not belong among the residents who slumped in limp, meek heaps around the walls of the lounge. Barely any of them spoke or betrayed any hint of the fascinating lives they must have led. I had seen ageing in the southern hemisphere, but it had never looked as hopeless as this. The worst thing was that, within a week, Rose too had had the spirit sucked out of her. She had given up bashing on the door of her room with a cane and demanding to be driven home; she had stopped commandeering the front office and using the phone to ask Chris to have her removed from "this dreadful place".

She had joined the ranks of those who were not quite there, unable to dress herself or brush her own hair, just staring vacantly and sadly ahead and not knowing where she was. The woman who normally insisted on applying a full face of make-up every day now wore only one sock and a jersey with food stains sliding down the front. It was heart-wrenching to see. It was also yet another reminder that perhaps it was time to stop chasing moonbeams. What would Rose and her fellow residents do if the years ahead of me, from my forties onwards, were miraculously handed back to them? They'd savour every second of glorious independence, that's what they'd do; they wouldn't waste a moment tormenting themselves over something that might never be. *I'll let it go soon*, I told myself. *Soon I'll get back on with life again.* The message came from all around: give it up, your time has passed. But still I kicked harder against it. I didn't realise how bloody-minded I was until I met infertility.

THIRTY-THREE

TWENTY-ELEVEN WAS THE year something I'd never heard of made its presence felt in my life. I didn't know what it was at first. I just knew that, suddenly, I was a lot more combative than I used to be. And, when I wasn't angry, I was irritable and perhaps a little irrational. The rest of the time I was quite normal, thank you very much. But it was unpredictable and difficult to call – which woman would be getting out of bed this morning? The calm, reasonable one or the one who has discovered the power of a good rant? I had no idea myself.

Not surprisingly, it caused a lot of arguments with Chris. They would start over trivial things, like the fact that I had said, "Please don't touch those plates on the bench" and he had said, "Okay" but not less than three minutes later, he had moved them. He never listened! Then his hackles would rise as he adopted his customary defensive position or, even worse, suggested I might want to calm down. After that, I would instantaneously self-combust – not about a pile of plates on a bench, but always, inevitably about infertility.

"Go on, admit it. You didn't even want me to be a mother! You can't have. Otherwise, why would you block me at every turn? Every bloody turn."

The difference was that, thanks to this unexplained change taking place within, I no longer got over-talked or easily placated. When we met, Chris had always dominated arguments, mainly because he was used to them and I wasn't. It was me who had the slow-burning fuse … until infertility came along and exerted its pressure. At the beginning of 2011, that's what I blamed – the build-up of tension caused by prolonged infertility. It had to be that. Wasn't it always?

But, if it was 'only' infertility, then why did I gradually realise that these seemingly random outbursts of foul temper were following a pattern? Things were definitely worse every time I skipped breakfast or lunch; going without food for any length of time had apparently become the equivalent of loosening a pin on a grenade.

Somehow, this didn't seem to be quite the same breed of anger as the 'infertility anger' had been. This wasn't always driven by pain and frustration; it was more like an inner shift, like suddenly, out of nowhere, at the age of forty-two I had discovered my voice. And I was damn-well going to use it. Meanwhile, not content with just having unattractive moods, I noticed a range of unappealing physical changes happening as well. For one thing, I seemed to have gotten a lot more hairy. There were long hairs growing at the back of my knees, in a place that I didn't think hair grew. And when I sat in direct sunlight, it highlighted an outbreak of downy fluff that seemed to have sprung from nowhere all across my neck. And chin. And jawline. Speaking of which, this seemed to be several inches lower than I remembered it. My face had started gradually, imperceptibly falling as long ago as 2005; it had now officially *fallen*. I would have preferred wrinkles, or laughter lines that suggested life had been fun, which it often had been. I felt like my droopy face, complete with downward creases at the edge of the mouth, was giving away my secrets, making it obvious that I must have privately cried a lot of tears. I didn't want people to see my downcast expression and suspect that, now and again, I still silently whimpered into the night because I would probably never have a child.

I didn't want to be reminded of sorrowful feelings myself when I looked in the mirror, for that matter. Hence, I began doing facial exercises, gurning and grinning madly for ten minutes twice a day. Maybe forty-two was the age it all fell apart. Is that what it was? I forgot words, too, sometimes

– I would go to search for an expression, or the name of something everyday and familiar, and it would be just out of reach. When I tried to find my way through the brain fog, it felt as confusing as the onset of a migraine. And sometimes at night, lying in bed before falling asleep, I appeared to be having palpitations as I became uncomfortably aware of my racing heartbeat taking over my chest. Again, I blamed these changes on stress. Damn infertility.

Then, one Saturday, I was contentedly browsing the shelves of an Oxfam bookshop and a red title in the health section jumped out at me: *Before the Change*. Oh no, maybe that's it, I thought. Maybe I'm about to go through the menopause. I slid the book out and realised that the sub-title said: *Taking Charge of Your Perimenopause*. What? There was a whole other stage before the change of life? Why had no one told me this? I instantly read the foreword and first chapter, still standing there in the shop. I wasn't falling apart after all. I was 'just' entering perimenopause. Delighted to read that I wasn't losing my mind, I forgot for a moment to consider what this meant: I was another step closer to the end of my reproductive life. That realisation would dawn soon enough; for now, I just wanted to know what this thing was and how to be rid of it. I paid £2.99 for the book and, for that tiny sum, received some of the most helpful insights of my life. How could there have been so much I didn't know about my own body, before infertility and before this?

I learned that perimenopause symptoms generally affected women between the ages of thirty-five and fifty as they began the slow, subtle decline that eventually led to menopause. The fundamental cause of symptoms was hormonal imbalance – it was described as being similar to experiencing a bad case of PMS, something I could personally vouch for. Irritability, joint pain, heart palpitations, bloating, sagging skin, facial hair, mood swings, anger, backache – I ticked them all off the list of symptoms, though I was relieved to see I hadn't yet reached the point where I was suffering the worst of it. Night sweats, irregular periods, panic attacks, weight gain and urinary incontinence might still lie ahead. I answered a list of questions to help determine my current status and it appeared I was just beginning the 'perimenopause transition'. A hormone-regulating diet, supplements, regular exercise and better stress management might be all I needed to alleviate my uncomfortable symptoms.

And one of the key points? Eat healthily and regularly to ensure blood sugar hormones are in balance – my body had already sent me that message but, as usual, I had been slow to translate it. I finally realised that, in short, what it wanted was essential fatty acids, and it wanted them now. I began with flaxseed oil, the number one 'Peri Zapper' of the ten outlined in the book. Having spent my twenties on one low-fat diet or another, it felt oddly subversive to swallow a tablespoonful of oil with breakfast every day. It might have been a 'healthy' fat, but I was still programmed to fear that it would add a stone to my midriff overnight. Of course, the fear proved groundless. What the oil actually did, over the course of a month or two, was gradually return me to myself. It was a relief to wake up in the morning and know that I had wrested back from my hormones control over my own moods.

My symptoms improved markedly and the anger settled down into a strong assertiveness; perimenopause had indeed brought forth a new voice. It would change the way I approached both infertility and my relationship with Chris. After eight years of trying to conceive, the ground was finally shifting and other events were about to cause additional shockwaves of their own.

※ ※ ※

Rose had escaped from the old people's home in time to spend Christmas 2010 with us at her own flat. Back in familiar surroundings, she was temporarily restored to her independent self, immediately sorting her mail, setting her hair and resuming the running of her empire from the telephone. However, she was still waging a stealth war against antibiotics, inventing a range of ruses to avoid taking her daily dose. No one knew where she was putting the tablets, but she was not swallowing them, despite Chris's best efforts at persuasion.

By March 2011, her original infection had returned, this time deteriorating into a potentially life-threatening condition. Rose was taken to hospital by ambulance and, having been her usual alert, chatty self upon admission, was reduced within days to a state of confusion, delusion and fear. Above all, she wanted to go home and did not understand why no one would take her. In her increasingly rare lucid moments, she developed an urgent interest in when Chris and I were going to get married. "I would rather like to see it," she told us. "You ought to think about it, you know." Rose never interfered in this way; we knew that she knew her time was running out.

One day, she looked across at me and said: "Now, when I die, I'd like you to have my wedding ring. It's the only one that's worth anything – you might be able to get some money for it. I'm told platinum has some worth." When I protested, she looked searchingly into my eyes and announced, "I think you're marvellous. Please, I want you to have it."

I felt guilty that I wasn't marvellous enough, that I argued endlessly with her son over infertility, that I berated him for things he hadn't done and refused to forgive him for things that he had. Saddest of all, I realised now that we would never climb the stairs to Rose's flat, open the door and present her with the little bundle that would be her third grandchild. I had pictured it over and over, the moment when she sat in her armchair with the high back and, beaming like a woman twenty years younger, cradled our child. Rose was getting weaker with every visit and I was now in perimenopause; there would be no child in her lifetime and probably none in mine. It dawned on me that Rose knew that before we did. At the start, she had encouraged us to become parents, sending articles and information that she thought might help. When I turned forty, she even phoned Chris and told him that I mustn't worry – after years of trying to conceive, her neighbour had just had her first baby at the age of forty-two. All sorts of things were possible these days! But over the past year or so, her tone had changed. "You don't want to become a father at your age, ducky," she told Chris. "It's hard work, you know. You'll be exhausted."

She began encouraging us to enjoy our child-free life. "You'd never get a minute to yourself, or any sleep, with a baby. You can have wonderful lie-ins now – and think of the travels you can take."

"See," I said to Chris. "Even your mum's given up on us."

"She doesn't mean it," he replied. "She's just doing it to protect us. She doesn't want us to get hurt, thinking about what we're missing out on. It's her way of trying to make us feel better."

Now Rose wanted us to get married and it sent a stab to my chest because I realised: here I was trying to have a family with this man and it had gone on for so many years that I no longer knew if I *could* marry him. I knew things about him now that I didn't know before and I wondered if he wasn't thinking the same. What horrors had infertility exposed in me? I had seen, through this prolonged challenge, that he wasn't the man I thought he was when we sat by the river in Bath on our second anniversary and I daydreamed about spending the rest of my life with him. When had I decided that he was a man who let me down when I needed him the most? What could I tell Rose when she lay there, only just with us now and wishing for an engagement? I just smiled and squeezed her hand. Even if she'd had another lifetime to listen, I couldn't have completely explained what prolonged infertility does to a relationship, or to a person. I was still finding out myself.

"You are happy aren't you, ducky?" Rose asked Chris with increasing regularity and urgency. "You have enjoyed your life, haven't you?"

"Yes Mum," he always replied. "I've had a wonderful life. You mustn't worry about me."

"But I do," she insisted. "I must know that you're happy."

During one visit, Rose no longer knew who I was, but she always knew Chris and she was still shrewd enough to see that his eyes weren't the same as they used to be, when they had twinkled and crinkled at women of all ages. When I looked at him, clasping her hand on the other side of the hospital bed, it was as if I *saw* him for the first time in years. He had seemed so blasé about infertility sometimes that I hadn't thought for a minute it could hurt him as much as it hurt me. But if you stopped to look, it was etched all around his eyes; he was in pain too, not just because he knew that Rose was slowly leaving us but because he had so wanted her to know his children. We were too late; we had taken too long.

After six weeks, they told Chris there was nothing more they could do for Rose; she was discharged to a care home, where she at least had a room of her own, with fresh air streaming through a door that opened onto a balcony. She was expected to live for a further two months. However, four days after her arrival Rose lost consciousness and we raced across London and through the Sussex countryside to see her one last time. She died early that afternoon, both of us talking to her and stroking her arms. She smiled when she went; it would have been wrong to wish her back.

It was the third time in my life that I had witnessed a death, but this was different. Like a stone being broken open, I suddenly felt something again. *So this is love. I remember.* I had been hardened shut by infertility and I didn't even know it. How long had I been numb to everything except frustration and anger? When I hugged Chris to comfort him, it was with a tenderness that had long been lost to us. A week after Rose's death, he handed me her platinum wedding ring. I have worn it ever since, on the third finger of my right hand. We don't know yet if the day will come when Rose will get her wish and the ring will be promoted to the left hand. It depends, as does so much, on whether we can recover from the fall-out that infertility leaves behind.

❦ ❦ ❦

Those two differing countdowns to the end – the onset of perimenopause and the fading away of so many lives on Rose's hospital ward – had a predictably profound effect. It was as if I was agitating to live, to just get on with things while I still could. At that moment, I didn't want to travel the world, scale a mountain peak or scuba dive on the Great Barrier Reef; the sum total of my aspirations – still – was to have a family. Once more galvanised into action, I cast the net wider and mounted one last assault.

Our sessions with Li Wei, and the hot herbal drinks, had come to a halt due, once again, to lack of funds. However, our kitchen remained littered with hints that we were trying to conceive. Chris was still taking his usual male fertility vitamins and eating bags of Brazil nuts, but, after further reading on my part, there had been two new additions to the regime. He was now trying Pycnogenol tablets, derived from French pine bark and credited with improving sperm morphology, along with liquid L-Carnitine, which had been found to improve motility. Neither of these potential remedies was cheap, but there was no point putting the money aside to save for fertility treatment – I would have been well into my late forties by the time we reached the target, if in fact we ever did.

Meanwhile, I had now been taking pre-conception vitamins for nearly nine years; of the other supplements I had tried along the way, only high-strength acidophilus had lasted the distance – and that was just because it made me feel better, not necessarily because I thought it could help me get pregnant. The flaxseed oil that worked so well for perimenopause symptoms had also been hurriedly swapped after I discovered there was conflicting advice about whether it was safe for use in pregnancy. It highlighted all over again how much time had passed since this began – of course perimenopause experts didn't expect a woman in need of flaxseed oil to still be trying to conceive. But here I was, still trying, and now swallowing safely-sourced fish oil every day instead of the flaxseed.

We were taking the right supplements, avoiding the right things and following what seemed to be the right advice, but I worried deep down that we still weren't doing enough of the main thing that we should have been doing – having regular intercourse throughout the month. Chris had not faltered since receiving his test results in 2008, something that was baffling to me after all the preceding years of problems but nevertheless a great relief. It felt like one burden at least had been lifted. Except, even with things running smoothly, we could manage only three or four attempts a month, all around the same week. It was just another factor lengthening the already unlikely odds of conception. I wanted better odds than that; I wanted to try every last thing before it was too late.

Secretly, I began exploring other options. I started Googling sperm clinics again and wistfully read through some of the profiles of potential donors. I could travel to Denmark, I could import it from America, I could go to a clinic in London. It was cheaper than fertility treatment; I might even be able to afford more than one attempt. Providing they took Visa.

I could do it alongside my continuing attempts with Chris, that's what I told myself. And the tests I would need to undertake before treatment might bring to light something we needed to know. It could help us on two levels. Couldn't it?

As far back as 2007, I had wanted to discuss the repercussions of sperm donation during my consultation with Janet Brown, but she had batted away the enquiry. I played the potential consequences around within my own head and, ignoring her admonishment to stop reading books, read as much about donor conception as I could. The idea still gave rise to instinctive guilt – was it selfish to ask this of Chris? Was it selfish to know from the outset that my child, assuming I could even manage to conceive him or her, would not know their biological father? Chris had said he was happy to consider it, before the consultation with Janet Brown, but he had never brought it up since or offered it as an option. As a matter of fact, he had barely offered anything as an option during the entire eight-and-a-half years, not that I could think of. It was more than starting to rankle. Despite our recent moments of tenderness, a new impatience surged up. It was as if I was being driven on, and away from Chris, by the sharp urgency known only by those who are reaching the end.

THIRTY-FOUR

ABOUT THE TIME I turned forty-three, I realised that what I planned to do was give infertility a decade of my life. A nice, neat ten-year package. *There. See that decade – I tried from start to finish.* The reasons to give up were beginning to far outnumber the reasons to keep going. It was autumn 2011 and I had already come through nearly nine years, but somewhere a voice said, 'Don't stop 'til you've done a full ten.' Perhaps it was just a pathetic way of trying to tidy up, to make order out of chaos by completing the challenge at that perfect, round number. Or perhaps I really thought my body still could conceive, sustain and bear a child. Not perhaps. I did believe that. It was the *combination* of the two of us that I was really having my doubts about. There was something toxic between us, something wrong, that prevented us conceiving together. But apart? Who knew what we could do apart? Our relationship might still have existed, at least on the surface, but the inquest into its demise had already begun.

The arguments flared from anywhere and everywhere. If I forgot about the previous nine years, Chris and I got along just fine. We went out together and laughed and shopped and walked and talked, like we always had. But if I remembered, if I thought back over what had happened, I could barely look at him.

"I dread coming home from work," Chris accused in the middle of a row one October night. "You don't see how miserable you look, sitting there. I see you sometimes, before you know I'm here, and you look like the unhappiest person on earth. That's how much you despise it, living here with me. You can't stand to see my face every day – go on, admit it!"

"Oh! I dare to look a bit sad in the privacy of my own lounge and still it's got to be all about you," I snapped. "Of course it does. Have you even been here for the last nine years?"

Chris threw back his head and flung his palms to the ceiling. "I know. I know what's happened."

"No you don't. You haven't got a clue. You're still wondering why I might have the nerve to look a bit worried. For God's sake Chris, I'm forty-three. Do you have any idea what that means for a woman?"

He sighed, exasperated, his face red and hot, eyes cold and blue. "I know it's hard, of course I do. But I've done everything I can to help and you don't see the way you look at me. I can't take this anymore, I really can't."

"What?" I surged off the couch in disbelief. "*You* can't take it anymore?"

He rounded on me then, looking every inch the often-spiky man he had been when we first met.

"No Louise, I can't. You don't give me credit for anything – I've been taking my vitamins, buying supplements, eating Brazil nuts, doing my bit at ovulation. It's been hard for me too. I've done my best and it's just not happening. I don't see what more I can do."

"Hang on a minute," I broke in, straining to keep my voice under control. "Let me get this straight – you've been taking a few vitamins and eating a few nuts since 2008 and you think that's enough?"

"See, this is what I mean," Chris interjected. "There are men out there who wouldn't make this effort, they wouldn't be bothered either way. It's not been easy for me either. I don't deserve this!"

"Oh, how awful. You've stepped up for two-and-a-half years and you think that was hard work. Well. Where the hell were you in 2003, four, five, six and seven?" I angrily counted off the years on the fingers of one hand.

"I was here, trying, for all those years. On my own. Where the *hell* were you?"

"I don't bloody believe this," Chris shouted.

The upside of being forty-three was that I no longer automatically retreated, or perhaps crumpled into tears, when confronted with such an outburst.

"Go on then. Tell me," I challenged evenly. "Tell me what you did, actually physically did, to help us have a family in the first five years?"

"You know I contributed! Really, Louise, I couldn't have done more – I went to the doctor with you, I took a test."

"That was in 2005," I exclaimed. "Go on then – what else?"

Chris paused; I could almost see his mind working, scratching around in slow motion for an answer.

"I went to acupuncture," he finally offered.

"And did you arrange any of that yourself? Did you even bother to read anything about this or come up with any ideas that might help?"

He stopped pacing the lounge floor. "No. If you put it like that, I don't suppose I did."

In earlier years, it might have stopped there. But now all the thoughts I had unwittingly boxed up were escaping into the open, along with all the doubts and niggles I had stupidly ignored because I couldn't let them be true. I couldn't let myself give up on this and start again. There wasn't time! I was thirty-seven, thirty-eight, thirty-nine. I was forty. I had to make it work. And, anyway, it wasn't the worst relationship in the world. He wasn't a *bad* man.

Chris was running his hands through his hair now; only the sides, though, he never liked to mess up the top. That was another thing. He paid far too much attention to his looks and not enough to the things that really mattered. *He's a middle-aged man, for goodness' sake.*

I continued my unrelenting interrogation.

"And when you needed to take another sperm test, what did you do? How long did it take? How many years did you waste fannying around?"

"That's not fair," Chris protested. "He told me I had enough sperm to fertilise the whole of the UK."

"And I told you *over and over* that we needed to know more than that. Why didn't you listen to me? Why? Why didn't you at least do a bit of research about it? Something. Anything!"

Chris began to speak and I cut him off. "Because the sun rises and sets in your butt, that's why. You couldn't possibly be anything except bloody perfect, could you?"

"That's not true! I know you think I'm an arrogant sod, but that's not how it was."

It was as if I had been taken over by another voice; I couldn't seem to stop the words that spilled from my mouth.

"Even your mother said it – 'no son of mine is going to have sub-standard sperm'. You both *automatically* thought it would be me because everything about you is so damn wonderful. Why bother to take a test when we all know it's me who's the flawed one?"

"It wasn't you. I didn't think that about you – I'd never think that about you." Chris's voice became husky and low. "If anyone's flawed it's me."

"If it wasn't me," I said flatly, "then why didn't you take that test? Why did you let it slide? You left me waiting for nearly three years." Finally, I started to cry. "You don't do that to someone you love. You can't have loved me, not really."

I slumped back down onto the couch.

"Lou, that's not true. That will never be true. I love you more than anything, I always have and I always will." Chris walked over and reached for my hand, but I refused to let him take it. "I've been a fool," he said, voice shaking now. "Oh, don't push me away. Sweetheart. Please."

"And I've been an idiot," I muttered. "Believing your promises."

Suddenly, I understood something I had known since the day we visited Rose and she had made the 'no son of mine' comment, and Chris had laughed.

Now I finally said it: "You thought fertility was just a women's thing, didn't you?" I looked him straight in the eye, searching. "Just affecting women. Nothing to do with you."

Chris sighed sadly. "I wouldn't have put it quite like that but, okay, yes. I suppose maybe I did think it was mainly a women's thing. There's some truth in that."

I gasped. "You just left me to it, scrabbling round on my own. I told you. I kept telling you. No wonder you didn't listen."

So it was true. Why was I surprised? It was far from the only thing I hadn't wanted to be true. There was worse still to come to the surface. Much worse. Perhaps the only thing holding back the floodgates now was that, deep down, I couldn't bear to know what I was about to uncover.

❧ ❧ ❧

I was starting to think a lot about the life I might have lived if I hadn't mucked everything up. I didn't seem able to stop trawling our relationship history for evidence of transgressions and misdemeanours. This must be what happens when the initial shock of an accident or a tragedy wears off – you start the hunt for something to blame. *There was nothing anyone could have done.* Wasn't that the platitude designed to make you feel better after the worst had happened? *You mustn't blame yourself – there was nothing anyone could do.* Oh, but there was plenty we could have done. That was the problem; I was spoilt for choice about where to look for something to blame. Inevitably, because it was after all the age-old, most basic way to resolve infertility, the searchlight often fell on sex itself. What might have happened if we'd been able to have it regularly and consistently? Sex and lies. Those were the two scars I scratched at, causing new welts in the process, but unable to stop until … until what? What was it I wanted?

It got my back up now whenever Chris said "we did our best" or "we've tried our hardest" or "I don't know what more we could have done" or "we've just been unlucky". One of his favourite expressions was, "Other people can have children at the drop of a hat." He knew a lot of men who had got women pregnant after having sex only once. He regularly mentioned that on those months when we had sex just the one time. It was enough for other people, we were just unlucky that it didn't happen for us.

That autumn, we were strolling through Hyde Park when we passed a perfectly-formed nuclear family of four, throwing bread to the ducks on the Serpentine.

"I sometimes think life is intrinsically unfair," Chris complained as we walked by. "It's so easy for people like that – they want to have a family so, whoosh, they have a boy, then a girl. Whatever they want just falls into place for them."

"I get what you mean," I replied. "But you can't know that. They might have had IVF to conceive those kids."

"I doubt it," he said. "Life just falls into place for those type of people."

I was unable to resist it, poking at the scar that couldn't heal.

"I'm not sure if we can really complain," I retorted. "Since we let months of my thirties go by without even having sex. Really, how did we expect to have a family?"

I laughed sarcastically at our own uselessness.

Chris instantly protested, a torrent of words that travelled faster along the path than we did. "Unfair … hard on me … critical … not on … really!" He was reminding me again of how many times we had made love throughout my thirties. "Many times!" he insisted. "There were many times."

I watched him unravelling on the path, pacing and sighing and tutting, and it was like observing someone rather than being *with* them. How long had there been this disconnect between us?

I argued back, almost by rote, even though I knew there was no point saying anything else. I often didn't bother anymore; it was futile. In my private thoughts, I increasingly diverted the focus to the only thing I could be sure of, which was myself. All these accusations that were starting to simmer up from our past seemed to be carrying the same message: *you can't rely on him.* In my mind, I was already cutting Chris out of my plans. But he was still there, in our bed at night, and I was still there and I didn't really know why anymore.

❦ ❦ ❦

I was sure there must have been normal, contented days in late 2011 but I couldn't remember them. I had to look back through my diary to be reminded of all the perfectly ordinary things that happened, to realise that not every day was tainted by the creeping dread that I would probably never be a mother. Unless I took drastic action. Now. Yesterday. Last year. When I was forty. When I was thirty-seven.

It took my diary to remind me that I filled in a form asking to be excused from jury service, we met real estate agents and solicitors about Rose's flat, we went to lunch with one of my clients and it took seven hours.

In November, around the time an elderly lady was putting in an offer on the flat, we stayed there for a week and passed a lot of our time having sex in the single bed that was still made up, ready for us as it always had been. We made love twice one day and then, on our last morning, once again "for luck" before returning to London. Maybe Chris is right. Maybe he only remembers the good times and I only remember the bad. I wrote it in my diary, though, so it did happen even if I didn't remember it eighteen months later: 'Did ovulatory for luck

412

and had breakfast in bed.' We made love again at home the next night; we had been for a walk in Kew Gardens during the day and Chris stood in the centre of a stone pavilion and pulled comical faces while he sang *Bread of Heaven* in a soaring tenor, as distinctively beautiful as his speaking voice. A group of Spanish tourists walked by and giggled en masse. I thought sunset over Syon House and the River Thames looked like a Turner painting. But why didn't I remember these things? My diary, as it turned out, was full of them. Days browsing together in bookshops and galleries in central London; drinking hot chocolate in basement coffee bars and walking to Covent Garden to spend £4.50 on a packet of biscuits from the southern hemisphere.

There was one other thing. I did remember it, but I wish I hadn't because it's so embarrassing. On December 2, we went to two Christmas markets in the evening and, all the time we were browsing the stalls and cradling hot drinks and listening to groups of school children singing carols, I thought I was pregnant. Definitely. For sure. I was feeling permanently nauseous, to the point where I couldn't bear to take even one bite of the steak and stilton pasty that I normally would have pounced on and which Chris's gloved hand now wafted before me. "Urgh," I groaned. "I think I'm going to be sick."

It must have been all that sex we'd had in the single bed and beyond. Finally – finally – it must have worked. A part of me always believed, deep down, that there would be a last-gasp great escape. That in later years we would tell people, "Oh, we thought it was all over. We'd given up. I mean, I was forty-three. Forty-three! But it happened. And we couldn't believe it." I knew also that someone would reply, "See, the minute you give up, the minute you relax, then that's when it happens." I'd let that slide, though, in my fantasies because who cared? I had my beloved child, didn't I, against the odds, and that was all that mattered. Yes, the universe, or God, or whatever it was that I possibly no longer believed in, wouldn't really let me go all the way through life without becoming a mother. Didn't things always come good in the end, if you just hung on long enough? These are the fairy tales you tell yourself, hugging them close like the most potent of secrets, just to keep going for another day, another month, another year.

What actually happened that December was not quite romantic enough for inclusion in a classic fairy tale. It doesn't quite fit that, two days after the Christmas markets, the heroine got her period and that a couple of weeks later she realised the cause of her constant nausea had not been a miracle conception. No. It was the daily ingestion of fish oil, giving rise to an unpleasant and well-documented side effect. Again, I was not pregnant. Again I cast aside a 'cure' – even if this one was only meant as a panacea for perimenopause – and looked around for another. From now on, I would get my essential fatty acids from coconut oil. According to Google, the only fertility advisor I could now afford, it was not only damn good at balancing hormones, it was also fantastic for getting people pregnant and even for increasing sperm counts. Chris started taking coconut oil, too. It came in solid form and we carved ribbons of it out of the jar each morning and laid them across the top of our breakfast bowls. We would each eat it because we – still – wanted to have a child together and then later in the day we might argue and berate each other as we – I – trawled back over all that had gone wrong between us. That's how much sense this makes.

❧ ❧ ❧

In the absence of the sex, there were always the lies to row about. It had come to my attention, nearly ten years later, that if Chris had been honest when we met, then I never would have gone out with him. He told me he was forty-two. He told

414

me his performance anxiety was a post-divorce blip. These were the two points I honed in on as I travelled across London on the tube, playing a now-regular game of *When Did I Fuck Up My Life?* This was how I filled the journeys, starting from the present time and rewinding until I found the crucial error, the faulty placement that had sent the house of cards crashing down. *I should have left him in Switzerland, after Janet Brown and after my birthday.* No, the real problem was earlier than that. *You gave him too many chances in 2005 and 2006.* Rewind, rewind. *Well, none of that would have happened if...*

Rewind some more. *It was when I met him and he lied and I let it go.* But why did I let it go? *Because of the position I found myself in, when I was thirty-three.* And on it went, back and back and back, through Jai and Dana and every relationship I'd ever had; but the more I picked at it, the more it seemed that every error was in fact a compound error, always built in some way on the mistakes that had gone before. I got nowhere on my tube journeys, except all the way back to the day I was born. Maybe that was it: I had come crashing into the world uninvited and my timing had been off ever since. That sounded about right. Timing. *That* was how I had fucked up my life.

There was someone at work, the year before I paired up with Chris. Right away, when I first saw him, I understood. Here he was, at last. We shared furtive eye contact across the office for months; the rumour was we liked each other. Then one day, he came over to my desk, picked up one of my magazines and casually began leafing through it. And I didn't know what to do so I kept on typing. I kept on typing. After a few minutes, he put down the magazine and walked off. What if I had said something? What if I had even just looked up and smiled? That, right there, could have been the moment and I missed it. He was five years younger than me and funny and good-looking ... and what? Nothing happened. But I thought about all those missed chances now and I wondered, would I have become a mother, if I'd taken them? Any of them?

There was also someone I'd been friends with since we were twenty year olds; there was my first love, who still lived in our home town, and there was always – always – what might have been with Jai. In one fleeting thought, three potential fathers who would have been the kindest, gentlest of dads. And somehow, the timing had never been right; I had missed my connection with all of them. It seemed I was always two paces ahead or two paces behind of what mattered.

And then, one Thursday night, I finally, gradually, dug it up, the ominous thing that lay hidden beyond all the questions I had taken to asking.

"I *know* you wish you were still with Jai instead of me," Chris snapped during the latest post-mortem. "How come he's so untouchable? I don't understand it. He left you for your best friend, I'd never do that to you. Never."

"Thanks," I said drily, "for reminding me. He obviously didn't think I was worth it either. I get it."

"That wasn't what I meant, sweetheart. I just meant that I care about you – you must see that. Of course you're worth it, that's the point."

I eyed him angrily. "Ha! You don't think I'm worth anything. You didn't even take a sperm test for me, or stick up for me with Janet Brown or—"

"Honestly!" Chris cut me off. "We can't keep going back over this. We've got to put it behind us and move on."

"Bloody hell. Of course you'd say that."

He looked confused, wary and furious all at once.

"You don't get it at all," I said. "I will *never* get to move on from this. For the rest of my life, I'll be childless. It doesn't ever stop. I won't have children, I won't have grandchildren either – it's with you forever. You think I can conveniently forget all this, just wander off as if it never happened? Yep. I bet that would suit you. Brush it all under the carpet and carry on."

Chris spat his words at the ceiling.

"I'm sorry those things happened. I am. But I can't keep apologising for them. I didn't mean for any of them to happen, but we can't keep talking about them, they're gone."

"Gone? They'll *never* be gone."

And then I saw in a flash the great, gaping disparity between us. It was so evident, so obvious, that after a while you got used to it and just stopped seeing it. But here it was, the manifest explanation as to why I was heartbroken and bereft and Chris was not: parenthood would never be officially *over* for him; it was only me now reaching the end of the road, me who would soon have no choice but to stop.

I interrupted his protests, eruptions and denials, all now spitting like angry fireworks around the room.

"Do you know what really pisses me off? I'll go through the rest of my life never being a mother and you – you'll go off and meet someone younger, maybe you'll get some money from somewhere and you'll have fertility treatment and, bam! – *you* will get to be a dad."

"Oh, please. That's not going to happen. Really!"

"Yeah, but it could happen and you know it. You've always had all the time in the world. That's why I've been running round like a mad thing trying to fix this and you just sit back and watch."

Chris wheeled away as if pushed off balance. "This is beyond belief. Why must you think these things of me? That's not what I want – I only ever wanted to be a father with *you*."

"Ha. You didn't act like it."

Now, as well as winding time back and morphing all the permutations, I was fast forwarding and scratching in my

417

own projected notches on the timeline. I was talking as if our relationship had ended, but where in this game was the end? It wasn't noted anywhere on my timeline, the great break-up.

Suddenly, the questions I should have paid more attention to much earlier, if I hadn't been so consumed by infertility, came surging into the foreground. I could feel the pressure rising in my chest, like it always did when something, somewhere within, was trying to get my attention, to issue a warning.

I spoke quietly now, although every nerve was taut and alert. "Why didn't you tell me the truth?" I asked. "At the beginning?"

"What?"

"Why did you let me think you were forty-two when you were actually forty-eight? Why would you do that?"

"Oh! Not this again." Chris slapped his thigh in frustration. "This is absurd. You could have left if it was so awful. Anyway, I did tell you the truth, you know I did."

He was pacing again, agitated; why could he never keep still?

"You waited until you knew I loved you," I retorted. "And you *didn't* tell me the truth – you said you were forty-seven."

"You make me feel so useless," Chris accused. "I walk down the street and I don't know who I am anymore. I can't believe I'm this horrible man you paint me as. Why must you think so little of me?"

The argument raced off down that dead-end byway, out of control. Was I really so unfair? Was it me? Was I just imagining things? *No! No. Don't stop now. Something's not right.* My chest constricted further.

"You lied about the sex thing as well," I interjected. "Blatantly."

"I can't keep apologising for these things. You're the one who stayed with me all these years. You must be getting something out of it!"

"Why did you do it?" I persisted. "I just want to know why you would do that."

Eventually, tortuously, it filtered out: "I thought you'd laugh at me. I thought you'd leave me. I didn't want to lose you."

I would have softened then, in earlier years, but the muffled note of warning kept driving me on. There was *something else to know*, something I couldn't quite grasp. The tension in my chest now all but crushed the air from my lungs.

"In other words, you got me into this relationship on false pretences," I whispered.

"It wasn't supposed to be like that. I swear! I just wanted to be with you and I didn't know how to tell you ..." He put his head in his hands. "I was a fool. I didn't want to lose you."

"So you lied to keep me?"

Then, all at once, it charged into view, with shocking ferocity, the force from just out of sight. Bile rose into my throat as I realised – finally – what this was really all about.

He lied to keep me.

"Oh," I gasped, reeling now as the full impact hit. "No!" I looked over at Chris in horror. "You *knew*. You knew all along."

"What? What do you mean?"

I clutched at my stomach, stunned, disbelieving. "You knew you had fertility issues." My voice began to shake, along with my insides, my hands, my legs. "That's why you didn't want to take that follow-up sperm test. That's why you dragged it out for so long. You already knew."

"No! No, this is all wrong." Chris moved across the room towards me. "You don't know what you're saying."

"You thought I'd leave you. It was just like the other things – you didn't want to lose me, so you didn't tell me the truth." I paused, almost unable to breathe. "Just so you know," I added in a hoarse whisper. "You don't know me very well. I'd never have left you for that."

"Please!" Chris pleaded. "You've got to listen to me. I did *not* know. I suspected I had duff sperm – yes – but everyone thinks that about themselves. I wouldn't keep something like that from you. I wouldn't."

I thought of all the attempts I had made, all the avenues I had gone down, all the people I had turned to for help. And he had known it was largely worthless, every effort?

"You knew how much I wanted to be a mother," I stammered, backing away. "Oh my God. You thought … That's why … You knew! I can't believe you knew."

I turned and ran down the stairs and out onto the street.

THIRTY-FIVE

IT WAS A MARK of how enmeshed our lives had become, and how isolated we were from everyone else, that the only place I had to go was Rose's empty flat. It didn't make much of a statement, leaving a man only to take up residence in a property that was technically owned by him. In my twenties, I would have booked into a hotel. I had good wages, then. And savings, and credit cards with available credit. I would have eaten chocolate and read magazines in the bath; I could afford to disappear then. And if I couldn't, well, there were always friends and family. Now it was all gone – bar the fledgling business with its one laptop and broken chair – and my dignity and sense seemed to have departed with it. Nine years of infertility and this was where I had ended up. I looked around and hoped I would have made a better fist of things if I'd actually had children. No wonder no one wanted to be born to me; they must have known what a mess I was going to turn into. *Stop it! It's just cells, just sperm meeting egg. You don't get chosen.*

"Oh shut up," I said to the empty lounge.

The sound of my mobile phone ringing stabbed through the silence. Chris again. Another shrill beep to let me know he'd left another shrill message. He'd forgotten. How many times had I reminded him? The message facility on that phone didn't work – he could deliver as many of his speeches as he liked; I'd never get to hear a word of it.

I stood up and stared out of the window, wondering what it was that I planned to do next. I should have grabbed my passport before I left, that's what I should have done. *You can't afford an air ticket anywhere.* I needed to go home; that's what I needed. *You're scared of flying.* I felt an ache where my family used to be; I needed to be with my family. *What? So you can hold everyone else's babies while they all stare at you? Like a barren zoo exhibit?* This was typical. I had consciously set out to expand my life circle and all I'd done was contract it. After nearly ten years, all that was left was me, standing alone in a lounge I had no right to be in.

How could he have done it? Did he really do it? Did he know, before he met me, that he might need help to have children? It had been hours and the bile was still trapped in my throat.

The front door rattled, the sound of a key in a lock. Did the flat's buyer have a key yet? No. She couldn't have. I ran to the mirror and frantically wiped at my tear-tracked face; it might be the estate agent. Hell! That was even worse.

The door swung open in a rush. "Sweetheart! Are you here?"

Oh. I certainly had a talent for overlooking the obvious.

Chris ran down the narrow hall towards me. "Thank God. I've been so worried about you. Why didn't you answer my calls? I've left so many messages."

"I've told you hundreds of times," I said, flatly addressing my remarks to the floor. "I can't pick up messages on this. If you ever listened to me, you'd know that."

"I was upset," he replied. "I was too upset to remember. I do listen to you, I do. But you've got to believe me – *I didn't know.* I wouldn't lie to you about that, I swear."

I sat down on the couch, vaguely aware that I was moving in slow motion. "You never told me," I said, "why you didn't have children with your wife. When you were in your thirties."

Chris crouched down in front of me and placed his hands on my knees, his head almost dropping into my lap. "She never wanted children," he said quietly. "I didn't think I would ever have a family of my own, but then there was you."

"Yes, exactly. Then there was me."

I couldn't look at him, not just his face but any part of him. "You're even weaker than I thought."

He abruptly stood up and crossed the lounge, sinking dejectedly into an armchair opposite me. "Please," he sighed. "Please stop saying these things."

It became another of our Talks That Last All Night. I'd loved this, when we first met, the fact that we could talk on the phone for seven or eight hours, right through the night, and never run out of things to say. Now his words were just tricks, designed to trap me.

He continued to deny it, over and over, but I couldn't stop thinking that if he could keep significant information from me twice, then he could do it a third time.

"Look," I said. "There's nothing to lose now. Please, I'm asking you – if you ever loved me at all, then tell me the truth. Did you already know what those sperm tests were going to show?"

"No!" he protested again. "No. I swear, I'd never had fertility tests in my life. I'm sorry I dragged my feet – I don't know why I did that – but it wasn't because I knew. I was scared, maybe, of what it would show but I didn't know."

"You're in your mother's flat," I said ominously. "Remember that."

"I'll swear it on anything and in front of anyone." He surged forward in the armchair. "I know I've given you cause to doubt me and I don't blame you, but you know who I really am and you know I wouldn't keep this from you. I'd never do that to you! I know how much you want to have a family, and you deserve to have one." The flood of words slowed to a mournful trickle. "I'm only sorry I couldn't give you that."

I looked over at him, properly – neither defiant nor challenging, like I so often seemed to be – and noticed the sadness all around his eyes. Just then, matching banks of tears broke loose and spilled down each of his cheeks.

"I'm so sorry," he whispered. "I know I've been no use to you, I know I must drive you mad. But I don't do any of these things on purpose, I promise you. I'm just a shambles sometimes, you know what I'm like. I don't mean to be. I want so much for you, so much more than this."

I left my entrenched position on the couch and sat on the arm of his chair, hugging his shuddering, defeated shoulders.

"I've mucked up plenty of things, too," I said gently. "It's not just you."

"But you've tried so hard ... I so wanted to give you a family."

"Well, maybe no one could've done that. We don't know if I ever could have had children. It might have been impossible, right from the start."

I almost began to tell him then about an HSG, about how I should have gone back to the doctor and insisted on having one – how I could have done that, instead of just sitting around waiting for him to take a sperm test. But some lesser instinct stopped me. If I told him, I knew that, sooner or later, he would throw it back at me; we were like opposing drivers in a car crash, negotiating and apportioning blame for the accident. It was as if I couldn't bear to hear that it was as much my fault as his. Anyway, why should I make it easy for him? He didn't even know what an HSG was. If he'd shown any interest at all, he would have known about these things. Besides, I'd already mentioned it years ago. Hadn't I?

Eventually, I made a much easier concession – I admitted that he was right; I should have called things off at the start if I wasn't happy about what I'd learned.

"I should have at least called time-out," I continued "and I didn't do that. I wasn't as strong as I could have been either."

"No," Chris broke in. "You were just kind. You stood by me, you always did."

"Well ..." I hesitated, not sure myself what had really happened. "It wasn't as simple as that. I didn't know how to deal with it and I didn't really get it right." I shook my head.

"No. I stayed for my own weird reasons – I can't blame anyone else for that."

What it amounted to, at the end of 2011, was that the messy, frayed cord which held us together was rapidly unravelling and all we knew how to do was follow it back to the place it started. Gradually, and without realising it, I had come to regard our relationship as some sort of failure. How could I work out if the only reason I thought that was because we hadn't managed to have children together? Would I still have regarded it as a failure if we'd had kids, even though it would have been the same relationship in every other regard? I didn't know anymore where infertility began and ended. It had seeped right through us and all between us. I was pretty certain that, if I'd been running around after three children in 2011, there wouldn't have been time to even remember that Chris once pretended he was forty-two. But now every little thing took on such importance. It was like listening to a black box recording after a plane crash and saying, "There! There's where it all went wrong." Why was I so fixated on trawling for clues? Was it going to make me feel better for the rest of my childless life that I had pinpointed all the places I went wrong? No. Probably not. But it didn't stop me doing it.

Now I had begun to doubt Chris so much that I actually believed for a while he might have lied about whether he was fertile. A tiny part of me still wondered, even then, if my suspicions weren't right. He was good with words; what if this was just another story he'd told me, nothing but promises woven in the air? Like a web that would hold me there. This note of caution joined all the other warning voices that had sprung up in the wake of our infertility. You would have thought that was the lowest point you could reach. Strangely, though, it wasn't that incident that really showed us what we had become.

❦ ❦ ❦

It happened between Christmas and New Year, sparked because I was subdued, quiet and introverted, once again missing family and children. "I can't take this," Chris snapped. "You're upsetting me now. Whatever I do, I can't make you happy."

"It's not about you," I said.

But he didn't believe me, and somehow it escalated until I said the second most horrible thing I've ever said to anyone. I was thinking it and then the words flew from my mouth: "Well, at least your mother can see what a tosser you are now!"

Chris bellowed then, his voice like a sledgehammer banging all around.

"You're just a fucking *leech*. Why don't you get out then? Go on. Get out! Just fuck off."

A leech was worse than an expletive; it made me feel small, like when I was a child and we had no money and sometimes you could see that people looked down on us for it. Enraged at the accusation, I pulled at my jersey with the moth holes in it and kicked the floor with my ten-year-old slippers.

"Where are all the diamonds then if I'm such a fucking leech? Where are they? Where's the holidays, the car, the designer clothes, the two hundred pound highlights? Where is *any* of it?"

I was shrieking, out of control, and I could tell that, too late, he wanted to shut it down, take back what we had said to each other. I whirled around the flat, gesturing at the kitchen where I did all the cooking, the lounge where I did all the vacuuming and dusting, the bathroom where I did all the cleaning and laundry, the office where I did all his online banking, filing, invoices, paperwork for the sale of Rose's flat …

"That's how much of a leech I am! You can bloody do everything *yourself* from now on. Except you don't even fucking know how to," I yelled before once again departing our flat.

I trudged to the park and sat alone on a mist-shrouded bench, too cold to sit there but too proud to get up and walk home.

426

It was as if Chris and infertility had morphed, become one and the same, and despising one was the equivalent of despising the other. But a leech? He thought I was a leech. Had I, after nearly ten years, become nothing but a person who bled other people dry? Who stuck with someone because of what they could give me? What exactly was it that he thought I was getting? It didn't feel like anything I had ever consciously sought out.

It was true that Chris had helped support me when I started the business, but I thought that was partly because we had agreed the new direction might lead us out of the state of limbo that infertility had become. It was a way of seeking movement where there was none. Now it had led us here, to these insults that crossed every line.

This time, it took two days to return to neutral territory. When we finally talked, calmly at last, we agreed: this was it. We could not go on taking chunks out of each other. It had to stop – the shouting, the swearing, the blame. We made a pact; if it ever happened again, then we would part for good. I knew that, this time, we both meant it. After nine years of trying to start a family, I was on the brink of having no children and no partner either. I dreaded deep down that it could only end as it had begun – with just me, a household of one.

THIRTY-SIX

OUR TENTH ANNIVERSARY FELL in April 2012. We must have given ourselves a shock at the end of 2011 because it followed a period of relative harmony. Anyone who saw us spending Valentine's Day together in central London two months before our anniversary might have thought we were a shiny new couple, attentive and interested in each other, not battered and bruised after nine years of infertility. That day, we didn't speak about children or ovulation or fertility treatments; we just enjoyed each other's company and laughed about how all my favourite places in London were also Chris's favourites. "We're still companionable, aren't we?" I joked, because that had always been one of 'our' words. "Of course," Chris agreed. "It doesn't matter what happens, we're always companionable." He leaned over then and kissed me on the nose, like he always had.

That January, we had spent two weeks together, emptying Rose's flat and sorting through her possessions. It was nearly nine months since she died, but we'd kept everything exactly the same, as if she might walk back through the door any day. That was the other thing we shared: we were both sentimental. It was one of the things that got us into a lot of trouble, especially where finances were concerned. After the flat sold, Chris received an inheritance that was large enough to pay off all of his loans and credit card debts, and for the first time I realised how the financial pressure had also been bearing down on us. We'd randomly thrown a lot of money at our fertility problems over the preceding nine years, perhaps choosing the wrong things in which to invest our hopes but nevertheless doing what seemed right at the time. Two hundred pounds here, one hundred and fifty there; it had all drip-fed away, eventually totalling much more than it would have cost for the fertility treatment we couldn't currently afford. We didn't think it would add up to that much; we didn't think it would be nine years.

Now Rose had gifted us a precious piece of breathing space and we both visibly unwound. I had been so consumed with the primary concern – being left childless – that I had forgotten infertility is not that one-dimensional. It insidiously permeates each level of your life, from finances to friendships, and ties every strand up into knots for you to fret over, deep down beneath the other layers of worry.

"I didn't realise I'd feel so relieved," I told Chris after his debts had disappeared. "It must have been on my mind more than I thought."

"I used to lie awake at night and it was all I could think about," he confessed.

"You didn't tell me that."

"I didn't want you to worry, sweetheart. You've got enough to deal with. No point both of us lying there in a cold sweat."

I wondered what further knowledge we each secretly protected the other from. He didn't tell me that he couldn't sleep because of our finances and I didn't tell him that some-times, when he was at work, I sat down on the couch and wept because I was so scared I would never be a mother.

Chris still took a romantic view; he thought we'd been together for ten years because of love, pure and simple. I wasn't so sure; sometimes I wondered if a break-up was just another of the things that he would never get around to doing, while it was probably more a matter of stubbornness on my part – I was simply too bloody-minded to quit. Still, it must have been something more that made me buy an anniversary card with space to write four of my fondest memories from the past ten years. I wrote them easily and I could have written twenty more without stopping to think. Did they outweigh, though, some of the other events that I wished had never happened? I thought that a person should probably have reached *certainty* by their tenth anniversary but there was still something about the fact that we hadn't had children together. It made us feel 'less' even though we were probably 'more' after all we'd endured together as an infertile couple. I didn't think it through that clearly; I just felt a little unsure, unsettled, by no means certain that we would reach our eleventh anniversary.

On the face of it, though, I woke up in the morning and said a cheery, "Happy Anniversary! Love you."

It was a Sunday; we read the papers in bed together then fell asleep in the afternoon sun. That night we walked arm in arm down familiar streets to a restaurant set amongst the grand houses that overlooked the tree-lined village green. We sat at a first-floor window and watched the sun set over the dog walkers and the families and the evening drinkers, all sharing the triangular patch of grass below. Since infertility, we had rarely allowed ourselves to spend money on this type of outing; it felt special, decadent even.

By the time we finished dinner, we were the only ones left in the restaurant; we moved to a two-seater couch at the back of the room and lounged contentedly, admiring the lights that now twinkled in the distance against the blue black sky. It was easy to forget that we had ever shouted at each other, that our differences had ever separated us. I rested my head on Chris's shoulder.

"Imagine if we lived in a house like this," I said. "If this was our lounge and that was our view."

"I could play my music as loud as I liked."

"Yeah," I laughed. "No loony Lorna living beneath us."

"Oh, don't. You're going to make me feel ill."

Loony Lorna, our downstairs neighbour, had taken something of a shine to Chris over the past three years; her monologues were now addressed entirely to him and she was given to thrusting various body parts in his direction, on the premise of demonstrating how she used to belly dance on stage.

"Wasn't she telling you the other day about the time she performed nude in the West End?" I teased him.

"Stop it," he ordered with a chuckle.

"It's always women of a certain age who go all funny around you. Have you noticed that? They always treat me like I'm not even there, but they can't get enough of you."

"Urgh, what a depressing thought. That can't be true. Anyway, you're the only one I see."

"Hmm, it's just a shame I don't fancy you as much as ancient belly dancers do."

We walked back home laughing, joking, content.

As well as being our tenth anniversary, it was Day Thirteen. The thirteenth day of my cycle, the one on which I very often appeared to ovulate, even now. 'Wouldn't it be perfect,' I thought, 'if we came through all of this and finally conceived our child on our tenth anniversary?'

The thought seemed so right; what more fitting sign could there be that perseverance pays off? So, it looked like I still believed in signs then. Significant happenings on significant days.

I wished Chris was the kind of man who could be relied upon to throw me on the bed after such a romantic night out and declare that he'd thought of nothing else, all the way through dinner. I knew, though, that if I wanted to mark our tenth anniversary in this way, it would be up to me to take the initiative. Oh well, things had been going smoothly. There was that one brief blip in January, but … no, that was nothing. He'd just need a hint, that was all.

When I finally settled on a way to get the message across, he was a bit taken aback. "I wouldn't have eaten all that pudding and drunk all that coffee if I'd known," he said.

"Okay. Well, don't worry about it then."

"No, no, I'll still try. I mean, I want to try."

"Can you *please* stop using that word?" I screwed up my face. "It makes me feel like you think I'm Lorna or something."

"Sorry. I know it's a bad choice of word. It just slips out – I don't mean it the way it sounds. Of course I don't have to try, not with you. I love being with you, you must know that."

My stomach tightened a little at the return of this word, 'try'; it was the word of a nervous man. It was the word people resorted to when they were asked to accomplish something at overwhelmingly long odds: "Well, I'll give it a try. That's all I can do."

I was about to remove my make-up for the night as I usually did; I looked in the mirror and left it on. Anything to help, anything not to remind him that he was about to go to bed with forty-three-year-old me. I was acting a role now, like I did when I consulted fertility experts and smiled and made light-hearted remarks and attempted to portray myself as calm and collected when, really, my insides had long ago disintegrated. Now I was the casual lover, going to bed without a care in the world, without a thought in my head; *there's no pressure here, nothing for you to worry about.* I laughed and snuggled – was this natural enough, was *I* enough to take the word 'try' out of his vocabulary?

We made a valiant start, but I could sense it almost immediately, the shift in him that transformed me from a partner of ten years to a terrifying challenge, an alien creature thrown between his sheets. I might as well have been absent; he was not making love to me, he was alone in his head facing down this thing he sometimes called a demon. He ground against my body, over and over, not looking at me, not seeing me, not taking a peek to see how I was doing. I was a blow-up doll, a sex surrogate, a crash-test dummy; two of those things didn't have feelings. That's how he treated me when this happened – like an inanimate object. I reassured him, tried to help, suggested we take a break – all the usual things. However, in the end, it turned out to be me who couldn't try any longer. It hit with a force that made me want to run: *this has to stop.*

"No," I said. "I can't do this anymore."

Chris rolled off me, probably relieved, and I urgently scrabbled around for my clothes. My hands stumbled onto a pair of track pants and a sweatshirt at the end of the bed; that would do, anything to cover me up. I sat up and hauled them on, wanting to go outside and walk the streets in the dark, wanting to go anywhere except back to my own bed.

It felt wrong, not just for me but surely for both of us. Then there was the sense of rejection – I wasn't enough, I would never be enough – and swimming all over everything was grief. I would never have children, I couldn't even try to make a child on my tenth anniversary. All these lost chances.

"I think it was the gravy and the red wine," said Chris. "It was too rich, all together like that."

I remained silent. "Come on, sweetheart," he urged. "It's not you, please don't think it's you. It was just a rich meal, that's all – I'm not used to it. And it was so hot up here tonight. Look! The sweat's pouring off me."

I tucked the sweatshirt into the pants; my midriff was chilled.

"Come on," Chris repeated. "I've been doing so well – I've made love to you every month since 2008 …"

Except it wasn't love-making; sometimes he didn't even touch me, just climbed on, like a person preparing to do push-ups at the gym, did his bit then climbed off again. It was always quicker, if he didn't have to actually touch me. When it really came down to it, there was only one reason I brushed aside that uncomfortable fact: because afterwards, I'd stick a pillow under my hips – he didn't know, but I used one of his whenever I could – and will his sperm to swim to my eggs, if I still had some. It was like bartering – here, I'll trade you a dollop of self-esteem for two mils of your sperm. Had it really come to that?

On some days, duty done, Chris had shown off and said crass things about the strength of his manhood, swaggering like a stud farm stallion.

Now, he was still talking. "We can try again tomorrow. You'll still be ovulating tomorrow, won't you?" Silence. "I'm happy to try again now. You know I am – I'm more than happy to have another go. We can always try again tomorrow. Lou?"

"No," I said quietly. "We can't."

I didn't know what else to say to him yet; I just knew that there – on our tenth anniversary – that was it. Even me, perpetually slow on the uptake, couldn't ignore that number. Ten. The return of this issue, the timing of it, was so obvious I might as well have been hit over the head with a concrete slab. We had been together ten years and he was no closer to admitting the existence of this problem – and therefore no closer to doing anything about it – than he had been in year one. It was always the gravy or the wine or the pudding or the heat or the noise outside the window. I realised something: I had given more thought to finding a solution to this over the past ten years than he had. *He* didn't have a problem; he was Don Juan, just like everyone in the office thought he was. I realised something else: this issue he said didn't exist had taken up almost as much of my energy as infertility had. It had repeatedly diverted the focus from what really mattered.

I disappeared for a day, under the duvet, temporarily defeated. Chris emerged at the top of the stairs every now and again to tell me what a great relationship we had. I felt too heavy to get up, until the next day when he went to work and, after he shut the door, I quickly began to feel lighter. By the time he came home again, I'd worked it out, what I was going to do.

"Oh, not this again," he interrupted when it became clear that I wanted to talk about The Sex Issue.

"Please," I said, "don't let your ego take over. We need to sort this out."

Chris threw up his hands, rolled his eyes. "This is unfair! I thought I was cured. I *am* cured. I don't know what happened on our anniversary. It was just one of those days. You've said it yourself – it's natural to have days like that."

This was a familiar diversion, away from the destination I was trying to reach. "How can you still not understand it?" I didn't wait for an answer. "Anyway, there's no point discussing it. What I wanted to tell you is that I don't think it's a good idea to have sex again, not—"

"Really Louise. How am I ever meant to get over this if you won't let me try again?"

Don't get drawn in now, you're nearly there.

"That's just it," I continued, throat constricted with too many emotions. "It's your problem to sort out. I should have said this at the beginning, but I'm saying it now – I can't sleep with you again until you've at least tried to do something about it." I stared intently at the wall ahead, knowing that tears would spill the moment I blinked. "I don't care if you can't completely overcome it, but I just need to know that you've tried."

He stared at me, part horrified, part uncomprehending. "You need to get a Plan B," I concluded shakily. "For both our sakes."

Chris didn't accept it, not immediately. I could tell that he thought I was just making a point, that I'd give in after a while and life could return to normal. I didn't really mean it – he didn't really have to confront this issue. He still seemed to believe that was the case, even when I told him it felt like I had become collateral damage because of his denial. It dawned on me then that he didn't really know me; what he knew was a woman in her thirties, and then her forties, who wanted to have children. The woman he knew was prepared to make any number of compromises if that's what she had to do to have a family. I didn't recognise her. She was a lot more desperate than I'd ever been. She traded things she never should have traded, just in case she could become a mother.

Maybe it was closer to the truth to say it turned us both into collateral damage. My mother's voice again: "You reap what you sow." How had we done this to each other? How had we done it to ourselves? And, where, I started to wonder, did children fit into this? Was there such a thing as being wanted too much?

⁂

Three days after our tenth anniversary, my niece Freya gave birth to a baby boy. There it was unfolding before me, my parallel life, the one in which I hadn't made bad choices and bad compromises. When the 'new arrival' photo came through, I had never seen such a touching image of a mother and new-born; for a moment I glimpsed what it would have felt like if I had been thirty-four and had a son of my own. Just for a moment, then it was gone. I was learning not to play games of 'if only' but I let myself think it: the baby days should have been long behind me by now. If I was as fertile as most of my family, my oldest child would be eight-and-a-half.

I wondered if perimenopause had brought with it the voice of the crone because I was increasingly shooting down these games I'd taken to playing. *Of course a new-born baby looks cute. Wait 'til you haven't slept for six months, then see how lovely you think it is.* I often tried to think of all the worst bits of parenthood – the squabbles and the tantrums and the overwhelming *suffocation* of it all. *You wouldn't have the tolerance for it, not now.* I couldn't tell if it was just self-preservation or if maybe the hormones that had hit in my thirties were starting to fade

436

away, no longer screaming quite so loudly: Reproduce! You must reproduce.

A month after our tenth anniversary, Chris and I, still sleeping in the same bed but not *sleeping together*, went to the May Fair on the same green that we'd looked out across that anniversary night. The other residents of our local area were clearly on better terms with fertility than we were – the lanes between stalls were jammed with strollers and buggies, while armies of escaped toddlers staged sit-ins in the middle of the path or haphazardly zoomed in and out under tables of second-hand books and toys. Groups of ten-year-old boys jostled and pushed each other, like a solid wave of destruction, followed by groups of ten-year-old girls who shrieked and giggled in their wake.

I realised I had become 'old' because the teenage girls bothered me. They still travelled in cliques – that was nothing new – but nine of them stood there, forming a louche circle, and every single one was wearing just their tights, not even cut-offs or a mini-skirt over the top. Every so often they pouted, en masse, into the tiny camera lens of a smartphone.

"Crikey," I said to Chris. "Aren't they embarrassed that everyone can see their knickers? I used to have bad dreams that I went out dressed like that."

We laughed about how old and uptight we were, not prepared to leave the house with everyone seeing our pants.

"I swear I wouldn't have even done that in my teens," I added.

The whole scene equated to mayhem set to a hundred different soundtracks, all at maximum volume. I could barely hear what Chris had to say about it all, but he was wearing the grim expression of one bent on escape.

Finally, spat out the side of the cyclone and into a quieter area at the back of the display tents, I could finish what I was saying.

437

"Maybe it's just as well I never had teenage daughters," I told him. "They would have hated me – refusing to let them out the door without a skirt on."

"It's appalling," Chris agreed, sounding even older than me, which he was. "I don't understand how their parents have allowed them to leave their houses looking like that. No one seems to realise what's normal anymore."

"Well," I replied. "I guess we've never had to do battle with a teenage girl."

We ducked and swerved along the pavements, through the crowds of families still heading for the green, and found sanctuary through the door of a coffee shop, gasping as if we'd just come up for air. We drank our peppermint tea – another old and fussy choice – and traded tales of Incidents We Had Witnessed at the May Fair. When it was my turn to contribute something, I sat back in my chair and thought deeply for a moment. I needed to word this carefully after the nine years we'd just endured, perpetually chasing fertility.

"Do you know what? When we were at the fair, I looked around and, I never thought I'd say this, but I kind of thought … maybe … well, maybe we've got off lightly."

I paused, unsure if I really was going to say it. "Not having kids."

Chris's head shot up and he instantly abandoned the excavation of his carrot cake. "Phew," he sighed. "I'm so glad you said that. I was thinking exactly the same thing. It was hell, wasn't it?"

We both laughed, relieved and perhaps surprised to be in agreement. I confessed properly then: "What I was actually thinking was 'thank *goodness* we didn't have children'."

Chris visibly relaxed in his chair. "I did wonder if maybe we're not a bit too old for all of this."

"Me too. Wow. I never thought I'd say that."

"*I* never thought you'd say that."

"It's tricky isn't it?" I pondered. "How do you tell if it's just other people's kids that bug you? Mind you, they'd always be round all the time, I suppose. I'd need earplugs, I'm sure of it."

"I'd need to live in a separate house," Chris joked. "That noise was like nothing I've heard – and I spent most of the seventies at prog rock gigs."

"What are we doing?" I giggled. "We're ancient."

We headed off in the direction of the river, springing over the ground. It was the first time since my twenties that I saw families with young children and thought: 'I'm glad that's not me.'

※ ※ ※

I was forty-three-years-old, I was no longer having sex, I was already in the grip of perimenopause and I was starting to wonder if having a baby was such a great idea after all. Naturally, I did not give it up. I did not abandon all efforts at conception and embark on a new chapter, in which I found my place in the world as a mature, single, childless woman. No. I still kept on – and on – trying to have children. A child. Even I could see that *children* plural was beyond the boundaries of belief. Apart from deciding that I would devote ten years to this, I had also begun to understand that I was not going to stop while there was a chance, even the speck of a spit of a chance, that I was still fertile. Ha! *Still fertile.* Who said I ever *had* been fertile? There was the question again: *if you'd been with a different man, would it ever have happened?* In a warped sort of way, I hoped the answer was no because otherwise it meant I'd thrown away my fertility with the choices I'd made. It was a disloyal thought but I picked away at it anyhow.

I wondered if Chris did this, too, or whether he really wasn't that bothered about having a family. The thing was, I couldn't tell if he'd still choose me, if he was offered a do-over, and I suspected I might have thrown my chips in elsewhere if I was offered the same. There it was, the biggest reason not to continue. Even worse, some of the *reasons for continuing* really should have counted as reasons against. I could tell already that part of the drive to keep going was because I didn't want any more 'if onlys' in my life. I did not want to look back when I was fifty-five years old and think, 'Well, maybe if you'd hung in there for a bit longer. Maybe if you hadn't given up, you might have been a mother. Oh well, too late now.'

It was amazing how, after such a long period of time, a 'family' became a vague, unformed idea, almost mythical, like something that didn't actually exist. I had to remind myself, you are trying to bring a *person* into the world. Their little life has to feel secure in your life. I thought about that often; whether the desire to be a mother was fuelled by what I could get or by what I could give. I knew exactly how it felt to be an unplanned and unwanted child, but I'd never considered the opposite: what was it like to carry so many years of someone else's yearning? That didn't sound like much fun either, especially if you ended up with far older parents than you might have wished for, a mother and father who drank peppermint tea and insisted that you wore a skirt over your tights. Also, the old fogeys weren't a hundred per cent sure if they still desired each other that much, but that was apparently okay because they *sure wanted you*.

My whole life, I had promised myself that my children would know they were wanted; they would never have to wonder what was so wrong with them that their parents – the people who created them – had cast them aside. They were not to have any doubts, my children; they would walk around in the world *knowing* that their mother had welcomed them since the first moments of their existence. I thought this would be a good thing. Now I was confused. The only fact I was sure of was that it wasn't their love I was looking for.

What I wanted was to give them *my* maternal love, the desire to care for them that currently had nowhere to go. It still seemed enough, knowing that. And Chris would be a good and kind father, I still thought that, even though it felt as if infertility had wedged us apart, staring at each other from opposite sides of a deep canyon. It would be temporary wouldn't it? We'd get over it wouldn't we?

I reached a conclusion that would probably make actual parents sigh deeply or even hoot with laughter: I didn't care if I never had sex again; I was quite prepared to swap my sex life for motherhood. So. I did it. Every month, I bought three or four baby food syringes from Boots and Chris would disappear to the bathroom to provide a 'sample', which I then injected into myself, with the help of some pre-conception lubricant. It was an every-second-day pursuit throughout ovulation, although sometimes we used only two syringes a month and never more than four. The odds were as ridiculous as we were. As I was. I now knew that there would be around 1.5ml of sperm on the first day, 1ml on the second and 0.5ml on the third. Secretly, I fretted that we fell short of the optimum 2-5ml. It couldn't have been further removed from when we first met and Chris played me Nick Drake songs and read lines of poetry from a battered book.

A decade later, it was just as well we were not also measuring resentment by the mil. First of all, the syringes didn't always work that well. Sometimes the plunger refused to budge, stuck fast by an airlock, and I had a syringe inside me but no way of expelling its contents. I pinched and stung myself as I grappled, trying to break the deadlock without spilling our last bit of hope out onto the sheets. Why, oh why, didn't he ask about Viagra? Why didn't he research some of the 'support rings' that were now available? He could order one online. No one would even have to see him. What could I conclude except that I wasn't worth it to him, and neither was our future.

441

Still, each month I would ask: "Would you mind doing a sample today?" and I resented that too. It felt like another humiliation, all this asking. If he wasn't interested in doing this, why didn't he just say so? I kept getting the image of me running a marathon while carrying Chris on my back. Sometimes he would climb off, but only to erect a barrier on the road, making it more difficult to reach the finish. That's what it felt like, always striving forward while someone else did his level best to pull me back.

We had made a pledge not to shout at each other, so my resentments emerged in hissed complaints, always around ovulation when I was reminded of how difficult he was making this, now that sex was indefinitely on hold. Each month, he issued the same promise: I *will* do something about it. Each month I warned: this is pushing us further apart.

"I give you my word," he replied. "I'm going to do something about it. I've told you, I'm going to do something."

After five months without sex, Chris borrowed my laptop and found two web pages open: an American sperm bank site and a dating site full of southern hemisphere men. The second one was an accident, but I didn't tell him that. Or that I'd clicked on several profiles anyway, just so I would know what life might be like if we didn't make it. He responded by immediately logging into Amazon and ordering a book on self-hypnosis. "See?" he said. "I've done something about it. I want to be with you – you must know that."

He also asked about the sperm bank site and I confessed that I wished I'd been strong enough to seriously consider the donor process when I was younger.

"I tried to ask Janet Brown about it," I added. "I did try, but she berated me for even bringing it up. I just wanted some proper information, that was all."

I still had many mils of resentment for Janet Brown. I had

turned on the radio one day and there she was, an earnest counsellor's voice proclaiming how crucial it was that infertile women were nurtured and supported at a time when they were feeling so vulnerable and fragile. I changed channels before I became the hysterical caller who phoned in and shouted, "What a load of shit." She was just another spiky barrier on the road during this damn endless marathon.

"I'd let you try a donor," Chris said suddenly. "I'm happy for you to do that."

"You'd *let* me?"

"I didn't mean it like that. I just mean I'm happy for you to try. I know you want to give this one last go. I'm happy to pay for it if you want to try."

Instead of being grateful, I was annoyed. "I'm a month off forty-four and you say this now?"

Chris looked baffled, irritated.

"Why didn't you say it earlier?" I challenged. "We were supposed to talk about it with Janet Brown, then she slapped me down and I didn't see you jumping in to explain that you backed me up."

"Ach!" he spat. "We can't keep going over this. I've told you I'm sorry for that. I can't keep saying sorry."

"Well maybe you should. You've waited until I'm practically in the menopause and then you've said, 'Oh, I'll help you now.' Of course you're 'happy' to be part of it now – you *know* it's too late."

"This is ridiculous," Chris snapped. "I don't know why this should turn into an argument when all I wanted to say was that I'd support you."

"Ha!"

He said it again: *we can't go on like this.*

I ignored him. "Just tell me," I asked, "did you even want to have a family?"

"Of course I did! I thought it would happen, I genuinely did. I know maybe this seems a bit late to you now, but I thought it would happen."

"I think you knew exactly what you were doing. How else do you explain all the messing around?"

Chris pressed the heel of his palm to his forehead, grimacing as if in pain. "I don't know. I don't know. I just thought it would happen. Maybe I was naive, but I did. You can't mean these things you're saying, I know you can't – you wanted me to be the father of your children. You must think I'm okay."

The festering mils of resentment exploded well beyond optimal level. I found myself dredging up the sludge that had been lying far below in the dark.

It spilled out before I could even register the thought. "I don't want my children to have a father like *you*. I want them to have someone *strong*, someone they can rely on."

"Well, that's it then." Chris's voice was as hard and hostile as I'd heard it. "You've never said that before. I can't be with someone who thinks that of me."

THIRTY-SEVEN

DURING MY TEN-YEAR wrestling match with infertility, I said the three worst things I had ever said to anyone. Number three: "I don't want my children to have a father like you." Number two: "At least your mother knows what a t***** you are now." And at number one, a phrase I won't even repeat because it actually, almost, wished harm on another. I said all three things to Chris – spewed them out really – and still he didn't throw in the towel, like a disgusted, defeated opponent might have done. Despite the words I wounded him with, he stayed there and slugged it out, hoping there could be a way to break the deadlock, both between ourselves and infertility.

"We all say things we don't mean when we're angry," he told me when I apologised later for the first, second and third worst things I had ever said. He held grudges with other people, but never with me. Instead of appreciating this, I became increasingly suspicious: did he want to stay with me so badly because he was afraid to start a relationship with someone else, knowing he'd have to tell them that sex might not be on the agenda? Was I just the convenient option? It seemed so improbable that he could still love me, like he did once, before we had each seen the worst in each other. Because, if nothing else, infertility had given us a good, long time to examine each other's flaws. I suspected that the only reason I didn't turn away from this mutual display of weaknesses was because I didn't know where else to go. Infertility had been tearing up my life plans for nearly a decade and I still hadn't adapted; I still kept trying to pick up the original life plan and piece it back together. This plan required a partner. Was that why *I* stayed?

Or was it just that I didn't know where to go next, now that my plan had been torn into shreds?

The scenery changed after the row about the sperm donors. It was as if all the arguments that had gone before had erupted like volcanoes, but they'd finally blown themselves out and we were left, the two of us, surveying the wasteland that remained. Maybe this was what happened when you took sex out of a relationship; there wasn't the passion anymore to power a volcano.

It had been nearly six months since the termination in physical relations. Three weeks before this milestone that I had never wanted to reach, I turned forty-four. I made the same wish on my birthday that year as I made every year: *please may this be the year I become a mother.* I didn't even add an ironic laugh to make it seem less ridiculous. I would continue inserting sperm via syringe, determinedly seeing it through to the bitter end.

As the six-month anniversary of our celibacy rolled around, Chris had still produced only one book on self-hypnosis by way of a prospective Plan B. He had not actually read it; it sat unopened on his side of the bed for weeks, until I picked it up and studied it from cover to cover in case it could help with fear of flying. It was like the sperm test issue all over again, with 'tomorrow' the magic word.

Whereas once I might have raised my voice or sworn in frustration, I now spoke to Chris in the manner of a line manager during a performance appraisal.

"I'm very disappointed that you have not made any attempt to resolve this problem."

"I would have appreciated it if you had been more proactive."

"I want you to be aware that if too much time passes, we will not find a way back from this."

One Saturday afternoon, I showed him an article I had found online about the invention of a support ring that had transformed the sex lives of injured and disabled men. "I'd have preferred it if you'd done the research yourself," I said. "But here it is, if you want to read about it and consider trying it."

"I will," he said, instantly relieved and enthusiastic. "I'll order one today."

Two more cycles-by-syringe followed; no support ring arrived in the post.

During the second of those cycles, Chris hurried upstairs into the bedroom, bearing a plastic jug containing his latest 'sample'. "It looks in much better form," he declared happily. "It's a real improvement."

Did he really believe this was all I wanted? His sperm in a measuring jug? This wasteland we were left with after infertility; how could he not know it was the loneliest place of my life?

"Great," I intoned. "Just what every woman dreams about."

"Don't be like that," Chris said. "I've offered to make love to you. I've said I'll try – many times."

"And I've told you I'm not your crash-test dummy. But what have you done about it? Nothing. Nearly eight months … and nothing."

"That's not fair. I went off and bought that book – there! – on self-hypnosis."

"But you haven't even read it."

"I am going to read it. You know I'm going to read it."

"And that ring I showed you, the one you said you were going to order—"

Chris flared then, face like the molten rock of old. "I can't take any more of this," he shouted. "I really can't take any more of this."

"Ha." I gave a sarcastic laugh. "That trick doesn't work anymore. You're going to have to think of something else."

"Ach! This is absurd."

I put the cap back on the conception gel, placed the near-empty tube in its box and returned it to my bedside table.

"What's absurd is that all you had to do was click one button on your laptop to order a product that could have made life so much better for both of us, and you didn't do it."

"Well, you should have kept me up to the mark on it. Anyway, I *am* going to do it. You know I am."

"It was two months ago!"

I got up, no longer concerned about lying still for at least thirty minutes, hips raised in perpetual hope that the sperm might finally reach its destination.

"You didn't click that button because you care more about your ego than you care about me. It's obvious."

Even this came out in the matter-of-fact manner of the line manager. We had reached the stage where I knew Chris's strategies too well to even be bothered arguing with him; it was like watching from afar, yet at the same time seeing him in close-up.

I went downstairs and started clearing out the storage room, which I calculated was just big enough to hold a single bed. It was time to reclaim a scrap of ground, even if my new territory measured no more than three steps down and two steps across.

By the time Chris returned from work later that night, I had pushed and squeezed and dragged the spare double mattress down the tight spiral staircase from its usual resting place under our bed. I could barely manoeuvre it between the ceiling and the stairs and it was equally too large for my new room, each side curling unwillingly up a wall and turning my resting place into a clumsily-constructed cocoon.

When he saw it, Chris exclaimed, "Sweetheart!" as if our earlier stand-off had never happened. "You shouldn't have brought that mattress down the stairs on your own. You could have hurt yourself."

"I've travelled the world on my own," I said archly. "I think I can get a bed down some stairs."

"I know, but you don't have to – I'm here to help you with those things. You only have to ask." He raced on, no pause between thoughts. "But why have you done this? I don't understand …"

"We're not a proper couple and—"

"But we are. We are a proper couple. Don't sleep down here. Please don't sleep down here, I'll miss you."

"Well, maybe I miss you," I said. "And maybe you've done nothing about it."

I grandly declared that I was reclaiming my dignity and shut my bedroom door. Although I was forty-four years old, with little to show for it except the draughty box that I was now bundled into, I felt a similar frisson to when I'd bought my first home – three bedrooms, garden, picket fence – at the age of twenty-three. Independence. When had I given it away? It was only just occurring to me that I had.

There was so much to fret about when chasing fertility that I had been overwhelmed by the fears and the concerns and the stark spectre of childlessness. I hadn't stopped to consider that it was also the first time in my life that I had *needed* a man. I had long been accustomed to life in a fatherless home, where women took care of everything; I paid my way in the world from the age of seventeen, if I had a problem I solved it with little input from anyone else. Independence I could do. I just didn't know how to do *dependence*. It seemed suddenly that I had overdone it, this alien thing. I had encountered infertility and I'd gradually traded away everything I had: my career, my finances, my interests, my family, my friends. And I had relied on Chris – depended on him as I had always depended on myself – to help me get it all back.

I lay on the distorted mattress on the floor, thoughts swooping and diving. *Who said having children would fix everything anyway? Stupid! You were stupid to think that.* Too many thoughts crowded and jostled for attention, darting to the surface and disappearing again before I could fully grasp them. Why had I let it come to this? *What other choices did I have? It's not like I could get* myself *pregnant.*

Here it was, the defining point, wrapped up in the most basic biology: getting pregnant was the only thing I had ever encountered that I could not achieve on my own. With or without Chris, it still look two, it still *needed* two. I didn't know where to draw the boundaries in these new surroundings. I didn't know how this interdependence worked. Somehow I had become so subsumed that his weaknesses had become my weaknesses and his futile diversions my futile diversions. I wondered if it worked the other way, too, if my weaknesses had morphed into his. I was unsure, even then, how likely that was – he didn't seem to have *wanted* a family as much as I did, to have been as involved. My thoughts looped back yet again to conception by sperm donor – although who was to say I had any viable eggs left? – and instantly I resented it. *If he'd tried harder, I wouldn't have to even consider this.*

The door handle creaked and rattled, as if being in use had caught it unawares, and the door shuffled open, catching on the edge of my mattress.

"Sweetheart? Are you still awake? This is silly, I miss you, can't we talk about this?"

I groaned into my pillow.

"Please," Chris said. "I've never turned you away like this. I've always wanted you, you must see that."

I balefully dragged myself upwards until I was leaning against the wall. "No. If you wanted me so much you'd at least have tried to find a solution."

"Ach! You're being really unfair." he protested. "This is just a fear I've got – you said you understood that. Look at me, I've never complained about your fear of flying. I've always supported you with it."

"What?"

"Well, when you couldn't fly back and forth to Switzerland, I never said one word about having to go by train instead. I didn't mind that you were afraid."

"You what?"

"We all have fears, you said it yourself—"

"You think it's the same?"

"Yes. No, I …"

"We've not had sex for eight months – eight months – and you think that's the same as me not wanting to get on a plane? Even though you say you want to have a family with me?"

Chris sank down to his haunches beside the mattress and reached for my hand, speaking in a rush of words.

"No, no! I see now it was a stupid comparison. I didn't mean that it was the same, I'm just a bit lost and—"

I disentangled my hand, pulled the duvet up under my chin. "I *have* supported you about your fear," I broke in indignantly. "For absolute years. And at least I've tried all sorts with planes – even though fear of flying isn't going to stop you from having children, is it? Or make you feel like the least desirable man in the world."

Suddenly, I realised what the past decade had finally come down to. "If this is the rest of our life together, then I don't want it."

I spoke in muted tones while Chris's reply already cascaded around us, gaining in volume all the time. "Listen!" I interjected firmly, trying to stem the flow. "You need to listen."

The room was silent and I continued before I lost momentum and thought better of it.

"I might have to give up on a family, but I am *not* giving up on a proper relationship. One that includes sex. If I'm not going to have children, then I'm damn well going to have some fun instead."

How long had I been planning this life I was going to have, after infertility? It was nine years and eleven months since we first started trying to have a baby together. Could it be that, at the end, it wasn't the lack of a family that forced us apart but the lack of something strong enough to take its place?

I might have been deemed 'older' in biological terms, but surely I was still young enough to feel a spark of attraction now and then, to still desire and be desired? I couldn't remember what it felt like, to be alive like that. These days, I barely looked in the mirror because who was there but the woman whose boyfriend was content to make love to her via syringe? I didn't want to see my reflection in case it gave reason to say, "Well, look at that. No wonder."

It was so belittling, feeling undesired, that I found myself making up stories about it, both for myself and others. Every time I inserted a syringe, I was not alone in our bedroom – I was in Switzerland with one of my *men who might have been* and a scenario that I had long ago daydreamed into being was unfolding scene by scene, like a cherished movie.

The monthly syringes were like a drug that I both relied on and despised, each delivering an injection of simultaneous hope and failure. I was buying them from Boots so regularly that I invented another story to explain that away: "Dispensers for the cat's medicine," I told the girl behind the counter, worried that she would see my regular syringe runs, and the endless packets of conception vitamins that we still bought, and piece together the real picture.

It was bad enough that I was infertile; I couldn't bear for anyone to know that not only could my partner not make love to me, he didn't actually want to. For it gradually became clear: the status quo suited him perfectly. Was this what he had wanted all along? No children. No lovemaking. A sterile life. I didn't realise what I was choosing, ten years ago. I thought it was as simple as sitting in Pizza Express and deciding on names for the babies you were going to have. What I wanted, more than anything, was to reach back through the years and show that girl where it ended. Then I'd reach back another decade and make sure that my twenty-three-year-old self also understood how it felt to be forty-four years old when winter has arrived and the conception gel and syringes sting like ice against your body. I was about to be officially admitted to the Ten-Year Club. It was nearly December 21, 2012. Time for the world to end.

THIRTY-EIGHT

WHEN THEY HEAR THAT you can't have children, some people will say, "Oh, you should just adopt," in much the same way as they might say, "Oh, you've run out of milk? Well, hey, just go to the corner shop to get some more." I can't imagine being one of those people, the ones who don't know what adoption is. Because before infertility stalked me for a decade, it was adoption that refused to let go. When I started trying to have a family of my own, I thought I might – finally – be rid of it. I was going to create some blood ties, I was going to tell my children every detail of their birth stories. It wouldn't matter so much then that I didn't know a thing about the day I was born – except that it was probably also the day I was taken away from my mother. Or was I? Did I get to stay a while? Could she bear to look at me or did she want to pretend I had never happened? I knew her name and that she turned seventeen two months before I arrived. I didn't know my father's name or if he knew I had arrived at all. Eventually, I reached the only conclusion that seemed possible – they must have left me, each of them, because I was defective, lacking, not worth loving. My adoptive father died when I was seven and that just proved I was right. Didn't the people I loved always leave? Wouldn't they have kept me if I was worth keeping? There was something about me that caused people to turn away, something *wrong*.

Even after I had got a bit older and learned to challenge such destructive thoughts, they could still sneak back in; the intruder who strikes when you are vulnerable. If you're not careful it becomes just another instinct, written right through the middle of you, like any other innate force of life: *I'm not good enough. I'm worth less than other people.* Mired in infertility, it infiltrated again and again. *You're too defective to be a mother. Who would want you for a mother?* I wondered sometimes if perhaps it wasn't best for everyone that I had not fallen pregnant, but it was a thought that could not be allowed to linger. Even so, it was an uncomfortable truth that much of the turmoil and confusion of infertility had its roots in my own birth.

It's part of the reason I kept going for so long, trying and hoping for a family, not just the yearning for blood ties but because I find it hard to let go of things. I didn't realise, until the past ten years, quite how much I hate to let go of people or things or situations; it terrifies me, as if every cell carries the memory of the initial letting-go, when I couldn't protect myself. When I had no say in the matter, except perhaps to cling to the familiar scent of my birth mother with tiny hands. I didn't know, until infertility, that I would do almost anything to avoid being cut adrift again. I hold on and hold on because some long-forgotten instinct takes over and insists that holding on is the safest thing to do. So I have held on to Chris, and to the distant dream of babies I might one day meet, well beyond the point when I should have let go. Somehow, each parting or ending feels intrinsically threatening, even if the choice to end something has been mine. It's like I can't tell the difference between letting go and *being* let go.

The truth is that what lies at the core of this infertility story is really adoption. But I've waited to acknowledge it, left it until last, because I wanted, more than anything, to leave it behind. I thought I was done with adoption, but infertility has turned me right back around and forced me to face it again. I confronted it in many guises along the way; it was there in my doubts about whether I would be a 'good enough' parent and it was there in the primal desire to somehow reattach the severed umbilical cord, to *know* and experience an unbroken bond between a mother and her child. It was there in the way

455

I kept trying and trying, each effort more ridiculous than the last. The final confrontation involves looking at adoption from a different angle altogether: should I, an adopted person, choose to adopt? It's the biggest question I've ever asked, partly because I come weighed down with experience of the subject. The people who say, "Oh, you should just adopt" are the ones who think adoption is a one-day-only event – you swap families, names, homes, maybe even countries, change your whole identity and then it is over. Done. They probably think infertility is like that, too. It happened, then it didn't happen.

These are the people who did not have to traverse years of infertility to properly understand that perhaps they held a romanticised view of 'family'. A blood family is a place I've never been, like the Paris of a would-be tourist's imaginings, the one with the Eiffel Tower and the moonlit Seine and no graffiti-scrawled outer suburbs. With adoption, it's the other way around. I know all about the grimy, ugly bits, the seedy parts of town where you wouldn't want to send anyone you loved. I know what it requires of you, and that a great adoptive mother is one of the strongest and most selfless women you will ever meet.

※ ※ ※

It took nearly six years of infertility before the fixation with blood ties began to wane. For so long, I had consoled myself with the thought, 'It's okay, I'll have a biological family of my own.' Then, as I approached forty, it became somehow less important, this sharing of DNA. It seemed the maternal surge that had overtaken me was too powerful to be restricted solely to my biological offspring. This about-turn was another thing I didn't see coming, another of infertility's little surprises.

From 2008 onwards, it wasn't just donor conception sites that I visited and wondered about. I researched adoption as well, tip-toeing around the perimeter of it while I read about the requirements of local authorities and agencies and lurked on forums where adoptive mothers and fathers discussed their journeys to parenthood. It was the wrong time; I was still too angry. I resented the idea of being grilled by home visitors, by social workers and adoption panels. They didn't turn up with their clipboards at the point of conception when the alcoholic down the road got herself pregnant. They didn't poke their noses into her life before sperm could meet egg; there was no, "Excuse me? Do you smoke? Aren't you a bit overweight? And, by the way, what does your ex-boyfriend think of you?" It rankled and stung that I was the one who would have to answer all these questions and more, just because my biological functions didn't work the way they should. It was clear I needed to get a lot less furious with infertility before I properly considered adoption.

More than that, though, I also wasn't too sure how an adoption panel and I would get along when it came to discussing adoption itself. Could I manage to keep demurely quiet and not rail against old perceptions, not say that all my life I've not been 'real' – 'Louise is not her *real* daughter', 'Louise is not her *real* sister' – and now I understand that what I'm signing up for is the inversion of that painful rebuff: 'Louise is not his *real* mother.' If these things upset and irritate me now, that would be nothing compared to the protective indignation I would feel on behalf of my adoptive children. *I'm done with hearing that we're all not real.* Could I stop myself from blurting that out?

And would I, or would I not, laugh when someone pointed out that I was adopted in the 1960s and that, these days, the term we use is 'biological'? 'He is not her biological son.' Because there is so much around adoption that has not moved on, so much that makes me vexed on my behalf and could now, for the rest of my life, potentially make me even more vexed on someone else's behalf. Why, for example, do people actually think it's funny to make 'jokes' about children who have been separated from their birth parents? Sometimes when you hear an adoption 'gag', it can feel, for a brief instant, like someone has stabbed your heart and soul with a pitchfork, one prong embedded in each. Yet these 'wisecracks' are considered so okay that Vince Vaughn's character even delivers a 'you're adopted!' jibe in the movie *Dodgeball*.

If I accidentally shared my thoughts on this with an adoption panel, would it be a positive or a negative; would they say, 'Sorry, we think you haven't come to terms with your own adoption' or, 'Good. We're glad you understand the territory'? Because I would want them to see, more than anything, that I get it; I know what it feels like to be adopted. I can't help wondering, now that I've been so spectacularly infertile, whether I'm being challenged to be involved with adoption all my life. It's not what I would have chosen at the outset. But would I be ready to fight these all-too-familiar battles on behalf of my adoptive children? Yes, in every heartbeat.

⁂

Today, it's five years since I first flirted, coy and cautious, with the idea of adoption. I'm not so angry now with infertility. Sometimes I even joke with it: 'Okay, I see what you wanted to teach me. You can leave now – your work here is done.' Infertility knows that I might not have stopped hoping entirely for a miracle conception, but adoption knows that I just want to offer a child a stable, loving home. Biology is not the issue when you have all this maternal love waiting to be given and you only want to do something positive with that force that still flows, even after ten years. I have imaginary conversations sometimes with my prospective children and, in my imagination, there is no distinction about whether they are my biological offspring; they are just little people who I love. I think of them and I think of the reasons why an adoptee might go on to become a great adoptive parent. For starters, you have a lifelong understanding of the unseen confusions that others might not consider – like how it feels to wonder about your birth parents, even just to know what they look like, to long for them to 'want' you, while at the same time feeling guilty that perhaps these instinctive yearnings convey ingratitude to the parents who came along and chose you. I understand that this so-called being 'chosen' won't always make you feel better. It's not personal, it's just nature.

I was given a dressing gown once, when I was about five, which had belonged to my birth mother. I didn't stop to think how this random item of clothing had come to arrive at our house. I wrapped the collar right around my head whenever no one was looking; it smelt of her, it brought her closer. If I was in trouble, I hid in my wardrobe with the dressing gown and inhaled the scent of my mother until I felt better. I couldn't help it that it was her essence which spoke of 'home'; it just did. These things have nothing to do with how much you love an adopted mother. I know that more than anyone, having had a lifetime's preparation in not taking it personally. Surely I'm ready now to see all of this from another side of the adoption triangle.

And yet. As an adopted person considering adoption, there are additional barriers to breach. There are times, as an adoptee, when you will do anything and go anywhere to avoid being rejected. Rejection. It's the bogey word you don't know you're being haunted by. It causes problems in relationships, romantic and otherwise; it might even turn up at a job interview, perhaps in the 'dream job' you suddenly decide you don't want or in the fantastical reasons you invent *not* to sit before an interviewer and explain where you see yourself in five years' time. Push it away before it pushes you away.

Don't risk it happening again. It's like having faulty wiring – you can't distinguish between the initial rejection, which really was threatening in its most primal sense, and later rejections, which might not be that threatening at all. There is a lot of rewiring to be done before you can confidently stand in front of an adoption panel, waiting for their judgment about whether you would be a 'good enough' mother. This is the sad irony: those who have experienced adoption themselves might also be the ones who find it hardest to stick with the necessarily gruelling process. Who wants to be rejected *by* their parents and *as* a parent? It's the wrong word, of course – rejection – but sometimes you instinctively take it for the truth.

As I sort through all the whys and what-ifs of adoption, I can hear tutting in the farmyard, where I grew up. "Tsk! All this navel-gazing. Just get on with it." I can imagine the earthy, robustly fertile women of my childhood leaning on a post-and-rail stockade, perhaps passing round flagons of cordial after cattle herding. "Hmph. That one thinks adoption's all about her." Tight lips and staccato nods of the head. "Too right she does – she didn't mention the poor child in question, not once." Shaking of the heads now. "Should be thinking about the child, that's what she should be thinking about."

The thing they wouldn't see is that, in picking apart all of these threads, I am thinking about a child. I can't get this wrong, not when I know first-hand what might be required. And, even then, I have seen only the most fortunate side of adoption. I was adopted when I was a baby; I didn't grow up consciously waiting for my 'forever family' to come for me. How much more might be required to support a child who has spent all of their little life just waiting to be loved? That's why the questions of an adoption panel are naught compared to the questions I ask myself. I want to reach out and wrap my arms around a motherless child as much as anyone. I want to reassure them, protect them, help them feel secure in the world.

I want to show them the joy of reading books, of running on the beach and of playing cricket on the sand. But that's nothing. That's just theory. It's the practical application that matters. It's whether I am ready for the 'testing out' that I remember so well in myself, the pushing and prodding at people to see whether they really meant it when they said they loved you. It's whether I can avoid the puppet-on-a-string response if my love is turned away, if every time, regardless of whether I'm tired or stressed or out of sorts, I can say, "It makes no difference. I'm still here and I'll always be here." If I have the slightest doubt about my ability to provide the most unconditional variety of love there is, then the kindest thing would be *not* to adopt. I don't know anything about parenting but I do know that.

⁂ ⁂ ⁂

As 2012 drew to a close and I ruefully joined The Ten-Year Club, there was one more crucial question to be answered. It was not just whether I was strong enough to make it through the adoption process, or even whether I believed, deep down, that I had enough of the 'right' type of love to give.

The biggest question was this: would I consider adoption as a single person or could Chris and I ever hope to return to the point where we could apply as a couple? We had been trying to start a family together for a decade and it seemed that infertility had exposed too many fragilities; our relationship had been dismantled, disappointment by disappointment. What was left to offer a child? What was left, even, to offer each other? It is infertility's parting shot, the rebuilding that needs to be done in its wake. I could probably answer the first two questions, but there was no foundation at all until I could answer the final, unspoken, question: what exactly were we left with, after infertility?

Thirty-nine

It was New Year's Day 2013. A decade to the day since Chris and I had romped in a flat in West Hampstead, laughing and giggling and still getting a kick out of indulging in that long-forbidden activity – *unprotected sex*. The risk of pregnancy! Having a baby. Were we really ready for it? It seemed such a bold step to take – *No going back now* – but also exciting; we were going to become parents together, create a new generation for each of our families. The fresh life we might have been forming, right at that moment, would bring with it a whole new future. New Year's Day 2003 had fizzed with hope, promise, expectation. I'm not sure if I even thought it was possible then, to have unprotected sex for a full decade and still not conceive. It wasn't the story I'd been told all my life. Ten years? I'd been afraid to have unprotected sex for ten seconds. If I had thought of 2013 at all on that day, it would have been in a blurry, abstract way; it was too far away in the future to feel relevant or real. I would have believed many things, but not that an entire decade could have passed without so much as a positive pregnancy test. No. I would not have accepted that version of events. In 2013, if it existed at all, I was a middle-aged mother on the school run.

The first day of the real 2013 was notable because it was light enough and warm enough and dry enough to actually have a pleasant walk outdoors. In west London, everyone had woken up to this surprising fact and the riverside paths and pavements were teeming with sunlight-seeking residents, emerging blinking and smiling from their usual winter incubations indoors. Chris and I joined them, looking like just another pair of friends making the most of the reappearance of the skyline.

"Do you remember what we were doing ten years ago?" I asked as we stood looking out, once again, across the River Thames.

Chris narrowed his eyes, creased up his forehead. "2003? Where were we living then?" A pause to consider. "It was West Hampstead, wasn't it? Yes, 2003 was West Hampstead. That was *before* we went on that trip to Australia."

I laughed. "We've practically had a different address for each different year."

"You'd got a bit annoyed with me on New Year's Eve."

"I did?"

"Yes, you accused me of flirting with a waitress. You said I was giving her crinkly eyes."

"Oh! That's right – you were."

"That's not fair. I didn't even know I was doing it, I would have been just the same if I was talking to a less attractive woman, or even a man."

"Ha. So you did think she was attractive," I joked.

"Sweetheart," Chris began with a chuckle, then stopped himself. "Can I still call you sweetheart?"

"I don't know."

He caught my eye, imploring, and I felt guilty for a moment that I would be back in the southern hemisphere by April and he didn't know it. I didn't want the big angsty, drawn-out goodbye; I just wanted to slip away quietly without any further turmoil for either of us. I knew he didn't have it in him to give me a hug and wave me off; he would have wanted to talk, again, to throw around all the words that he thought were going to save us.

"Let's just be realistic," I said, "but nice to each other at the same time."

Before he could ask what I meant, a voice interjected from the shingle path behind us. "Excuse me folks, can you help us out here?"

463

I turned to find two middle-aged men gazing hopefully in our direction. "Is this the way to Richmond-Upon-Thames?" It was the precise enunciation of an American tourist, who, it turned out, was on his way to see the wild deer grazing in Richmond Park.

"That's where we're heading," I said. "Want us to show you a shortcut?"

Immediately, we were introducing ourselves. "I'm Chris," said the elder of the men, "and this is my cousin, also called Chris. Makes it easy for folks to remember, I guess."

We both laughed, reaching across to shake hands. "I'm Louise and this, believe it or not … is Chris."

The three Chris's and I spent the rest of the day walking together and swapping travel stories. At one stage, as the elder of the Americans and I led the way across Richmond Green, the conversation turned to family and he asked if Chris and I had children.

The answer came quite naturally; there was no stab of despair or panic about what to say. "No. No kids," I answered. "We did try for quite a while, but it never happened."

"Aw," he said, "that's tough. I never thought I'd become a father myself; happened pretty late in my life, that's for sure."

And on we walked, up Richmond Hill to the park.

It hadn't knocked me off my feet or set me back, the type of inquiry I thought I had learned to dread. I was surprised at the ease of my reply. Maybe acceptance was sneaking in at last.

❦ ❦ ❦

In February, I began 'streamlining' my possessions, preparing to pack up my life once again and take it back to the other side of the world. Chris didn't notice at first, when it was just clothes and shoes being dispatched to a charity shop, but his interest was piqued when I started to sift through my collection of books. "You don't normally give those away," he noted, looking on as I bagged up a pile of paperbacks.

I couldn't bring myself to look at him. "I know, it's just … You know …"

He sat on the bed in 'our' room, where I still slept when the spare room became too damp, but where we had not 'slept together' again. Not since our anniversary in April 2012. The stalemate had lasted nearly ten months.

"You're going to leave me, aren't you?" Chris said suddenly.

"It's not that simple. We've kind of already left each other, wouldn't you say?"

He stood up and walked over to me, reaching out to touch my shoulder. "Sweetheart, I don't want to be like this any more than you do. I want to get *us* back too. I think about it all the time." His eyes softened along with his voice. "I miss you."

"Well, you can't miss me that much because you haven't done anything about it." I laughed as if I actually found it funny. "It's been nearly a year."

I had lasted the full decade trying to have a family, limping to the end of the line with cloudy syringes of sperm provided by this man who I now only 'liked'. Even I had realised by the arrival of the New Year that it would be ridiculous to continue advising him when it was the 'right' time for another syringe.

"I knew you'd given up on us when you didn't tell me you were ovulating last month," he said.

"You could have asked."

"I did ask."

"It was day twenty-five by then! Anyway, I'm forty-four – I probably hardly ever ovulate at the best of times."

I still took note of my cycle, though, still knew which 'day' it was. Some things were harder to let go of than others. Unexpectedly, my cycle was operating more smoothly than ever, now that I had discovered how to deal with perimenopause. After much experimenting, I was dosed up on krill oil and manuka honey and generally still had all the expected reproductive signs at all the expected times; I forgot sometimes that I was officially middle-aged.

Chris began to protest that he still wanted to help me have a child. "It's the least I can do," he said. "It would be absolutely wrong if you never became a mother. I want it for you more than anything."

I stopped sifting through the stack of paperbacks. "Huh. That ship's well and truly sailed – there was a time for trying and we missed it."

"But you're saying I can't make it right. How can I ever make it right if you don't let me try? Please let me at least try."

"Look," I said. "Even if it was possible, which it seriously, obviously isn't, it wouldn't be right. The two of us trying to have a baby when things are like this between us? The poor little thing would be stuck in this … this …"

Chris kept trying to draw closer to me and I kept leaning away. "What you're saying is that you don't love me anymore. That's what you mean, isn't it?" He came to a halt in the centre of the room. "I don't blame you, I know I've let you down."

"Well. I feel like you did."

"But I don't want to let you down!"

Chris, now seated again on the edge of the bed, was the usual flurry of jiggling legs and rushing words; in the end I just sat and watched him protest, feeling strangely calm, as if we had reverted to being mere colleagues, like we were in the beginning.

Eventually, even he began to run out of last straws to grasp at. "I don't have a leg to stand on," he said. "I'm just sorry – I didn't mean for any of this to happen. I'm so sorry, I really am."

Chris was still struggling to understand that the ground had shifted now that we were no longer trying to have a family together. How was he to know that I'd made compromise after compromise, just in case? That I was now reclaiming the things I had traded away in order to have children? I'd not even realised myself that I'd done it; it was like awakening from a ten-year bender and gradually realising, to your utter horror, what you'd done while you were 'under the influence'. And here was me, thinking I'd not succumbed, not become 'one of those people' who get obsessive about fertility. Just because I wasn't peeing on sticks for half of the month, or keeping spreadsheets that tracked my cervical secretions. No, infertility had changed me in much more insidious ways than that. I didn't even know how to say it to Chris: "Sorry darling, I've swapped personalities now." Because it was starting to feel as if the woman who had spent most of our relationship trying to have children with him was an imposter.

"You don't even know me. Not really." It was all I could think of to say, trying to explain my impending departure that day in the bedroom.

"What do you mean? Of course I know you – I know you better than anyone. Think of all the things we've been through together, everything we've shared."

"Yes, but I was different."

"What?"

"Before all this." Suddenly I was battling tears again. "Before I couldn't have children. I wasn't … I'm not … You didn't know me before, you don't know what I'm normally like." I shook my head. "Oh, you won't understand."

Chris's voice sounded tender and raw. "Lou, of course I understand. I feel like I've left myself behind somewhere too. It changes you, of course it does. Sometimes I feel like I'll never be the same again."

I turned my face away to hide the tears; I wanted him to think I was calm, indifferent. "I really want to get back to myself," Chris said. "I want *us* to get back to ourselves."

"That's what I'm trying to do," I stammered. "I wouldn't have put up with some of this stuff before, so I just want to—"

"Feel like you've returned to some semblance of yourself," he finished.

"Yes, exactly. I want to at least come out of this a bit stronger again."

Chris smiled. "See. You say I don't know you, but it's so *you* to say that. I love your spirit and determination, I always have."

"No you haven't." I managed a laugh. "I bet you think it's a major pain in the butt."

"Well," he replied. "Maybe you're the one who doesn't know me if that's what you think."

He was different, too; I knew it and I worried that I'd done it to him, caused him to become a more subdued version of himself. An air of resignation seemed to shroud him, taking the place of all the dreaming and hoping he used to do when we first met. Now he seemed not to look forward at all.

"I'm sorry," I said quietly. "About everything. I really do want you to be happy – whoever you meet after me. I mean it. I don't care who it is, I just want you to be happy."

"That's all I've ever wanted for you," he said. "And there won't be anyone else for me, not after you. I've always known that."

The leg jiggling had stopped; Chris was uncharacteristically still. Then, suddenly, he leapt to his feet, as if physically prodded into action.

"What am I saying? I'm a bloody idiot. An idiot! It's time I stood up and dealt with this once and for all."

"What?" I was taken aback by his sudden change in attitude.

"You don't have to stay with me, that's not what I'm saying. But I've been sleepwalking and it's time I damn well woke up. I'm going to sort myself out, I give you my word."

And he disappeared down the stairs and out the front door, as if running late for an appointment. Upstairs, I surveyed my pile of charity shop books and wondered what to do with them.

❧ ❧ ❧

Chris returned home later that afternoon. He didn't tell me where he'd been and I was too proud and stubborn to ask. I had resigned from my role as house initiator; if he wanted to drive anything forward, he could do it himself. I was disinterested and indifferent, or at least doing my best impression of both. Why did I care where he'd been?

"Nice afternoon?" I couldn't help myself.

"Yes. I've done something I should have done a long time ago."

"Well, that's good. Do you want chicken or fish tonight?"

"Either, don't mind … fish maybe?"

I turned to ferret around in the bottom of the fridge, hoping he would be the one who caved in and told me what was going on. *Don't ask, don't ask. You don't care.*

"I wasn't going to say anything yet …"

"Mmm."

"I've been to the surgery. I've made an appointment to see Doctor Bell."

"Oh. Aren't you feeling well?"

"I'm going to talk to him about Viagra."

I abandoned the fridge, leaving both the fish and chicken inside, as I spun around to face him. "You are not!"

Chris wore an injured expression. "I knew you wouldn't think I'd done it."

"Sorry. It was just a shock – I mean a surprise. When's the appointment?"

"Well, it's quicker if I ring first-thing tomorrow to get an on-the-day one. They said he'll be in tomorrow and I should be able to see him then, if I ring early enough."

I chortled; this was just another ploy, tomorrow would come and it would turn out that the day he planned to ring was actually the next tomorrow.

"I knew you wouldn't believe I'd do it," Chris complained. "That's why I wasn't going to tell you until I'd actually been."

"Well, time will tell, won't it?"

"Yes, it will. I know you don't care anymore, but it's time I did this anyway, whether you're still here or not. I can't spend my life running away from this. It's ridiculous. It's time I fronted up once and for all."

"Well, good for you – that takes a lot of courage. If you mean it."

The next day Chris was up two hours earlier than usual; I tried not to feel anything when I heard his voice on the phone, tried not to feel 'involved' in the step he was taking. I finally betrayed myself when he delivered a morning cup of tea, as he often still did.

"So? What happened?" *You fool, you couldn't even hold out until lunchtime.*

"I'm seeing him at 3.30. It's all arranged."

Chris looked unnaturally alert, like a person braced for a career-defining examination or like me, whenever I knew I was going to be boarding a plane later in the day.

I got out of bed and gave him a hug. "Well done. I know it's not easy."

"Thanks – that still means something to me, you know."

"Hmm?"

"That you think I've done something half-decent at last."

I gave a rueful smile. "Will you be okay? Do you know what you're going to say?"

"Yes, I'm ready. I'll just say it straight – it doesn't have to be such a big issue, I see that now. I'm only sorry it's taken me so long, I really am. I've been an absolute buffoon. A buffoon!"

I broke into laughter at his earnest use of such a stupid word, and he joined me, the two of us finally sharing a joke again in our battleground bedroom.

Epilogue

September 2013

WHEN I STARTED WRITING this book, part of me still thought there was a chance of the 'Hollywood ending'. I worried, even, that it would be too neatly scripted, too convenient, for the final chapter to reveal, after all that went before, the ecstatic news of a pregnancy. The triumph against the odds, the inspiring fight-back. But in the end, all I could write is this: I'm forty-four years old and, as far as I know, I've never been pregnant. I never did escape the Ten-Year Club, unless it counts that, soon enough, I'll be joining the Eleven-Year Club.

It was hardly romantic enough for Hollywood, but what happened in real life was this – the boy took Viagra (a Plan B) and the girl took him back. For now. To see how it goes.

Chris has read the whole of this book (or at least says he has) and jokes that the sub-title should be 'A decade of impotence and us'. He's happy with my version of events, although not happy that it happened, and wants both of the 'i' words brought out into the open. As for the other of those words, it's still too early to tell where prolonged infertility will ultimately send us as a couple but, for now, we're together. I worried when I took him back that maybe someone had just thrown me a crumb of love and I jumped on it. I told Chris as much during all the toing and froing we inevitably went through before finally settling back into our new, old relationship.

The truth is that there were times, while writing this book, when I intended it to be the world's longest 'Dear John' letter, a way of saying 'we can't be together and this is why'.

The unforeseen by-product was that reading it brought about a mellowing of the edges in both of us – we saw ourselves in these pages and got a life-changing jolt.

"Hell," said Chris, when he'd reached the end. "That Chris guy is a complete and utter tosser."

"Louise isn't any better," I said. "That's the whole point."

It wasn't until I actually wrote it down that we realised what we had been doing to each other all these years. We were both horrified; it wasn't what either of us consciously set out to do.

It's undeniable that infertility exposed great, gaping failings within each of us but, where the massive mistakes blew us apart, it turned out to be the smaller everyday kindnesses that drew us back together – the tea and biscuits that appear while you're working at your desk, the note on your keyboard that says 'keep going', or the favourite magazine that mysteriously manifests on your pillow. It might not sound much compared to all the blame and heat and drama of fertility problems, and maybe it won't be enough in the long term, but for now it's a starting point. That and the shared sense of humour that never quite got killed off, although I won't be laughing anytime soon about missed sperm tests or botched fertility clinic visits. Chris *does* laugh about smashed wine bottles and photo frames; that's his way of dealing with it.

I'm still working out whether it matters that neither of us *intended* to hurt the other – we might not have set out to cause anyone pain, but how many excuses can we each make for the pressure we were under? I'll get back to you on that – I don't yet know the answer. After spending a decade failing to have children together, it feels like we've got to make our two separate recoveries before we can be fully certain about the third recovery, of 'us' as a couple.

At least we realise exactly who the other is now; infertility could not have blown our insides further out if it tried. There are no secrets or pretences left, just two people who have seen further into each other than they might have wished. Having done so, it turns out we're not completely scared off by what lies in the hidden places. We still want to be friends, we still want the best for each other. It sounds so little to say about the person you are supposed to love – *I care for him, I want him to be happy* – but those two ordinary sentiments survived prolonged infertility, they lasted when so much else fell away; their sheer durability gave them a new value. Eleven years ago, we shared songs and poems and gushed about the person we thought we'd met. Infertility set us straight; it barged in and properly introduced us. Ironically, it would have been a great apprenticeship for parenthood.

⁂

It still takes my breath away to realise that, if I had conceived easily, my eldest child would be about to turn ten. All those formative years – infant, toddler, primary school pupil – would have gone by already; all those experiences we could have lived together, an eighth of an average lifetime. I wonder what type of little person they would have been, what they would have liked and disliked, what would have made them laugh. But I can never know them, except in my imagination.

I still struggle to write: I will not become a mother. I know, by now, that it's not going to happen naturally but the voice of 'what if?' won't quit. What if there's another way? What if it's not too late to pursue other avenues? Perhaps it's progress, of sorts, that that voice is now a lot quieter than the one that says, 'The time has passed, find something else to do with your life.' It's a huge decision to make, which voice to listen to, and there is barely any time in which to make it. I am nose to nose with so many cut-off points – the upper age limit for adoption in some countries, the upper age limit, even, for my own beliefs about when I will no longer have the stamina to be a parent.

The problem is that I can't take action, not yet. It wouldn't be fair to even consider inviting a child to join us when there is still so much rebuilding to be done. It's the final sting in the tail of infertility – once it's swept through your life, you look up and realise that it's washed away both certainty and confidence, the two things you need to make the very decisions you're left with, let alone to see them through.

In the aftermath, I question every decision I've ever made, the domino-fall of choices that led me here, to childlessness. I don't trust what I think is 'right' any more – what do I know? I spent ten years chasing conception and still didn't get myself pregnant. Maybe I won't really be reconciled to infertility until I can accept the feeling of powerlessness it bestows. I've never given myself up to it; I've fought it all the way, trying to wrest back control of my destiny. How can something as fundamental as the choice to become a parent be so far out of my own control? Then, niggling away underneath all this, is the guilty thought that I don't 'deserve' to say these things because I never, in an entire decade, underwent fertility treatment. I wonder if Chris blames me, the way I blame myself sometimes, for not being 'brave' enough to have IVF until we had tried other, gentler options, which soaked up the money we needed later. Then, almost before the thought has finished forming, I have fiercely dismissed it; why should I apologise for meeting infertility in the only place where I *could* meet it? See? I don't know what I think sometimes, now that certainty and confidence have disappeared.

The truth is that, in the aftermath, there are some days when I barely have the confidence to speak to other people. I used to work six days a week in one of the toughest industries there is; now I worry about whether I've said the 'right' thing, acted the 'right' way, in a passing conversation with the next-door neighbour. I feel intimidated by aisle-hogs in the supermarket and by road-hogs on the streets; I try to move over, keep out of their way, take the parking space furthest from the door. There are days when I feel like one big apology for a person. I think it's the isolation that did it – the staying off Facebook to avoid photos of other women's wombs, keeping out of offices because of the pregnancy talk, even living a hemisphere away from my own family, where there are babies, six recent arrivals at the last tally. In the past five years, I know exactly how many times I have socialised with others – I can count them out, uncomfortable event by uncomfortable event, because it has been such a rarity. I have needed to be alone to get through, away from the questions and the comments and the casual hurts that I feared might knock me over just as I stood back up. Maybe it was another thing I got wrong, but my instinct was to hide. Now the time has come to re-emerge; I've got to rejoin life and pretend I know how to live it, in this state that I didn't choose. I have to decide what my future will look like without a family in it. Me, who can't even remember how to pass the time of day with other people.

I've noticed an intriguing irony lately – the only other women who I hear speaking of these things, the missing confidence, the wondering where you've 'left' yourself, are mothers of small children, whose lives have also been sucked up by an outside force. I overhear their conversations on trains and in cafés and I marvel at how alike we feel. I would have resented it once – don't they realise how much I want what they so casually have? – but finally, gradually your perspective widens, affording a less painful view than the narrow, constricted focus of infertility. Sometimes it seems as if infertility and parenthood might be flip sides of the same coin. The other side of the coin could have tested us to breaking point, too. You see that, but of course you still wish that the toss of the coin had fallen your way.

This is the part where someone is supposed to talk wisely about 'moving on', that wonderfully vague thing we're all told to do when our heart has been broken or a door has slammed in our face. No one ever mentions specifics, they just say 'you need to move on now' as if we're all too stupid to work that out for ourselves. Even if there were specific instructions rather than just the clichéd sentiment, I'm not sure if there ever is a 'moving on' from infertility; if I remain childless, and maybe even if I don't, it will always be beside me. It will be there in the often-asked questions about whether I have children and in the missing milestones in my life. It will be there in the pictures on my walls – no first birthday photos, no school camp photos, no wedding photos and, eventually, no photos of grandchildren. There are so many spaces to fill, after infertility, that you start to realise there will never really be an 'after', more a different, and hopefully improved, way of coping with what will always be.

I'm short on useful solutions myself, when it comes to 'moving on'. All I know is that I want to take the maternal energy that swelled inside me and channel it into something positive. It still exists, in simplest terms as a deep desire to nurture, but what will I nurture? There are no childless women, either voluntary or involuntary, to look to amongst my family or friends. There are famous childless women but they are famous precisely because, most of the time, they've been doing something else with their lives all along. They've been succeeding, achieving, attaining, often making deeply worthwhile contributions, for years. I thought my 'worthwhile' contribution would amount to being a good parent. I've got some catching up to do after a decade of striving for something that didn't exist. I don't exactly know where to start, but I suspect learning how to let go of regrets might be a good place. For a time, while blindsided by infertility, it seemed that regret was the sole preserve of women in my position. Eventually it dawned on me that of course parents have their regrets, too, some of them equally deep-seated.

476

Maybe it's just a side-effect of ageing, this obsession with what could have, or should have, been done. I have hated infertility, despised it, loathed it, wanted it dead and buried. However, I can't allow myself to regret it. It was not the experience I would have chosen, but infertility was still *an experience*. I've got it under my belt now, mistakes and all, and I can let it go to waste in that place where broken dreams fester or I can sift out the parts that might be of use and piece them back together in a different shape. Maybe 'moving on' just starts with a positive intention.

I do have some ideas about how I might live without a family. My upbringing on the farm looms large in thoughts of the future; it might be animal care and conservation that I plough my energies into, or it could just as easily be natural healthcare. All I know is that it has to be something. Apart from anything else, I've lived a decade with infertility and I've got fed up with its company. I would like to tell it that I think we should spend some time apart; we need space to 'grow as individuals'. I feel fairly sure that it will be a bit clingy and refuse to let go of this one-sided relationship. I feel fairly sure that *I* will refuse to let go, not completely, not while I am still governed by a monthly cycle that surges and urges procreation, then crashes and mourns its absence. Sometimes I wonder if it wasn't just about hormones all along, that soon they will quieten down and I will return to my non-maternal twenty-something self.

I know, though, that if I remain childless, I will shed a tear at menopause when I realise that my unfertile, fertile life is over. If I reach old age, I will shed more of those private tears, only sometimes, when I rock in my chair and wish for grandchildren. It will never really be over, I know that, just as it is not over when someone dies and you mourn their loss at a funeral. These empty spaces last forever but they are spaces, not barriers.

Perhaps there will never really be life 'after' infertility, but there will be a life. I'm off to find mine and I hope that, if you've been touched by infertility, you will find yours too. More than that, I hope you will find true joy somewhere in this new life that neither of us planned to be living. That's my dearest wish, for all of us.

Acknowledgements

There is one person above all others to thank – Bink, for giving me the freedom to write this (and patiently continuing to support me when it took longer than I said it would). I'll always be grateful and I hope the time will come when I can repay you. Thanks also for blazing the trail and showing me it could be done – then handing over your desk space while I did it myself. There's so much I won't forget.

Thanks to my lovely brother, the real-life Ray, for taking such an interest and encouraging me to complete this project (even though he'll – hopefully – never get to read it or know what it's about). I thank my four other brothers and sisters, too, for the many ways in which they've all enriched my life – not least, by providing me with thirteen amazing nieces and nephews, who are the closest thing I have to children of my own.

I hope I'll one day write a book my mother can actually be allowed to read. I want to thank her anyway for being such an inspiration and for having the strength of spirit to single-handedly provide me with the type of childhood I'd have loved my own children to have. And Dad, too, for showing me the joy of reading and leaving behind his own writing, in the books which now sit on the shelf by my desk and motivate me onwards.

Thank-you to the real-life Rose, who could never possibly be forgotten, for her tireless interest, enthusiasm and spirited support. It made more of a difference than you knew. Thanks also to the real-life Maggie, David Taylor, Samuel and Li Wei, who all provided help and expertise when times were tough (and endless hugs, of course, for Dudley and Duke, my 'rescue dogs' and the only two boys who knew what to do).

I am grateful to all at Bryter Music (*www.brytermusic.com)*, Warlock Music and BMG, for kindly allowing me to reproduce the Nick Drake lyrics which have meant so much to us.

TEXT PERMISSIONS

Northern Sky, written and performed by Nick Drake, is taken from the album *Nick Drake – A Treasury* (www.brytermusic.com) and reproduced by kind permission of Warlock Music/BMG Rights.

RESOURCES

Books
A Child Against All Odds, Professor Lord Robert Winston (Bantam)

Before The Change: Taking Charge of Your Perimenopause, Ann Louise Gittleman, PHD, CNS (HarperOne)

Feeling Good: The New Mood Therapy, David D Burns, MD (Harper)

Mother Daughter Wisdom: Understanding the Crucial Link Between Mothers, Daughters and Health, Christiane Northrup, M.D (Bantam)

Taking Charge of Your Fertility: The Definitive Guide to Pregnancy Achievement, Natural Birth Control and Reproductive Health, Toni Weschler, MPH (Vermilion)

The Fertility Diet: How to Maximize Your Chances of Having a Baby at Any Age, Sarah Dobbyn (Simon & Schuster UK)

The Fertility Solution: A Revolutionary mind-body process to help you conceive, Niravi B Payne, M.S & Brenda Lane Richardson (Thorsons)

The Infertility Cure: The Ancient Chinese Wellness Program for Getting Pregnant and Having Healthy Babies, Randine Lewis, PHD (Little, Brown)

Why Am I So Tired? Is Your Thyroid Making You Ill? Martin Budd, N.D, D.O (Thorsons)

Women's Bodies, Women's Wisdom: Creating Physical and Emotional Health and Healing, Christiane Northrup, M.D (Bantam)

Television
Imagine: The Secret of Life, Alan Yentob (BBC One)

INDEX

482

483

Grief 152, 315, 331, 352, 433
See also Infertility: Emotion
Gynaecologist 253

Hair growth 397
Harley Street 35, 80, 89, 128, 133,
    183
Headaches 182
Healthcare, private 35, 80
Heart palpitations 398
Heat magazine 192
Henley-on-Thames 21, 42
Herbs
    See Acupuncture: Herbs
Hogmanay 6
Hormones 75, 239, 338, 398-9,
    414, 436, 477
    Imbalance 398-9
    Progesterone 48
Horses 7, 16, 176, 181, 184
    Falls from 179
    Showjumping 179
Hospital 49-50, 52-3, 57-60, 65
    Pathology 53
    Radiology 58-60
HSG test 301, 424
Hypnosis 168, 442, 446-7
Hysterectomy 368

Ian (landlord) 191, 201-5, 223, 225,
    277, 326-7, 368-70
Immaculate conception 151, 299
Impotence 244, 313, 471
    See also Performance anxiety
Infertility
    Acceptance (and) 464
    Advice from fertile people 350-6
    Aftermath 374, 403, 425-7, 446-
    53, 461-78
    Anger (and) 30, 136, 159-62, 211,

228-9, 255-8, 260-5, 274-6, 331,
343-5, 365-6, 384, 397, 403, 406-
12, 443-5, 458, 477
Anniversary, 4th 185
Anniversary, 5th 221
Blame (and) 410, 414-20, 424-5,
472, 474
Career (and) 37, 115-16, 358,
374-5, 380, 449
Comments about 14, 202-3, 263,
332, 349-56, 375, 413, 454, 456,
475-6
Doubts about continuing 100,
438-9
Emotion (and) 2, 45, 81, 96-100,
126-32, 151-63, 180, 200-1, 211-13,
233-6, 239, 244, 249-63, 271-5,
293-6, 307-20, 331, 337-45, 364,
377, 381-3, 400-3, 429, 433-5
Faith (and) 328-34, 347, 413
False hope (and) 22, 29, 34, 42,
76, 80, 101, 111, 116-19, 165, 177,
186, 191, 238, 287, 291-2, 321-2,
326-7, 331, 337, 361, 376-7, 387,
389-93, 395, 413-14, 431, 441,
444, 446, 458, 462
Family (and) 31, 321, 328, 348,
358-62, 378-83, 393-5, 422, 436,
449, 475
Fears for future (and) 1, 25, 47,
129, 131, 136, 154, 175, 214, 358,
449, 475
Finances (and) 35, 75, 87, 89,
115, 133-4, 150, 183, 185, 214,
220, 246-7, 249-50, 254, 259, 261,
307-8, 319-20, 322-3, 325, 335,
337, 357-9, 365-6, 371-4, 383-4,
387-8, 403-4, 428-9, 449
Fixation on solving 264, 276,
395, 405-6, 439-42, 455, 467
Friends (and) 32, 89-94, 100, 297-
8, 362, 449, 475

489

CPSIA information can be obtained
at www.ICGtesting.com
Printed in the USA
LVHW090035100720
660292LV00001B/106

9 780992 959500